MAYO CLINIC a-z 🧰 Health Guide

WHAT YOU NEED TO KNOW ABOUT SIGNS, SYMPTOMS, DIAGNOSIS & TREATMENT

2nd Edition

Edited by Sanjeev Nanda, M.D.

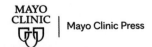

MAYO CLINIC | Mayo Clinic Press

MAYO CLINIC

Medical Editor Sanjeev Nanda, M.D.

Publisher Daniel J. Harke

Editor in Chief Nina E. Wiener

Managing Editor Anna L. Cavallo

Art Director Stewart J. Koski

Production Design Darren L. Wendt

Illustration and Photography Mayo Clinic Media Support Services, Mayo Clinic Medical Illustration and Animation

Editorial Research Librarians Anthony J. Cook, Edward (Eddy) S. Morrow Jr., Erika A. Riggin, Katherine (Katie) J. Warner, Morgan T. Wentworth

Copy Editors Miranda M. Attlesey, Alison K. Baker, Nancy J. Jacoby, Julie M. Maas

Indexer Steve Rath

Thanks to Mohit Chauhan, M.B.B.S., for contributing to the review of several mental health topics.

Published by Mayo Clinic Press

© 2023 Mayo Foundation for Medical Education and Research (MFMER)

For bulk sales to employers, member groups and health-related companies, contact Mayo Clinic, 200 First St. SW, Rochester, MN 55905, or send an email to SpecialSalesMayoBooks@mayo.edu.

ISBN 978-1-945564-13-0 (paperback)
ISBN 978-1-945564-72-7 (hardcover)

Library of Congress Control Number: 2022942475

Printed in China

INTRODUCTION

You face decisions about caring for your health every day. *Mayo Clinic A to Z Health Guide* is designed to be a handy medical reference to help answer your questions and guide those decisions.

This book is organized alphabetically, providing clear information on more than 150 common health conditions. Each topic answers key questions, such as: What is it? What's the cause? What are the symptoms? How is it diagnosed? What treatments are available? And what can you do in your daily life to prevent or manage it? You'll also find detailed medical illustrations to help you understand what's really going on.

This second edition of *Mayo Clinic A to Z Health Guide* covers an expanded range of topics, with added information on specific mental health conditions, cancer, COVID-19 and more. And each topic has been vetted and updated to help provide the most current expertise.

Every page includes facts and guidance based on what Mayo Clinic health care providers share with their patients every day. This information isn't a substitute for seeing a doctor. It's meant to help you understand various diseases and conditions so that you can communicate effectively with your health care team. Working together, you can address your individual needs and effectively manage your health.

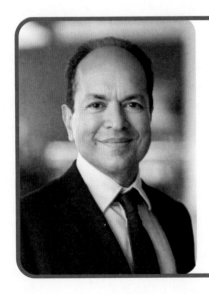

Sanjeev Nanda, M.D., is a consultant in general internal medicine at Mayo Clinic in Rochester, Minnesota. A passionate educator, he has helped create continuing medical education courses focused on fibromyalgia, medically unexplained symptoms and updates in the field of internal medicine. He has also received awards for excellence in teaching as an assistant professor at Mayo Clinic College of Medicine and Science. Dr. Nanda has a broad interest in medicine, with a particular interest in preventive health and lifestyle medicine.

TABLE OF CONTENTS

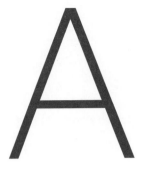

Acne

WHAT IS IT? Acne is a skin condition that occurs when hair follicles become plugged with oil and dead skin cells. It is most common on the face, neck, chest, back and shoulders. The pimples and bumps heal slowly. Often, when one pimple begins to resolve, others crop up.

Acne can cause emotional distress and can leave scars on the skin. The good news is effective treatments are available. The earlier treatment is started, the lower the risk of lasting damage.

WHAT'S THE CAUSE? Three factors contribute to the formation of acne:

- Overproduction of oil (sebum)
- Irregular shedding of dead skin cells
- Buildup of bacteria

An oily substance known as sebum lubricates your hair and skin. It travels up along the hair shafts and then out through the openings of the hair follicles onto the surface of your skin. When your body produces an excess amount of sebum and dead skin cells, the two can build up in the hair follicles and form a soft plug.

This plug may cause the follicle wall to bulge and produce a whitehead. Or the plug may open to the surface and darken, causing a blackhead. Pimples are raised red spots, often with white centers. They develop when blocked follicles become inflamed or infected. Blockages and inflammation that develop deep under the skin may produce hard lumps (nodules) or large, fluid-filled cysts that are painful to the touch.

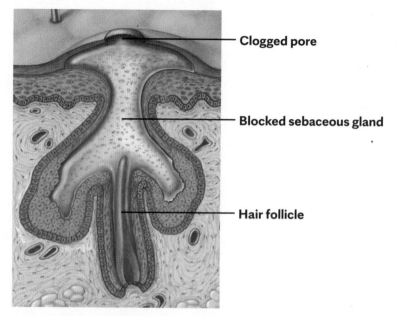

Clogged pore

Blocked sebaceous gland

Hair follicle

Acne develops when sebum — an oily substance that lubricates your hair and skin — and dead skin cells plug hair follicles. Bacteria can trigger inflammation and infection resulting in more-severe acne.

Risk factors

Factors that can trigger or aggravate acne include:

- **Hormones.** During puberty, hormones increase and cause the oil (sebaceous) glands to enlarge and make more oil. Pregnancy and use of oral contraceptives also can affect sebum production.
- **Certain medications.** Drugs containing corticosteroids, certain hormones or lithium are known to cause acne.
- **Diet.** Milk and carbohydrate-rich foods, such as bread and chips, which increase blood sugar, may trigger acne or make it worse.
- **Greasy or oily substances.** Contact with some cosmetics or lotions may trigger or worsen acne.
- **Family history.** You're at increased risk if your parents had acne.
- **Friction or pressure.** This includes pressure on the skin from items such as cellphones, helmets, tight collars and backpacks.
- **Stress.** Stress doesn't cause acne, but it may worsen acne.

TREATMENT Acne treatments work by reducing oil production, speeding up skin cell turnover, fighting bacterial infection, reducing inflammation or doing all four. It may take a while to see results, and your skin may get worse before it gets better.

Types

Treatment for acne includes:

Topical creams available without a prescription. These products may dry up the oil, kill bacteria and promote sloughing of dead skin cells. They are generally helpful for very mild acne.

Prescription topical creams. These treatments promote cell turnover and help prevent the plugging of the hair follicles. Topical antibiotics kill excess bacteria on the skin.

Antibiotics. A short course of prescription oral antibiotics to reduce bacteria and fight inflammation may be used for moderate to severe acne. Oral antibiotics are often used together with topical creams.

Isotretinoin. This medication is used for scarring cystic acne or acne that doesn't respond to other treatments. It is very effective but can cause a number of side effects and requires monthly checkups.

Oral contraceptives. Some oral contraceptives may improve acne that occurs in relation to menstrual cycles.

Laser and light therapy. Laser treatment damages sebaceous glands, causing them to produce less oil. Light therapy targets the bacteria that cause acne inflammation. More studies are needed, but these therapies may be options for people who can't tolerate other treatment.

Cosmetic procedures. Chemical peels and microdermabrasion are most effective when used in combination with other treatments.

LIFESTYLE Good skin care can reduce or control most acne.

- **Use a gentle cleanser.** Wash your skin with gentle, oil-free, water-based skin care products.
- **Avoid heavy makeup.** Use products labeled "water-based" or "non-comedogenic." Remove all makeup before bedtime.
- **Watch what touches your face.** Keep your hair off your face. Don't rest your hands or objects such as your phone on your face.
- **Limit sunlight.** The sun worsens acne in some people. Some acne medications may make you more susceptible to the sun's rays.
- **Shower after exercise or heavy physical labor.** Oil and sweat on your skin can trap bacteria, causing acne.

ADHD (attention-deficit/ hyperactivity disorder)

WHAT IS IT? ADHD is a mental health disorder that includes a combination of problems, such as difficulty sustaining attention, hyperactivity and impulsive behavior. This chronic condition begins in childhood and often persists into adulthood. However, sometimes it isn't diagnosed until the person is an adult.

Symptoms sometimes lessen with age. Many people never completely outgrow their ADHD symptoms, but they can learn ways to cope and be successful.

WHAT'S THE CAUSE? The exact cause of ADHD is unclear. Many factors may be involved in its development.

ADHD can run in families, and studies indicate genes may play a role. Certain environmental factors may increase the risk. So may central nervous system problems at key moments in a child's development. Maternal drug use, alcohol use, smoking during pregnancy and premature birth are other possible risk factors.

Although sugar is a popular suspect in causing hyperactivity, there's no reliable proof of this. Many things in childhood can lead to difficulty sustaining attention, but that's not the same as ADHD.

SYMPTOM CHECKER In some children, signs and symptoms are noticeable as early as age 2 or 3. They may include:

- Difficulty paying attention
- Frequently daydreaming
- Difficulty following through on instructions
- Difficulty organizing tasks or activities
- Frequently forgets or loses needed items
- Frequently fails to finish schoolwork, chores or other tasks
- Easily distracted
- Frequently fidgets or squirms

- Difficulty remaining seated and seemingly in constant motion
- Excessively talkative
- Frequently interrupts or intrudes

ADHD occurs more often in males than in females, and behaviors can be different in boys and girls. For example, boys may be more hyperactive and girls may tend to be quietly inattentive.

It's important to remember that most healthy children are inattentive, hyperactive or impulsive at times. It's typical for preschoolers to have short attention spans. Even in older children and teenagers, attention span often depends on the level of interest. And some children naturally have a higher activity level than others do. Children aren't diagnosed as having ADHD just because they're different from friends or siblings.

In adults, ADHD symptoms often include impulsiveness, disorganization, poor time management, problems focusing and restlessness. Many adults with ADHD also have at least one other mental health condition, such as depression or anxiety.

WHAT TESTS TO EXPECT There's no specific test for ADHD. A diagnosis generally includes a medical history and interviews or questionnaires. Information is generally gathered from several sources, including parents, schools and caregivers.

To be diagnosed with ADHD, your child must meet the criteria in the Diagnostic and Statistical Manual of Mental Disorders DSM-5-TR published by the American Psychiatric Association. A child diagnosed with ADHD may be given a more specific diagnosis (a subtype), such as predominantly inattentive type ADHD, predominantly hyperactive-impulsive type ADHD or combined type ADHD.

TREATMENT Standard treatments for ADHD include medications, education, training and counseling. These treatments can relieve many of the symptoms, but they won't cure ADHD. It may take some time to determine what works best for you or your child.

Stimulant medications
Stimulant drugs (psychostimulants) are the most commonly prescribed medications for ADHD. They're thought to boost and balance levels of brain chemicals called neurotransmitters. The medications can help

improve symptoms of inattention and hyperactivity — often quickly. Examples of stimulant medications include methylphenidate (Concerta, Ritalin, others), dextroamphetamine (Dexedrine), dextroamphetamine-amphetamine (Adderall XR) and lisdexamfetamine (Vyvanse). Medications are available in short-acting and long-acting forms.

Talk with your health care provider about possible side effects of stimulants. These drugs may increase blood pressure or heart rate, but studies show no increased risk of serious heart-related effects. Your provider may check for any heart condition or family history of heart disease before prescribing a stimulant.

Other medications

Atomoxetine (Strattera) and antidepressants such as bupropion (Wellbutrin, others) are used to treat ADHD. Clonidine (Catapres, Kapvay) and guanfacine (Intuniv) are other options. Atomoxetine and antidepressants work more slowly than stimulants. They may be good options if your child can't take stimulants for health reasons or if stimulants cause severe side effects.

Behavior therapy and counseling

A psychiatrist, psychologist, social worker or other mental health provider may provide behavior therapy, social skills training, parent skills training and counseling. The best results usually occur when a team approach is used, with teachers, parents, and therapists or physicians working together.

LIFESTYLE To help reduce problems or complications:

- **Provide structure.** Structure doesn't mean inflexibility or strict discipline. Instead, it means arranging things so that a child's life is as predictable, calm and organized as possible. Be consistent, set limits and have clear consequences for your child's behavior.
- **Follow a routine.** Put together a daily routine for your child with clear expectations for things like bedtime, morning time, mealtime, simple chores and TV.
- **Avoid distraction.** When talking with your child, don't multitask. Make eye contact when giving instructions.
- **Set an example.** Try to remain patient. Speak quietly and calmly. Reward good behavior and provide positive reinforcement.

Alcohol use disorder

WHAT IS IT? Alcohol use disorder is a pattern or habit of unhealthy drinking. It includes being unable to control how much you drink, needing to drink more to get the same effect, using alcohol even if it causes problems, and having withdrawal symptoms if you stop drinking.

Alcohol use disorder can range from moderate to severe. The focus on alcohol can become so intense that a person can't function at work, school or home.

WHAT'S THE CAUSE? No specific cause of alcohol use disorder is known. Alcohol affects everyone in a different way. Genetics, biology and social factors all may play a role.

Men are more likely than women to have an alcohol use disorder. Having an anxiety disorder or being depressed also may increase a person's risk of misusing alcohol. In some people, over time, drinking too much alcohol can affect the brain. The result may be cravings for alcohol.

SYMPTOM CHECKER Anyone can have alcohol use disorder. Drinking as a teenager increases the risk. An unhealthy pattern of drinking often starts when people are in their 20s or 30s.

Signs and symptoms vary from person to person. They include:

- Having more than two alcoholic drinks on most days
- Wanting to cut down on drinking but not being able to do so
- Having strong cravings for alcohol
- Hiding alcohol in different places
- Not meeting obligations at work, school or home because of use
- Drinking when it's not safe to do so, such as when driving
- Drinking to feel good or feel better
- Needing more and more alcohol to feel its effects
- Becoming nauseated, sweating and shaking when you don't drink

To screen for alcohol use disorder, a doctor may ask how often you drink and whether you or anyone around you is concerned about the drinking. A psychiatrist, psychologist or addiction counselor also may help make the diagnosis.

WHAT IS 1 DRINK?

One standard drink is any one of these:

- 12 ounces of regular beer (about 5% alcohol)
- 8 to 9 ounces of malt liquor (about 7% alcohol)
- 5 ounces of unfortified wine (about 12% alcohol)
- 1.5 ounces of 80-proof hard liquor (about 40% alcohol)

TREATMENT Admitting that drinking is a problem is the first step in treating alcohol use disorder. The next step is stopping use and safely detoxifying. This takes about 2 to 7 days. For some people, the detoxification happens in a hospital or residential treatment center.

Outpatient counseling

Individual, group or family counseling often is part of the plan for treating alcohol use disorder. With counseling, people learn how and why to avoid alcohol. They also get emotional support. And they gain coping skills to help fight the urge to drink.

Medication

Drugs that can help people with alcohol use disorder include:

- Acamprosate, which may balance alcohol-related brain activity, promoting longer sobriety
- Naltrexone (Vivitrol), which may reduce alcohol cravings
- Disulfiram, which may provide motivation not to drink because using alcohol while taking this drug can make a person sick

LIFESTYLE Once a person has stopped using alcohol, making lifestyle changes is key to staying sober and avoiding a relapse. Having a support system of family and friends to support recovery is important. Many people find that joining a self-help group such as Alcoholics Anonymous (AA) is valuable.

A person with alcohol use disorder may need to stay away from friends or social situations linked to drinking. Replacing activities that involve drinking with hobbies that don't center around alcohol can be helpful.

Allergies

WHAT IS IT? Allergies occur when your immune system reacts to certain substances — such as pollen, bee venom or pet dander — that don't cause a reaction in most people.

Your immune system produces proteins known as antibodies that help protect you from unwanted invaders that could make you sick or cause infection. In the case of allergies, your immune system mistakes a particular substance (allergen) as harmful, even though it isn't. So when you're exposed to the allergen, your antibodies react to it. They release a number of chemicals, such as histamine, that can inflame your skin, sinuses, airways or digestive system.

WHAT'S THE CAUSE? Substances that most commonly trigger allergies include:

- **Airborne allergens.** This includes pollen, animal dander, dust mites and mold.
- **Certain foods.** Examples include peanuts, tree nuts, wheat, soy, fish, shellfish, eggs and milk.
- **Insect stings.** Bee stings or wasp stings can trigger allergies.
- **Medications.** Examples include penicillin or penicillin-based antibiotics.
- **Latex.** It's a common cause of allergic skin reactions.

Risk factors

You may be at increased risk of developing an allergy if you:

- **Have a family history of asthma or allergies.** If you have family members with asthma or allergies, such as hay fever, hives or eczema, it's more likely that you'll have allergies.
- **Are a child.** Children are more likely to develop an allergy than are adults. Children sometimes outgrow their allergies as they get older. However, it's not uncommon for allergies to go away and then come back later.
- **Have asthma or another allergic condition.** If you have one type of allergic condition, you're more likely to be allergic to something else. And in a typical progression, someone with food allergies may later develop asthma and other allergies.

SYMPTOM CHECKER Symptoms may involve the airways, sinuses and nasal passages, skin, and digestive system. Allergic reactions may range from mild to severe. Severe allergies can trigger a life-threatening reaction called anaphylaxis, releasing a flood of chemicals that can cause the body to go into shock.

Types

Symptoms are dependent on the type of allergy.

Hay fever. Also called allergic rhinitis, hay fever may cause:

- Sneezing
- Runny nose and nasal congestion
- Watery or itchy eyes
- Itchy nose, roof of mouth or throat

Food allergy. Symptoms of a food allergy may include:

- Tingling mouth
- Swelling of the lips, tongue, face or throat
- Hives
- Anaphylaxis

Insect sting allergy. An insect sting may produce:

- Swelling (edema) at the sting site
- Itching or hives all over the body
- Cough, chest tightness, wheezing or shortness of breath
- Anaphylaxis

Drug allergy. Drug allergy signs and symptoms include:

- Hives
- Rash or itchy skin
- Facial swelling
- Wheezing
- Anaphylaxis

Skin allergy. Your skin may:

- Itch
- Redden
- Flake or peel

WHAT TESTS TO EXPECT To determine if you have an allergy, your health care provider may ask questions about signs and symptoms you commonly experience. If you have a food allergy, you may need to keep a detailed diary of the foods you eat. Your provider may recommend one or more of the following tests.

Skin tests. A doctor or nurse pricks your skin and then exposes it to small amounts of a possible allergen. If you're allergic, you'll likely develop a raised bump on your skin (hive) at the test location. In certain cases, an allergen injection (intradermal) test also may be recommended.

Blood test. The radioallergosorbent test (RAST) uses a blood sample sent to a lab. The test measures your immune system's response to an allergen by measuring the amount of allergy-causing antibodies in your blood.

TREATMENT Treatment depends on the type of allergy. The following approaches may be used.

Avoidance
It's important to identify and avoid your allergy triggers. This is a key step in preventing allergic reactions and reducing symptoms. If, for example, you're allergic to pollen, stay inside with windows and doors closed during periods when pollen is high.

Medications to reduce symptoms
Over-the-counter and prescription drugs used to treat allergies include antihistamines, nasal corticosteroids and decongestants. They're available in the form of oral medications, nasal sprays or eye drops. Your health care provider will advise you on the best medication.

- **Antihistamines.** They treat sneezing, itching and a runny nose. Newer oral antihistamines are less likely to make you drowsy.
- **Nasal corticosteroid sprays.** They help prevent and treat nasal inflammation, nasal itching and runny nose caused by hay fever. For people mostly bothered by nasal symptoms, they're the most effective hay fever medications. They're often the first type of medication prescribed.
- **Decongestants.** They relieve congestion. Don't use a decongestant nasal spray for more than two or three days at a time, though. Continued use can actually worsen symptoms, causing what's called rebound congestion.

Immunotherapy

For severe allergies or allergies not completely relieved by other treatment, your health care provider may recommend allergen immunotherapy. This form of treatment involves allergy shots. These are generally given on a regular basis over a period of months to years, to decrease your sensitivity to the allergen.

Another form of immunotherapy is a tablet that's placed under the tongue (sublingual) until it dissolves. Sublingual drugs are used to treat some pollen allergies.

Epinephrine

If you experience a severe allergy, your doctor may give you an emergency epinephrine injector to carry with you at all times. Used in severe allergic reactions, an epinephrine shot (EpiPen, Auvi-Q, others) reduces symptoms until you receive emergency treatment. If you've ever had a severe reaction, you should wear a medical alert bracelet (or necklace) to let others know in case you have a severe reaction and can't communicate.

LIFESTYLE Simple steps taken at home can help relieve symptoms for certain allergies. Try these therapies.

Nasal irrigation. This involves rinsing out your sinuses with a salt and water solution. You can use a neti pot or a specially designed squeeze bottle to flush out thickened mucus and irritants from your nose. Nasal irrigation is most effective for hay fever and other nasal allergies.

Improper use of a neti pot or other device can lead to infection. Use water that's distilled, sterile or filtered. Rinse the device after each use with distilled, sterile or filtered water, and leave open to air-dry.

Dust and dander elimination. If you're allergic to dust or pet dander, you can reduce exposure to these allergens. Frequently wash bedding and stuffed toys in hot water, maintain low humidity, and use a vacuum with a fine filter such as a high-efficiency particulate air (HEPA) filter. Replacing carpeting with hard flooring may also be helpful.

Moisture reduction. If you're allergic to mold, use ventilation fans and dehumidifiers to reduce moisture in damp areas, such as the bathroom, kitchen and basement.

ALS
(amyotrophic lateral sclerosis)

WHAT IS IT? ALS is a progressive neurological disease that causes loss of muscle control. It is often called Lou Gehrig's disease, after the famous baseball player who was diagnosed with it. This motor neuron disorder causes nerve cells to gradually break down and die.

The disease most commonly occurs in people between the ages of 40 and 75. In most cases, medical experts don't know why ALS occurs. In about 5% to 10% of people with ALS, the disease is inherited. Among people with inherited (familial) ALS, their children have a 50-50 chance of developing the disease.

Researchers are looking at certain environmental factors as possible triggers of the disease in some people. Smoking cigarettes appears to increase a person's risk of ALS. Some evidence suggests that exposure to lead or other environmental toxins may increase risk of the disease. However, no single chemical has been consistently associated with ALS.

In addition, people who've served in the military are at higher risk of ALS. The exact reason why is uncertain. It may have to do with exposure to toxins, traumatic injuries, infections or intense exertion.

SYMPTOM CHECKER ALS often begins with muscle twitching and weakness in an arm or leg, or sometimes with the slurring of speech. Early signs and symptoms include:

- Difficulty walking, tripping or difficulty doing your usual daily activities
- Weakness in your leg, feet or ankles
- Hand weakness or clumsiness
- Slurring of speech or trouble swallowing
- Muscle cramps and twitching in your arms, shoulders and tongue
- Difficulty holding your head up or keeping a good posture

As the disease advances, your muscles become progressively weaker. Eventually, the disease can affect your ability to control the muscles needed to move, speak, eat and breathe. The disease usually doesn't affect your senses or your thinking (cognitive) skills.

A

WHAT TESTS TO EXPECT ALS is difficult to diagnose early because it can appear similar to several other neurological disorders. A diagnosis is often made after ruling out other possible conditions.

Your doctor may order tests such as an electromyogram (EMG) and nerve conduction study to evaluate the electrical activity of muscles and nerves. Imaging tests may be used to look at the brain and spinal cord. Blood and urine samples may help eliminate other possible causes of your symptoms. Sometimes a sample of spinal fluid is taken for analysis.

TREATMENT No treatment can reverse the course of ALS. Treatment focuses on slowing the progression of symptoms, preventing complications and maintaining comfort. Devices that assist with breathing may become necessary at some point. Nutritional needs also are monitored.

Medications

Riluzole (Rilutek) is the primary drug used to slow the disease's progression. It may work by reducing levels of a chemical messenger in the brain (glutamate) that's often present in higher levels in people with ALS.

Edaravone (Radicava) is a newer drug approved by the Food and Drug Administration for the treatment of ALS. It may slow the loss of physical function by reducing free radicals in the body, which can damage cells.

Your doctor also may prescribe medications to provide relief from signs and symptoms such as muscle cramps and spasms, spasticity, constipation, fatigue, excess salivation, pain, and depression.

Therapy

Physical therapy can address pain, walking, mobility, bracing and equipment needs. Low-impact exercises are often prescribed to maintain cardiovascular fitness, muscle strength and range of motion for as long as possible. Appropriate stretching can help prevent pain and help muscles function at their best.

Occupational therapy can help you perform daily activities such as dressing, grooming, eating and bathing. Speech therapy may be prescribed to help maintain speech and to assist in alternative methods of communication.

Alzheimer's disease

WHAT IS IT? Alzheimer's disease is a progressive disease that destroys memory and other important mental functions. It's the most common cause of dementia — a group of brain disorders that results in the loss of intellectual and social skills.

Over time, Alzheimer's disease leads to significant brain shrinkage, resulting from two types of changes in brain tissue that are hallmarks of the disease: plaques and tangles.

Plaques are clumps of a protein called beta-amyloid that can damage and destroy brain cells in several ways, including interfering with cell-to-cell communication. Tangles refer to twisted threads of another protein (tau). The twisted strands interfere with the transport of brain nutrients and other essential materials.

WHAT'S THE CAUSE? For most people, Alzheimer's disease likely stems from a combination of genetic, lifestyle and environmental factors that affect the brain over a period of time. Less commonly, it results from specific genetic changes that virtually guarantee a person will develop the disease.

Risk factors

Factors that may increase your risk of Alzheimer's disease include:

- **Age.** Increasing age is the greatest known risk factor. Your risk increases greatly after you reach age 65. In the United States, nearly one in three people over age 85 have Alzheimer's.
- **Family history and genetics.** Your risk appears to be higher if a parent or sibling has the disease. Scientists have identified rare changes (mutations) in three genes that virtually guarantee a person who inherits them will develop Alzheimer's. People with such genetic changes may begin experiencing symptoms as early as their 30s. Fortunately, these changes account for less than 5% of cases.
- **Sex.** Women are more likely than men to develop Alzheimer's disease, in part because they live longer.
- **Race and ethnicity.** Studies show that dementia occurs at higher rates in older Black and Hispanic people than in older white people. More research is needed to understand why. Possible explanations include disparities in health care.

- **Early memory problems.** People with memory problems or other signs of cognitive decline that are worse than what might be expected for their age have an increased risk of developing dementia.
- **Past head trauma.** People who've had a severe or repeated head trauma appear to have a greater risk of Alzheimer's disease.
- **Lifestyle.** Some evidence suggests that the same factors that put you at risk of heart disease — such as lack of exercise, tobacco use, high blood pressure and high cholesterol — also may increase the chance that you'll develop Alzheimer's disease.

SYMPTOM CHECKER Brain changes associated with Alzheimer's disease can cause a variety of signs and symptoms. The most common include the following.

Memory difficulties. Everyone has occasional memory lapses. Memory loss associated with Alzheimer's disease is different in that it persists and worsens. People with Alzheimer's may:

- Repeat statements and questions over and over, not realizing that they've asked the question before
- Forget conversations, appointments or events, and not remember them later
- Routinely misplace possessions, often putting them in illogical locations
- Forget the names of family members and common objects

Disorientation. People with Alzheimer's disease may lose sense of what day it is, the season, or their location or current life situation.

Speaking and writing difficulties. It's harder to find the right words, identify objects, express thoughts or take part in conversations.

Troubles thinking and reasoning. Managing finances, balancing the checkbook and paying bills on time becomes difficult.

Troubles performing familiar tasks. Once-routine activities that require sequential steps, such as planning and cooking a meal or playing a favorite game, become a struggle.

Personality and behavior changes. Depression, anxiety, social withdrawal, mood swings, distrust in others, irritability or aggressiveness, and changes in sleeping habits may occur.

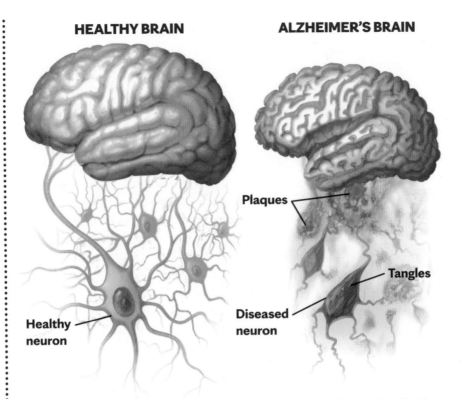

HEALTHY BRAIN

ALZHEIMER'S BRAIN

Plaques

Tangles

Diseased neuron

Healthy neuron

Plaques and tangles destroy brain cells. Plaques are clumps of a protein called beta-amyloid that damage brain cells in several ways. Tangles result from irregular twisting of a protein called tau that prevents the transportation of nutrients.

WHAT TESTS TO EXPECT There's no specific test that confirms you have Alzheimer's disease. Your health care provider will make a judgment based on information you provide and results of various tests.

To help distinguish Alzheimer's disease from other causes of memory loss, health care providers typically rely on the following types of tests.

- **Physical and neurological exams.** Your doctor will likely perform a thorough physical exam and check your neurological health by testing your reflexes, muscle tone and strength, sight and hearing, and coordination and balance.
- **Blood tests.** They can help rule out other potential causes of memory loss and confusion.
- **Mental status testing.** Certain tests may be used to assess your memory and other cognitive skills. Short forms of mental status testing can be done in about 10 minutes. If your provider thinks you may have a very early stage of Alzheimer's or another dementia, a more extensive assessment may be recommended.

- **Brain imaging**. Images of the brain are used to pinpoint irregularities related to conditions other than Alzheimer's disease — such as strokes, trauma or tumors — that may cause cognitive changes. New imaging applications, however, may enable doctors to detect brain changes associated with Alzheimer's disease.

TREATMENT For now, no treatment can halt the disease or check its course. The goal of treatment is to relieve and slow symptoms. A variety of medications may be used, depending on the symptoms present. Behavior modification strategies also may be helpful. Treatment can help individuals with Alzheimer's maintain their independence for a longer period of time.

Regular exercise is important to improve mood and maintain health. Exercise also helps promote sleep and prevent constipation. Good nutrition is important too. Individuals with Alzheimer's may forget to eat, lose interest in preparing meals or not eat healthy foods.

People with Alzheimer's disease commonly experience a mixture of emotions — confusion, frustration, anger, fear, grief and depression. A calm and stable home environment can help reduce behavior problems. New situations, noise, large groups of people, being rushed or pressed to remember, or being asked to do complicated tasks can cause anxiety. When a person with Alzheimer's becomes upset, the ability to think clearly declines even further.

PREVENTION

Studies show an association between lifelong involvement in mentally and socially stimulating activities and a reduced risk of Alzheimer's disease. Factors that may reduce your risk of Alzheimer's include:

- Higher levels of education
- A stimulating job
- Mentally challenging leisure activities, such as reading or playing an instrument
- Frequent social interactions

Scientists can't explain this link. One theory is that using your brain develops more cell-to-cell connections, which protects your brain against changes related to Alzheimer's.

Anemia

WHAT IS IT? Anemia is a condition in which you don't have enough healthy red blood cells to carry adequate amounts of oxygen. Having anemia may make you feel tired and weak.

Types

There are many forms of anemia, each with its own cause.

Iron deficiency anemia. It results from a shortage of iron in your body. Your bone marrow needs iron to make hemoglobin. This is the protein that gives blood its red color and that enables blood cells to transport oxygen. Iron deficiency anemia is often caused by blood loss, such as from heavy menstrual bleeding or an ulcer. Pregnancy, eating too little iron in your diet or problems absorbing iron may be other causes.

Vitamin deficiency anemia. Your body also needs folate and vitamin B-12 to make healthy red blood cells. A diet lacking in these and other key nutrients can decrease red blood cell production.

Anemia of chronic disease. Some chronic diseases — such as cancer, HIV/AIDS, Crohn's disease and other chronic inflammatory diseases — can interfere with the production of red blood cells.

Aplastic anemia. This rare anemia is caused by a decrease in the bone marrow's ability to produce red blood cells. Causes of aplastic anemia include infections, drugs and autoimmune diseases.

Bone marrow-related anemia. A variety of diseases, such as leukemia, myelodysplasia or myelofibrosis, can cause anemia by affecting blood production in your bone marrow.

Hemolytic anemia. This type of anemia results when red blood cells are destroyed faster than bone marrow can replace them.

Sickle cell anemia. This inherited anemia is caused by a defective form of hemoglobin that forces red blood cells to assume a crescent (sickle) shape. The irregular-shaped red blood cells die prematurely, resulting in a chronic shortage of red blood cells.

Others. Other rare forms include thalassemia and anemias caused by defective hemoglobin.

SYMPTOM CHECKER Signs and symptoms vary depending on the cause. Initially, they may be so mild they go unnoticed.

- Fatigue
- Weakness
- Pale skin
- A fast or irregular heartbeat
- Shortness of breath
- Chest pain
- Dizziness
- Cognitive problems
- Cold hands and feet
- Headache

TREATMENT Blood tests to check the number of red blood cells in your blood and their size, shape and color are used to diagnose anemia.

Treatment depends on the cause. Iron deficiency anemia, for example, is often treated with iron supplements and a change in diet. If the underlying cause of the iron deficiency is loss of blood — other than from menstruation — your health care provider may do some tests to determine the internal source of the bleeding.

Other forms of anemia may be treated with specific dietary supplements, blood transfusions to boost levels of red blood cells or a bone marrow transplant. For some uncommon anemias, such as hemolytic anemia and sickle cell anemia, medications may be used.

LIFESTYLE Most anemias can't be prevented. But you can help prevent iron deficiency anemia and vitamin deficiency anemia by eating a healthy diet that contains adequate nutrients, including:

- **Iron.** Iron-rich foods include beef and other meats, beans, lentils, iron-fortified cereals, green leafy vegetables, and dried fruit.
- **Folate.** This nutrient is found in citrus fruits and juices, bananas, green leafy vegetables, asparagus, legumes, and fortified breads and cereals.
- **Vitamin B-12.** It's found naturally in meat and dairy products. It's also added to some cereals and soy products.
- **Vitamin C.** Foods containing vitamin C — such as citrus fruits, melons and berries — help increase iron absorption.

Anxiety

WHAT IS IT? Being anxious from time to time is typical. Occasional anxiety is different from an anxiety disorder, which causes frequent, intense, excessive or persistent worry or fear about everyday situations. Anxiety disorders can interfere with daily activities and be difficult to control.

An anxiety disorder may start during childhood or the teen years and persist into adulthood. Examples include generalized anxiety disorder, social anxiety disorder (social phobia), separation anxiety disorder and panic disorder, involving recurrent panic attacks. A person can have more than one anxiety disorder.

WHAT'S THE CAUSE? The exact cause of anxiety disorders isn't fully understood. Life experiences such as traumatic events appear to trigger anxiety disorders in people already prone to becoming anxious. Inherited traits also can be a factor.

For some people, anxiety is linked to an underlying health issue. Medical problems associated with anxiety include heart disease, diabetes, thyroid problems and asthma. On occasion, anxiety can be a side effect of certain medications.

Factors that may increase risk of an anxiety disorder include:

- **Being female.** Women are more likely than men to be diagnosed with an anxiety disorder.
- **Trauma.** Children who endured abuse or trauma or witnessed traumatic events are at higher risk of developing an anxiety disorder at some point in life. Adults who experience a traumatic event also can develop anxiety disorders.
- **Stress.** A serious health condition, a big event or a buildup of smaller stressful life situations may trigger excessive anxiety.
- **Personality.** People with certain personality types are more prone to anxiety disorders than are others.
- **Other disorders.** People with other mental health disorders, such as depression, are more likely to have an anxiety disorder.
- **Family history.** Anxiety disorders can run in families.
- **Drugs or alcohol.** Drug or alcohol use or withdrawal can cause or worsen anxiety.

SYMPTOM CHECKER Signs and symptoms include:

- Feeling nervous
- Feeling powerless
- Having a sense of impending danger, panic or doom
- Having an increased heart rate
- Breathing rapidly (hyperventilation)
- Sweating
- Trembling
- Feeling weak or tired
- Trouble thinking about anything other than the present worry

TREATMENT A psychological questionnaire is often used to help diagnose an anxiety disorder and rule out other conditions. You may also have a physical exam to look for indications that your anxiety is linked to a medical condition.

The two main treatments for anxiety disorders are psychotherapy and medications. You may benefit the most from a combination of the two.

Psychotherapy

Also known as talk therapy or psychological counseling, psychotherapy involves working with a therapist to reduce your anxiety symptoms. Cognitive behavioral therapy is the most effective form of psychotherapy for anxiety disorders. It focuses on teaching specific skills so that you can return to activities you've avoided because of your anxiety.

Medications

Some of the more commonly used drugs for anxiety include:

Antidepressants. They influence the activity of brain chemicals (neurotransmitters) thought to play a role in anxiety disorders. Antidepressants used to treat anxiety include fluoxetine (Prozac), imipramine (Tofranil), paroxetine (Paxil, Pexeva), sertraline (Zoloft) and venlafaxine (Effexor XR).

Buspirone. This medication may be used on an ongoing basis. As with most antidepressants, it typically takes up to several weeks to become fully effective.

Benzodiazepines. These drugs are generally used only on a short-term basis for relieving acute anxiety. They aren't recommended for long-term use because they can be habit-forming. Examples include alprazolam (Xanax), chlordiazepoxide (Librium), clonazepam (Klonopin), diazepam (Valium, others) and lorazepam (Ativan).

LIFESTYLE There are steps you can take to control anxiety.

- **Keep physically active.** Be active most days of the week. Exercise is a powerful stress reducer and may improve your mood.
- **Avoid alcohol and other sedatives.** They can worsen anxiety.
- **Quit smoking and limit caffeine.** Both nicotine and caffeine can worsen anxiety.
- **Use relaxation techniques.** Deep breathing, meditation and yoga are examples of relaxation techniques that can ease anxiety.
- **Make sleep a priority.** Do what you can to make sure you're getting enough sleep to feel rested.
- **Eat healthy foods.** A nutritious diet may reduce anxiety, but more research is needed.
- **Socialize.** Social interaction and caring relationships can lessen your worries.

PANIC ATTACKS

A panic attack is a sudden episode of intense fear without an apparent or realistic cause. Panic attacks can be very frightening. When one occurs, you might think you're losing control, having a heart attack or even dying.

Panic attacks typically begin suddenly, without warning, and can occur almost anywhere at any time. They have many variations, but symptoms usually peak within 10 minutes. Symptoms may include a rapid heart rate, sweating, trembling, shortness of breath, hyperventilation, chills, and a sense of impending doom or danger.

One of the worst things about panic attacks is the fear you'll have another one. Because of this, you may avoid certain situations or not want to leave your home.

If you experience a panic attack, seek medical help. Panic attacks are hard to manage on your own. And they may get worse without treatment. Similar to other anxiety disorders, the main treatments are psychotherapy and medications.

Aortic aneurysm (abdominal)

A

WHAT IS IT? An aortic aneurysm is a bulging area in the aorta, the major blood vessel that runs from the heart through the center of the chest and abdomen. Aneurysms can develop anywhere along the aorta. Those that form in the lower section are called abdominal aortic aneurysms.

Abdominal aortic aneurysms often grow slowly and without symptoms, making them difficult to detect. As the aneurysm enlarges, you may notice a pulsating feeling near your navel, constant pain in your abdomen or on the side of your abdomen, and back pain. An aneurysm that ruptures can cause life-threatening complications.

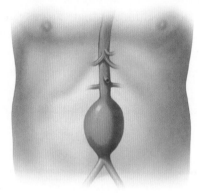

An abdominal aortic aneurysm occurs when the lower portion of the aorta weakens and bulges.

Risk factors

Factors that increase the risk of an abdominal aortic aneurysm include being older, being male, using tobacco, having atherosclerosis and having a family history of abdominal aortic aneurysms.

TREATMENT Treatment is often dependent on the size of the aneurysm. If it's small and you have no symptoms, your health care provider may suggest a watch-and-wait (observation) approach. If the aneurysm is large or growing rapidly, you'll likely need surgery. For a medium-sized aneurysm, discuss with your provider the benefits and risks of waiting versus having surgery.

With more-invasive surgery, the damaged section of the aorta is removed and replaced with a synthetic tube. Less invasive procedures involve insertion of mesh support at the aneurysm site to reinforce the weakened aortic wall.

Appendicitis

WHAT IS IT? Appendicitis is an inflammation of the appendix that typically causes pain in the lower right abdomen. In most people, the pain begins around the navel and then moves to the right lower abdomen. As the inflammation worsens, the pain generally increases.

Appendicitis typically results from a blockage in the lining of the appendix that produces an infection. As bacteria multiply, the appendix becomes inflamed and swollen and fills with pus. If not treated promptly, it can rupture.

Other signs and symptoms of appendicitis include nausea and vomiting, loss of appetite, low-grade fever, constipation or diarrhea, and abdominal bloating.

TREATMENT Treatment for appendicitis usually involves surgery to remove the inflamed appendix (appendectomy). Before surgery you may be given a dose of antibiotics to prevent infection. Your health care provider may want to perform some tests to confirm that appendicitis is the cause.

Tests used to help confirm the diagnosis include:

- A physical examination of the painful area
- A blood test to check for a high white blood cell count, indicating infection
- A urine test to make sure that a urinary tract infection or kidney stone isn't causing the pain
- Imaging tests, such as an abdominal X-ray, ultrasound exam or computerized tomography (CT) scan, to rule out other reasons for the pain

An appendectomy may be performed with open surgery or done laparoscopically. In general, laparoscopic surgery allows for faster recovery and healing with less pain and scarring.

It isn't appropriate for everyone, though. If your appendix has ruptured and infection has spread beyond the appendix or you have an abscess, you may need open surgery. Open surgery allows the surgeon to clean the abdominal cavity.

Arthritis

WHAT IS IT? Arthritis is inflammation of one or more of your joints, causing pain and stiffness. Severe arthritis, particularly if it affects your hands, can make it difficult to perform daily tasks. Arthritis of weight-bearing joints can keep you from walking comfortably. In some people, joints may become twisted and deformed.

The most common types are osteoarthritis and rheumatoid arthritis.

Osteoarthritis

Osteoarthritis involves wear-and-tear damage to the joint's cartilage — the hard, slick coating on the ends of bones. Enough damage can cause bone to grind directly on bone, producing pain and restricting movement. The wear and tear can occur over many years, or it may be hastened by a joint injury or an infection.

Rheumatoid arthritis

In rheumatoid arthritis, the body's immune system attacks the lining of the joint capsule, a tough membrane that encloses all the joint parts. This lining, known as the synovial membrane, becomes inflamed and swollen. The disease can eventually destroy cartilage and bone within the joint.

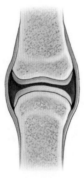 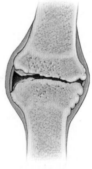 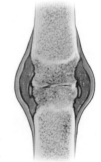

Healthy joint　　　　**Osteoarthritis**　　　　**Rheumatoid arthritis**

Osteoarthritis involves wearing away of the cartilage that caps the bones in your joints. With rheumatoid arthritis, the synovial membrane that protects and lubricates joints becomes inflamed. This can lead to joint erosion.

WHAT'S THE CAUSE? Factors that may put you at increased risk of arthritis include:

- **Family history.** Some types of arthritis run in families. You may be more likely to develop arthritis if your parents or siblings have it.
- **Age.** The risk of many types of arthritis increases with age.
- **Sex.** Women are more likely than men to develop rheumatoid arthritis.
- **Previous joint injury.** People who've injured a joint, perhaps while playing a sport, are at increased risk.
- **Obesity.** Carrying excess pounds puts stress on joints, particularly the knees, hips and spine. Obese people are at higher risk.

SYMPTOM CHECKER Depending on the type of arthritis you have, your signs and symptoms may include:

- Pain
- Stiffness
- Swelling
- Redness
- Decreased range of motion

WHAT TESTS TO EXPECT During a physical exam, your health care provider likely will check your joints for swelling, redness and warmth, and how well they move. Additional tests may include:

Laboratory tests
Analysis of different types of body fluids may help pinpoint the type of arthritis you have. Fluids commonly analyzed include blood, urine and joint fluid. To obtain a sample of your joint fluid, a needle is inserted into the joint space to withdraw fluid.

Imaging tests
They're performed to identify problems within the joint.

- **X-rays.** X-rays can show cartilage loss, bone damage and bone spurs. X-rays may be used to track progression of the disease.
- **Computerized tomography** (CT). A CT scan takes X-rays from many different angles and combines the information. CT scans can visualize both bone and the surrounding soft tissues.

- **Magnetic resonance imaging (MRI).** An MRI can produce more-detailed cross-sectional images of soft tissues such as cartilage, tendons and ligaments.
- **Ultrasound.** This uses high-frequency sound waves to show soft tissues, cartilage and fluid-containing structures. It is also used to guide needle placement for joint aspirations and injections.

Arthroscopy

In some cases, a doctor may look for damage in the joint by inserting a small, flexible tube (arthroscope) through an incision near the joint. The arthroscope transmits images from inside the joint to a video screen.

TREATMENT
Arthritis treatment focuses on relieving symptoms and improving joint function. You may need to try several different treatments, or combinations of treatments, before you determine what works best for you.

Medications

The medications used to treat arthritis vary depending on the type of arthritis. Commonly used arthritis medications include:

Analgesics. They help reduce pain, but have no effect on inflammation. Examples include acetaminophen (Tylenol, others), tramadol (Ultram, others), and opioids containing oxycodone (Percocet, Oxycontin, others) or hydrocodone.

Nonsteroidal anti-inflammatory drugs (NSAIDs). NSAIDs reduce both pain and inflammation. Over-the-counter NSAIDs include ibuprofen (Advil, Motrin IB, others) and naproxen sodium (Aleve). Some NSAIDs are available only by prescription. Others are available as creams or gels, which can be rubbed on joints.

Counterirritants. Some creams and ointments contain menthol or capsaicin, the ingredient that makes hot peppers spicy. Rubbing these preparations on the skin over your aching joint may interfere with the transmission of pain signals being sent from the joint.

Disease-modifying antirheumatic drugs (DMARDs). Often used to treat rheumatoid arthritis, DMARDs slow or stop your immune system from attacking your joints, to prevent further damage. Examples include methotrexate (Trexall, others) and hydroxychloroquine (Plaquenil).

Biologics. Typically used in conjunction with DMARDs, these genetically engineered drugs target various protein molecules involved in the immune response. Examples include etanercept (Enbrel) and infliximab (Remicade).

Corticosteroids. These include prednisone and cortisone, which reduce inflammation and suppress the immune system. Corticosteroids can be injected directly into a sore or inflamed joint. This allows the medication to go directly to the area needed without affecting the entire body. Relief can last for several months, and injections can usually be given 2 to 4 times a year.

Therapy

Physical therapy can be helpful for some types of arthritis. Exercises can improve range of motion and strengthen the muscles surrounding joints. In some cases, splints or braces may be needed.

Surgery

If other treatments don't help, a doctor may recommend surgery. During joint replacement surgery (arthroplasty), the damaged joint is removed and replaced with an artificial one. Joints most commonly replaced are the hips and knees. In some cases, only part of the joint needs to be replaced.

Joint fusion may be used for smaller joints, such as the ankle, wrist and fingers. The ends of two bones in the joint are removed and the bones locked together until they heal into one rigid unit.

LIFESTYLE To lessen symptoms of arthritis, consider:

- **Weight loss.** If you're obese, losing weight will reduce the stress on weight-bearing joints.
- **Exercise.** Regular exercise helps keep your joints flexible. Swimming and water aerobics may be good choices because the buoyancy of the water reduces stress on weight-bearing joints.
- **Heat and cold.** Heating pads and ice packs may help relieve pain.
- **Yoga or tai chi.** The slow, stretching movements of these therapies may help improve joint flexibility and range of motion.
- **Massage.** Light stroking and kneading of muscles may increase blood flow and warm affected joints, temporarily relieving pain.

Asthma

WHAT IS IT? Asthma is a condition in which the airways narrow, swell and produce extra mucus. This can make breathing difficult and trigger coughing, wheezing and shortness of breath. For some, asthma is a minor nuisance. For others, it's a major problem that can lead to a life-threatening asthma attack.

It isn't clear why some people develop asthma and others don't. It's probably due to a combination of environmental and genetic (inherited) factors. Exposure to substances that trigger allergies (allergens) and irritants can cause signs and symptoms. Asthma triggers include:

- Airborne allergens, such as pollen, dander, mold and dust
- Respiratory infections, such as the common cold
- Physical activity (exercise-induced asthma)
- Cold air
- Air pollutants and irritants, such as smoke
- Strong emotions and stress
- Sulfites and preservatives added to some foods and beverages
- Acid reflux from gastroesophageal reflux disease (GERD)

SYMPTOM CHECKER Signs and symptoms range from minor to severe and vary from person to person. They include:

- Shortness of breath
- Chest tightness or pain
- Trouble sleeping caused by shortness of breath or coughing
- A whistling or wheezing sound when exhaling
- Coughing or wheezing attacks worsened by a cold or the flu

WHAT TESTS TO EXPECT Tests that measure lung function are used to diagnose asthma. They include:

- **Spirometry.** This test estimates the narrowing of your bronchial tubes by checking how much air you can exhale after a deep breath and how fast you can breathe out.
- **Peak flow. This** measures how hard and fast you can breathe out. Lower than usual readings are a sign your lungs may not be working as well as they should be.

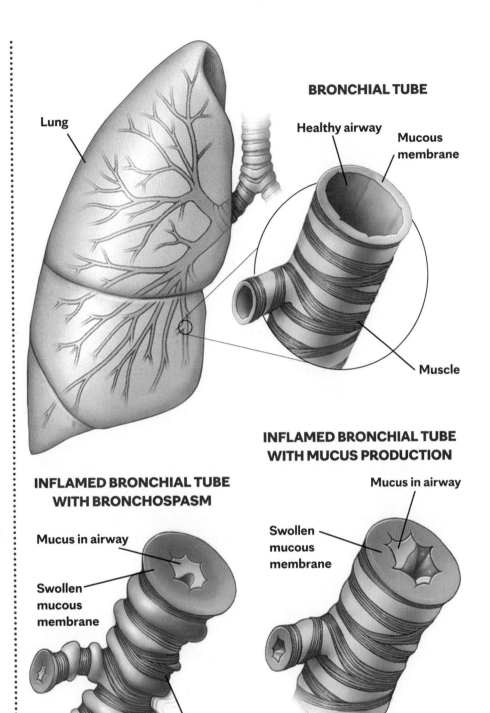

BRONCHIAL TUBE

Lung

Healthy airway

Mucous membrane

Muscle

INFLAMED BRONCHIAL TUBE WITH MUCUS PRODUCTION

Mucus in airway

Swollen mucous membrane

INFLAMED BRONCHIAL TUBE WITH BRONCHOSPASM

Mucus in airway

Swollen mucous membrane

Tightened muscles (bronchospasm)

With asthma, the inside walls of lung airways become inflamed and swollen. Airway muscles may tighten (bronchospasm), and membranes in the airway linings may secrete excess mucus.

TREATMENT Prevention and long-term control are key in stopping asthma attacks before they start.

Treatment usually involves learning to recognize your triggers, taking steps to avoid them and tracking your breathing to make sure your daily asthma medications are keeping symptoms under control. In case of an asthma flare-up, you may need to use a quick-relief inhaler. The right medication for you depends on a number of things, including your age, your symptoms and what seems to work best.

Long-term control medications

Long-term control medications reduce the inflammation in your airways. These medications are the cornerstone of asthma treatment.

Inhaled corticosteroids. They include the medications fluticasone propionate (Flovent HFA, others), budesonide (Pulmicort Flexhaler, others), ciclesonide (Alvesco), beclomethasone (Qvar Redihaler) and mometasone (Asmanex). You may need to use these medications for several days to weeks before they reach their maximum benefit.

Leukotriene modifiers. These oral medications include the drugs montelukast (Singulair), zafirlukast (Accolate) and zileuton (Zyflo). They relieve asthma symptoms for up to 24 hours.

Long-acting beta agonists. These inhaled medications, which include salmeterol (Serevent) and formoterol (Foradil, Perforomist), open the airways. It's recommended they be taken in combination with an inhaled corticosteroid.

Combination inhalers. Medications such as fluticasone-salmeterol (Advair Diskus), budesonide-formoterol (Symbicort) and mometasone-formoterol (Dulera) contain a long-acting beta agonist along with a corticosteroid.

Theophylline. Theophylline (Theo-24, Elixophyllin, others) is a daily medication that helps relax the muscles around the airways. It's less commonly used today.

Quick-relief medications

These medications are taken for rapid, short-term symptom relief during an asthma attack — or before exercise. They include:

Short-acting beta agonists. These bronchodilators act within minutes to ease symptoms. They include albuterol (ProAir HFA, Ventolin HFA, others), levalbuterol (Xopenex) and pirbuterol.

Anticholinergic agents. Like other bronchodilators, ipratropium (Atrovent HFA) and tiotropium (Spiriva, Spiriva Respimat) act quickly to immediately relax your airways, making it easier to breathe.

Oral and intravenous corticosteroids. Medications such as prednisone and methylprednisolone relieve airway inflammation. They're taken only on a short-term basis to treat severe symptoms.

Allergy medications

If your asthma is aggravated by allergies, allergy medications — including allergy shots, antihistamines and decongestants — may help control symptoms.

LIFESTYLE You can do several things on your own to maintain your health and lessen the possibility of an asthma attack.

- **Use your air conditioner.** Air conditioning reduces the amount of airborne pollen from plants that finds its way indoors. It also lowers indoor humidity and can reduce your exposure to dust mites.
- **Decontaminate your decor.** To reduce dust in your home, encase pillows, mattresses and box springs in dustproof covers.
- **Clean regularly.** Clean your home at least once a week.
- **Maintain optimal humidity.** If you live in a damp climate, use a dehumidifier.
- **Reduce pet dander.** If you're allergic to dander, avoid pets with fur or feathers.
- **Cover your nose and mouth.** If your asthma is worsened by cold or dry air, wear a face mask.
- **Get regular exercise.** Regular exercise strengthens your heart and lungs, which helps relieve asthma symptoms.
- **Maintain a healthy weight.** Being overweight can worsen asthma symptoms.
- **Monitor your breathing.** Regularly measure and record your peak airflow with a peak flow meter.
- **Manage gastroesophageal reflux disease (GERD).** Acid reflux that causes heartburn may damage lung airways and worsen asthma symptoms.

Autism spectrum disorder

WHAT IS IT? Autism spectrum disorder is a condition related to brain development. Having autism can make it hard to communicate and interact with other people. Autism includes a wide range of symptoms, and they are more severe in some people than in others.

WHAT'S THE CAUSE? No specific cause of autism spectrum disorder is known. Genetics and environmental factors both may play a role. No reliable study has shown any link between vaccines and autism.

Some things are known to increase the risk of autism spectrum disorder. Boys are four times more likely than girls to develop it. In addition, having a sibling or parent with autism also is a risk factor for autism.

SYMPTOM CHECKER Signs of autism spectrum disorder are usually seen by age 2. Each person's pattern of behavior is unique. The range of symptoms includes:

- Poor eye contact
- Lack of facial expression
- Lack of speech or delayed speech
- Use of a robot-like or singsong voice
- Repetitive behavior, such as rocking, spinning or hand-flapping
- Unusual fixation on specific routines, rituals, objectives or activities
- Inability to express or understand emotions, pick up social cues, and make or keep friends

For some people, symptoms of autism spectrum disorder make interacting more difficult, but they can still handle many life skills on their own (high functioning). For others, having autism makes it very hard to communicate and to live independently (low functioning). Some children with autism have trouble learning. Others learn quickly but have trouble communicating and adjusting to social situations.

TESTS TO EXPECT Autism spectrum disorder is diagnosed by interviewing the person and family. An autism specialist, who may be a child psychiatrist, psychologist or other specialist, does this evaluation and may watch the person play or interact with others.

Tools commonly used by autism specialists include questionnaires and interview rating scales. To be diagnosed with autism spectrum disorder, a person must have trouble with social communication and repetitive behaviors. Those symptoms must start in early childhood and affect daily functioning.

TREATMENT Autism spectrum disorder is a lifelong condition. The care plan for someone with it may address social, language and behavior problems. It may include:

- Behavioral training to teach new skills and reduce problem behaviors
- Educational therapies to improve social skills, communication and behavior
- Family therapy to improve how the family interacts
- Therapy for physical and sensory needs

Medication

There is no drug that specifically treats autism. But some medications may help control symptoms and may be helpful to use along with other types of therapy. These include:

- Psychostimulants to control hyperactivity
- Antidepressants for anxiety
- Antipsychotics for severe behavioral problems

Research hasn't shown that alternative and complementary therapies (also called integrative therapies) are effective for autism spectrum disorder. Some of them may reinforce negative behaviors or be harmful.

LIFESTYLE To reinforce the care from a specialist, working with loved ones on behaviors at home is key. Someone with autism may benefit from:

- Consistent schedules and routines
- Set times to go to bed and get up
- A consistent schedule and structure for meals and snacks
- Structured playtime
- Descriptions and examples of social skills provided by others
- Examples of how to act in certain places or situations
- Praise from others for positive behaviors

B

Back pain

WHAT'S THE CAUSE? Back pain is a common complaint. Most people in the United States will experience back pain at least once during their lives. It's one of the most common reasons people go to the doctor or miss work.

Back pain often develops without a specific cause that's easy to identify with a test or imaging study. Conditions commonly linked to back pain include:

Muscle or ligament strain. Repeated heavy lifting or a sudden awkward movement may strain back muscles and spinal ligaments. If you're in poor physical condition, constant strain on your back may cause painful muscle spasms.

Bulging or ruptured disks. Disks act as cushions between the individual bones (vertebrae) in the spine. Sometimes, the soft material inside a disk may bulge out of place or rupture and press on a nerve (herniated disk).

Compressed nerve. A herniated disk or a bone spur presses on a spinal nerve, causing pain in the lower back. The compression may also cause numbness in the affected leg. Most commonly, the sciatic nerve is affected (sciatica).

Arthritis. Osteoarthritis in the spine can lead to a narrowing of the space around the spinal cord, a condition called spinal stenosis.

Osteoporosis. Porous and brittle bones in the spine (vertebrae) can cause compression fractures, resulting in back pain.

SYMPTOM CHECKER Back pain symptoms may include:

- Muscle ache
- Shooting or stabbing pain
- Pain that radiates down the leg
- Pain accompanied by numbness or tingling in a leg
- Limited flexibility or range of motion of the back
- Inability to stand up straight

WHAT TESTS TO EXPECT Diagnostic tests aren't always needed. If there's reason to suspect a specific condition may be causing your pain, a health care provider may order one or more tests.

Tests used to diagnose back pain include:

- **X-ray.** An X-ray shows the alignment of your bones and whether you have arthritis or broken bones.
- **Magnetic resonance imaging (MRI) and computerized tomography (CT).** These imaging techniques can reveal herniated disks or problems with bones, muscles, tissue, tendons and nerves.
- **Blood tests.** These can help determine whether you have an infection or other condition causing your pain.
- **Bone scan.** In rare cases, a doctor may use a bone scan to look for bone tumors or compression fractures caused by osteoporosis.
- **Nerve studies.** An electromyography (EMG) test measures the electrical impulses produced by nerves and the responses of your muscles. It can confirm nerve injury caused by herniated disks or narrowing of your spinal canal (spinal stenosis).

TREATMENT Most back pain gets better with a few weeks of care and attention at home. If self-care therapies aren't effective, you may need stronger medications or other treatments.

Medications

If mild to moderate back pain doesn't get better with over-the-counter pain relievers, your doctor may prescribe a muscle relaxant. Be aware that muscle relaxants can cause dizziness and may make you sleepy.

For short-term relief of severe pain, opioid medications may be prescribed for a short period of time — usually a week or less — with close supervision by a doctor.

For nerve-related back pain, drugs such as gabapentin (Neurontin, Gralise, Horizant), pregabalin (Lyrica) and duloxetine (Cymbalta) are sometimes used. Low doses of certain antidepressants — particularly tricyclic antidepressants — may be used for chronic pain.

Physical therapy

Treatments such as heat, ultrasound, electrical stimulation and muscle-release techniques applied to your back muscles and soft tissues may reduce pain. A physical therapist also can provide instruction on specific exercises that may increase flexibility, strengthen back and abdominal muscles, and improve posture. The exercises can help prevent pain from returning.

Injections

If other measures don't relieve your pain and if the pain radiates down your leg, you may receive an injection of an anti-inflammatory medication such as cortisone into the space around your spinal cord (epidural space). A cortisone injection helps decrease inflammation around the nerve roots, reducing pain. The relief may be temporary.

In some cases, numbing medication and cortisone are injected into or near structures believed to be causing pain, such as the facet joints of the vertebrae. Located on the sides, top and bottom of each vertebra, these joints help stabilize the spine.

Surgery

If you have unrelenting pain or progressive muscle weakness from nerve compression, you may benefit from surgery. Otherwise, surgery usually is reserved for pain related to a structural problem that doesn't respond to other measures.

Lifestyle

A short period of bed rest is OK, but more than a couple of days may do more harm than good. Continue your daily activities as much as you can tolerate. Light activity, such as walking and daily activities of living, is usually OK. If an activity increases your pain, stop doing that activity. It's also important to maintain a healthy weight because extra weight strains your back muscles. In addition, try and lift smartly, letting your legs do most of the work.

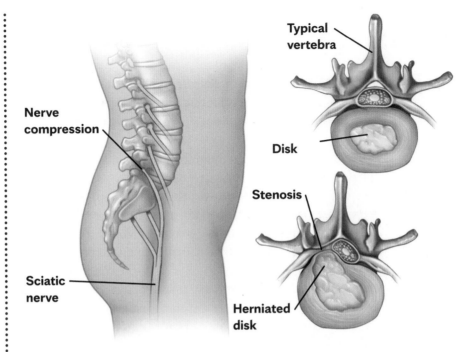

Back pain can occur for many reasons. Often, it stems from a muscle or ligament strain. Sometimes, back pain is related to one of the following conditions.

Herniated disk

A herniated disk describes a problem with one of the rubbery cushions (disks) between the bones (vertebrae) that form the spine. A spinal disk is a bit like a jelly doughnut — a softer center encased within a tougher exterior. Sometimes called a slipped or ruptured disk, a herniated disk occurs when some of the softer "jelly" pushes out through a crack in the tougher exterior and presses on a nearby nerve.

Sciatica

Sciatica is the name for pain that radiates along the path of the sciatic nerve — which branches from the lower back through the hips and buttocks and down each leg. Sciatica occurs when the sciatic nerve becomes pinched, usually by a herniated disk in the spine or a bony overgrowth (bone spur) on the vertebrae. Typically, sciatica affects only one side of the body. Some people also experience numbness, tingling or muscle weakness in the affected leg or foot.

Spinal stenosis

Spinal stenosis describes a narrowing of the open spaces within the spine, causing pressure on the spinal cord and the nerves that travel through it. Spinal stenosis occurs most often in the neck and lower back, producing neck or back pain. Compressed nerves in the lower (lumbar) spine can cause pain or cramping in the legs when standing for long periods of time or when walking. Bending forward or sitting down usually eases the discomfort.

Bipolar disorder

B

WHAT IS IT? Bipolar disorder is a mental health condition that causes extreme, unpredictable mood swings, including low periods (depression) and high periods (hypomania or mania).

In a period of mania or hypomania (which is less severe), you might have extreme energy and self-esteem, or you might be highly distracted or unusually irritable. When you become depressed, you may feel hopeless or low-energy and have less interest in what you usually enjoy. These ups and downs are known as episodes. They may last for days, weeks or months, and they can affect your ability to function.

Bipolar disorder was formerly called manic depression. There are several types, based on how long symptoms last and how severe they are.

WHAT'S THE CAUSE? People with bipolar disorder have physical changes in their brains, although no specific cause is known. A person's risk of bipolar disorder is higher if a sibling or parent has it. A very stressful event, such as death of a loved one, is another risk factor.

Lack of sleep, stress and unhealthy use of drugs may affect whether someone develops bipolar disorder. They can also trigger an episode.

SYMPTOM CHECKER People with bipolar disorder have periods of depression, mania or mixed moods. To be diagnosed with bipolar disorder, you must have experienced at least one 7-day period of elevated mood with at least three of these symptoms:

- Inflated self-esteem
- Less need for sleep and more energy
- Racing thoughts
- Distractibility
- Increased goal-directed activity
- Talkativeness
- Impulsivity
- Hypersexuality

The mood swings of bipolar disorder should not be due to medications, substance use or another illness.

WHAT TESTS TO EXPECT No test on its own can show if you have bipolar disorder. To make a diagnosis, your health care team will need to learn about you and your symptoms. This may include:

B

- Giving you a physical exam and lab tests to check for medical problems that could be causing symptoms
- Referring you to a psychiatrist, who will talk to you about your thoughts, feelings and behavior patterns
- Having you keep a daily record of your moods, sleep patterns or other factors that could help with the diagnosis and finding the right treatment

TREATMENT Getting treatment for bipolar disorder is important, because people with it may not realize what a big impact their episodes have on those around them. During an emotional high period, you may have poor judgment and place yourself in risky situations. In a low period, you may stop caring for yourself and could be at risk of self-harm or suicide.

Adults

People who have bipolar disorder usually take medications to stabilize their moods. They include:

- Lithium (Lithobid)
- Antipsychotics, such as olanzapine (Zyprexa), risperidone (Risperdal), lurasidone (Latuda), asenapine (Saphris), quetiapine (Seroquel), ziprasidone (Geodon) and aripiprazole (Abilify)

A psychiatrist might also prescribe an antidepressant to help with depressive episodes. For anxiety, a short-term treatment with a benzodiazepine may be added.

You may be tempted to stop taking medication if your symptoms don't improve right away or if you feel side effects. But it's important not to stop or change your treatment unless your doctor suggests a change. Some drugs need time to build up in the body. If you stop medication, you're at risk of having episodes again.

People with bipolar disorder also usually see a counselor for therapy. Talking with a therapist can help you identify unhealthy thoughts and behaviors, cope with a life crisis, or explore what triggers mood swings.

Types of psychotherapy commonly used include:

- Cognitive behavioral therapy
- Interpersonal and social rhythm therapy
- Individual therapy
- Group therapy
- Couples or family therapy

Children

The patterns of symptoms in children and teens may be different from those in adults. Some children also have other mental health conditions, such as attention-deficit/hyperactivity disorder (ADHD).

A child psychiatrist who has experience with bipolar disorder usually guides the care of a child with the condition. Treatment is based on a child's symptoms, medication side effects and other factors. It generally includes:

- **Medication.** The same mood-stabilizing drugs are often prescribed for children and adults with bipolar disorder.
- **Psychotherapy.** This type of therapy can help children and teens manage routines, develop coping skills, address learning difficulties and resolve social problems. It may also help strengthen family bonds and communication.
- **Psychoeducation.** Learning the symptoms can help the child's family understand how signs of bipolar disorder differ from typical behavior for a child's age and other factors.
- **Support.** Teachers, school counselors, family and friends can support the child and the family to encourage success.

FAMILY AND FRIENDS CAN HELP

It may not be easy to talk about bipolar disorder. But there's a much better chance to get the treatment you or your child needs, as soon as it's needed, when your family and friends know about the condition and know the signs of an episode beginning.

Talk to your family and friends. Help them learn about your condition so that they have accurate information. It could help save your life someday.

Blood clots

WHAT'S THE CAUSE? Blood clots can occur under many different circumstances and in many different locations. Those that form in response to an injury or a cut are beneficial because they stop potentially dangerous bleeding. But a number of conditions can produce blood clots that can be life-threatening.

Deep vein thrombosis is a condition in which a blood clot forms in a deep vein, usually in a leg. It's a serious problem because the blood clot can break loose, travel through the bloodstream and lodge in the lungs, blocking blood flow. This is called a pulmonary embolism. (A blood clot that forms in a brain artery can produce a stroke. See page 341.)

Many factors can increase your risk of developing deep vein thrombosis. Smoking, having a blood-clotting disorder, being off your feet for bed rest and being overweight are all factors. Additional factors include injury or surgery to your veins, use of estrogen found in birth control pills and hormone replacement therapy, and having heart disease.

SYMPTOM CHECKER A blood clot that forms in a leg may produce the following signs and symptoms:

- Swelling in the affected leg. Rarely, swelling in both legs.
- Pain in the leg that often starts in the calf and may feel like cramping or soreness.

Signs and symptoms of a pulmonary embolism include:

- Unexplained sudden onset of shortness of breath
- Chest pain that worsens when you take a deep breath or cough
- Feeling lightheaded or dizzy, or fainting
- Rapid pulse
- Coughing up blood

TREATMENT The goal of treatment for deep vein thrombosis or a pulmonary embolism is to get rid of the clot. Medications are most commonly prescribed. Other treatments also may be used depending on the type and size of the clot and its location.

Blood thinners. Anticoagulant medications, also called blood thinners, decrease the blood's ability to clot. They don't break up existing blood clots, but they keep them from getting bigger. They also help prevent the development of new clots. These medications, which include the drug heparin, are often given by injection. After starting heparin injections, your treatment may be followed by an oral blood thinner, such as warfarin (Jantoven), dabigatran (Pradaxa) or rivaroxaban (Xarelto).

If you're taking warfarin, watch how much vitamin K you're eating. Vitamin K can affect how warfarin works. Talk with your health care provider or a dietitian about your diet.

Clot busters. For severe deep vein thrombosis or a pulmonary embolism, or if other medications aren't working, your doctor may prescribe medications to break up the clot. A range of medications may be used, including thrombolytic agents. Thrombolytics are administered in a hospital and given through an IV line or a thin, flexible tube (catheter) placed directly into the clot.

Filters. If you can't take medications, a filter may be inserted into a large vein (vena cava) in your abdomen. The filter prevents clots that break loose from lodging in your lungs.

Clot removal. If you have a large clot in a lung, your doctor may suggest removing it. This is generally done via a catheter that's threaded through your blood vessels.

LIFESTYLE To help prevent blood clots from forming:

- **Avoid sitting or standing too long.** If you've had surgery or you've been on bed rest, try to walk as soon as possible. If you sit a lot, try to walk around every hour or so. If you're on a plane, stand or walk occasionally. You can also exercise your lower legs by flexing your heels and toes.
- **Get regular exercise.** Exercise lowers your risk of blood clots.
- **Lose weight and quit smoking.** Obesity and smoking increase your risk of deep vein thrombosis.
- **Wear compression stockings.** These tight-fitting stockings help prevent swelling associated with deep vein thrombosis and reduce the chances that your blood will pool and clot. They're available in a range of colors and textures.

Brain aneurysm

WHAT IS IT? A brain aneurysm is a bulge or ballooning in a blood vessel in the brain. It often looks like a berry hanging on a stem. A brain aneurysm can leak or rupture, causing bleeding into the brain (hemorrhagic stroke). An aneurysm that ruptures is life-threatening and requires prompt medical treatment.

Many brain aneurysms, however, don't rupture or cause symptoms. They're often detected during imaging tests for other conditions.

WHAT'S THE CAUSE? A number of factors can weaken an artery wall and increase the risk of an aneurysm. They include:

- A family history of aneurysms
- Older age
- Smoking
- High blood pressure (hypertension)
- Hardening of the arteries (arteriosclerosis)
- A condition at birth that increases blood pressure or interrupts blood flow
- Drug misuse, particularly the use of cocaine
- Head injury
- Heavy alcohol consumption

SYMPTOM CHECKER An unruptured brain aneurysm may not produce any symptoms, particularly if it's small. An unruptured aneurysm that's large may press on brain tissues and nerves, possibly causing:

- Pain above and behind an eye
- A dilated pupil
- Change in vision or double vision
- Numbness, weakness or paralysis of one side of the face
- A drooping eyelid

A ruptured aneurysm may produce several signs and symptoms:

- Sudden, extremely severe headache
- Nausea and vomiting

- Stiff neck
- Blurred or double vision
- Sensitivity to light
- Seizure
- A drooping eyelid
- Loss of consciousness
- Confusion

In some cases, an aneurysm may not fully rupture but leak a slight amount of blood. This leaking (sentinel bleed) generally produces a severe headache. Immediate treatment is important because a more severe rupture almost always follows.

WHAT TESTS TO EXPECT If you have a sudden, severe headache or other symptoms possibly related to a ruptured aneurysm, you'll undergo tests to determine if you have had bleeding in the brain. If bleeding has occurred, your emergency care team will determine the next steps.

If you have symptoms of an unruptured brain aneurysm, you may undergo one or more tests, including computerized tomography (CT) or magnetic resonance imaging (MRI) of the brain. Sometimes, dye is released into brain arteries before CT or MRI scans are taken to help identify an aneurysm. Your cerebrospinal fluid also may be examined to look for red blood cells, indicating bleeding.

TREATMENT The most common treatment options for a ruptured brain aneurysm are surgery to close off the aneurysm or a less invasive procedure. With the less invasive procedure, a catheter is threaded through the body to the aneurysm. A wire device is then implanted to disrupt blood flow and cause blood to clot.

A catheter or shunt may also be used to drain excess fluid and lessen pressure on the brain. Medications also may be prescribed to help prevent complications.

Treatment for an unruptured brain aneurysm generally involves a procedure to clip and seal off the aneurysm. In some cases, risks of such a procedure may outweigh the potential benefits. Other options include careful observation and medications and lifestyle changes to control high blood pressure.

Brain tumor

WHAT IS IT? A brain tumor is a mass of abnormal cells in the brain. Different types of brain tumors exist. Some are noncancerous (benign) and some are cancerous (malignant). Brain tumors can also result from cancer that begins in another part of the body and spreads to the brain (metastatic).

Benign brain tumors tend to grow more slowly than cancerous tumors. These tumors are still serious and possibly life-threatening. A benign tumor can press on parts of the brain, causing various symptoms. Benign tumors need to be monitored to be sure they're not growing.

WHAT'S THE CAUSE? Factors that may put you at increased risk of a brain tumor include:

- **Age.** Brain tumors are most common in older adults. However, a brain tumor can occur at any age.
- **Exposure to radiation.** People who've been exposed to ionizing radiation are at increased risk of a brain tumor. Ionizing radiation includes radiation therapy used to treat cancer and radiation exposure from atomic bombs. Radiofrequency radiation from cellphones hasn't been linked to brain tumors.
- **Family history.** A small number of brain tumors occur in people with a family history of brain tumors or genetic syndromes that increase the risk of brain tumors.

SYMPTOM CHECKER Signs and symptoms of a brain tumor vary greatly and may include:

- New onset or change in pattern of headaches
- More-frequent and more-severe headaches
- Unexplained nausea or vomiting
- Vision problems
- Gradual loss of sensation or movement in an arm or a leg
- Difficulty with balance
- Speech difficulties
- Hearing problems
- Personality or behavior changes
- Seizures

TREATMENT If a health care provider suspects a brain tumor, a number of tests and procedures may be recommended. Treatment depends on the type, size and location of the tumor. Some benign tumors may be monitored with imaging scans.

Surgery
If the tumor is located in a place that's accessible, surgery may be done to remove as much of it as possible. Some tumors are small and easy to separate from surrounding brain tissue, making complete surgical removal possible. In other cases, the tumor can't be separated from surrounding tissue or it's located near sensitive brain areas, so only a portion is removed.

Radiation
Radiation to kill the cancer cells may be focused on the area of the brain where the tumor is located or applied to the entire brain (whole-brain radiation). Whole-brain radiation is most often used to treat cancer that's spread to the brain from other areas.

Radiosurgery
Multiple beams of radiation are focused on a very small area. Each beam of radiation isn't particularly powerful, but the point where all the beams meet — the tumor — receives a very large dose of radiation. Radiosurgery is typically done in one treatment.

Chemotherapy
The chemotherapy drug used most often to treat cancerous brain tumors is temozolomide (Temodar). Other drugs may be used depending on the type of cancer. In another type of chemotherapy, after removal of the tumor the surgeon places one or more disk-shaped wafers in the space left by the tumor. The wafers slowly release a chemotherapy drug over the next several days.

Targeted drug therapy
Targeted drug treatments focus on specific features or functions of cancer cells. One type of targeted therapy stops the formation of new blood vessels, which cuts off the blood supply to the tumor. Another type blocks an enzyme that plays a key role in the growth of cancer cells.

Breast cancer

WHAT IS IT? Breast cancer is the uncontrolled growth of cells in the breast. After skin cancer, it's the most commonly diagnosed cancer in women in the United States. While it's more common in women, breast cancer can occur in anyone.

Parts of the breast where cancer begins include:

- **Milk ducts.** Breast cancer most often starts in the lining of the milk ducts. The ducts are the tubes through which milk flows to a reservoir under the nipple.
- **Milk-producing lobules.** Lobular breast cancer (lobular carcinoma) starts in the lobules of the breast, where breast milk is made.
- **Connective tissue.** Less commonly, breast cancer may begin in the connective tissue that's made up of muscles, fat and blood vessels. This type of cancer is called sarcoma.

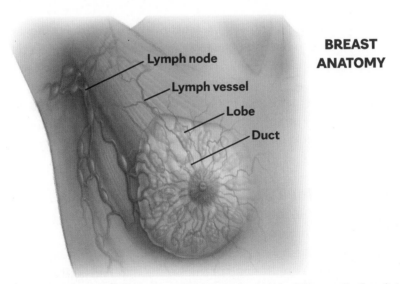

BREAST ANATOMY

Each breast contains 15 to 20 lobes of glandular tissue. The lobes are further divided into smaller lobules that produce milk for breastfeeding. Small tubes (ducts) conduct the milk to a reservoir that lies just beneath the nipple.

WHAT'S THE CAUSE? Breast cancer develops when gene changes (mutations) cause some cells in the breast to grow out of control and divide faster than healthy cells. The cancerous cells then form a lump and can spread to a lymph node or other parts of the body.

About 5% to 10% of breast cancers are caused by changes in genes that are inherited. People with mutations in genes called BRCA1 and BRCA2 have a much higher risk of both breast and ovarian cancers.

Women and older adults generally have a greater risk of developing breast cancer. Other risk factors include:

- A personal history of certain breast conditions, such as lobular carcinoma *in situ* or atypical hyperplasia of the breast
- Having a family history of breast cancer
- Having radiation treatments to your chest
- Being overweight
- Getting your first period before age 12
- Beginning menopause at an older age
- Having your first child after age 30
- Having never been pregnant
- Taking postmenopausal hormone therapy (estrogen and progesterone)
- Drinking alcohol

More than 80% of breast cancers are sporadic, meaning they are not due to inherited gene changes. The cause may be related to a person's lifestyle, environment and other factors such as hormones.

Risk factors for breast cancer in men include having more than one copy of the X chromosome (Klinefelter's syndrome), liver disease, and testicle disease or surgery.

SYMPTOM CHECKER If you find a lump or notice a change in your breast, make an appointment with your health care provider. Signs and symptoms of breast cancer can include:

- A breast lump or thickening that feels different from tissue around it
- A change in the size, shape or appearance of the breast
- Changes in skin over the breast, such as dimpling
- A newly inverted nipple
- Peeling, scaling, crusting or flaking of skin around the nipple (areola) or the breast itself
- Redness or pitting of the skin over the breast, like the skin of an orange
- Discharge from a nipple, particularly in men

WHAT TESTS TO EXPECT Several tests and procedures are used to diagnose breast cancer, including:

Breast exam
The breasts and lymph nodes in the armpit are checked for lumps or changes.

Mammogram
An X-ray of the breast is done. If a mammogram shows an irregularity, you may need to have another mammogram to evaluate.

Breast ultrasound
This test uses sound waves to make images of structures in the body. If you have a breast lump, you may have an ultrasound to see if the mass is solid or a fluid-filled cyst.

Biopsy
A biopsy is the only sure way to diagnose breast cancer. Tissue is removed from the breast with a special needle. The sample can be tested to find out if the cells in it are cancer. If they are, the lab can determine how aggressive the disease is and if it might respond to certain types of treatment.

Breast magnetic resonance imaging (MRI)
Images of the interior of the breast are made with use of a magnetic field and radio waves. Before having an MRI, you may receive an injection of dye. This test does not involve use of radiation.

Molecular breast imaging (MBI)
This test uses a radioactive tracer and special camera to find breast cancer. On the images, tissue that contains rapidly growing and dividing cells, such as cancer cells, looks brighter than less active tissue.

TREATMENT Once you've been diagnosed with breast cancer, your health care provider will review the results of imaging tests and the report on the biopsy. That information helps your medical team anticipate how the cancer may act and what treatments might be most effective.

Treatment for breast cancer depends on the extent (stage) of the disease, how aggressive the cancer appears to be (grade) and the tumor's size. Knowing whether the tumor is sensitive to hormones also helps your doctor decide the best way to treat it or prevent cancer from recurring.

Stage

The stages of breast cancer range from 0 to 4. If a person has stage 0 disease, it is noninvasive or has not spread outside the milk ducts or lobules where it started. Stage 4 disease is metastatic. That means it has spread to other areas of the body.

Grade

Breast cancers are graded on a 1 to 3 scale. Grade 3 cancers look the most different from typical cells and are generally the most aggressive.

Hormone sensitivity

Some breast cancers respond to naturally occurring hormones — estrogen and progesterone. They have receptors that catch these hormones in the body. Other cancers don't have these receptors. Your doctor may test cells from your tumor to see if they have receptors and, if so, which ones.

Types of treatment

Most people with breast cancer undergo surgery. They may also receive other treatment after surgery, such as chemotherapy, hormone therapy or radiation. In certain situations, chemotherapy may also be used before surgery.

Breast cancer surgery. Operations used to treat breast cancer include:

- Lumpectomy, in which only the tumor and a small margin of healthy tissue around it are removed
- Mastectomy, in which all of the breast is removed
- Sentinel node biopsy, in which a node or nodes closest to the tumor are removed and tested for cancer

Some women with cancer in one breast choose to have their other (healthy) breast removed. This may be because they have a genetic predisposition to the disease or a strong family history of it.

Radiation therapy. Radiation uses high-powered beams of energy, such as X-rays and protons, to kill cancer cells. External beam radiation of the whole breast often is used after a lumpectomy.

Chemotherapy. In chemotherapy, drugs are given that destroy fast-growing cells, such as cancer cells.

Hormone therapy. If your breast cancer is sensitive to hormones, you may be treated with drugs to block hormones from attaching to cancer cells or to stop your body from making estrogen after menopause. Surgery or medication can be used to stop hormone production in the ovaries.

Targeted therapy drugs. Newer drug treatments are available for breast cancer that attack specific changes in the cells. For example, if your tumor produces too much of a protein called human epidermal growth factor receptor 2 (HER2), you may be given a drug to stop the tumor from making so much.

Immunotherapy. Another area of active research is immunotherapy for breast cancer. This type of therapy mobilizes your own immune system to fight the disease. Immunotherapy might be an option if you have triple-negative breast cancer. That means the cancer cells don't have receptors for estrogen, progesterone or HER2.

LIFESTYLE There's no certain way to prevent breast cancer, but there are things you can do to lower your risk:

- Talk to your health care provider about the benefits and risks of screening for breast cancer.
- Do regular breast self-exams, and tell your provider right away about any changes you notice.
- If you drink alcohol, use it in moderation (for healthy adults, up to one drink a day for women and up to two drinks a day for men).
- Exercise at least 30 minutes on most days of the week. Talk with your provider about including strengthening exercises 2 to 3 times a week. This can lower your cancer risk overall.
- Before taking hormone therapy in menopause, talk with your provider about the benefits and risks, considering your age and other health factors.
- Maintain a healthy weight. If you're overweight, ask your provider about healthy ways to lose weight.

- Eat a healthy diet. A Mediterranean diet may reduce risk of breast cancer. People who follow it choose healthy fats, such as olive oil, over butter and fish instead of red meat.

If you have certain risk factors for breast cancer, your doctor may recommend other options to help prevent the disease, such as:

- **Selective estrogen receptor modulators and aromatase inhibitors.** These drugs block estrogen and can reduce the risk of breast cancer in women with a high risk of the disease.
- **Preventive surgery.** Surgery to remove healthy breasts or ovaries, or both, may be an option for some people who have BRCA1 or BRCA2 gene changes.

HOW TO PERFORM A SELF-EXAM

A breast self-exam is a good way to become familiar with the look and feel of your breasts. You may want to ask your health care provider to show you how to do it. The steps are as follows:

- Face forward and look for puckering, dimpling, or changes in size, shape or symmetry in your breasts.
- Check to see if your nipples are turned in (inverted).
- Inspect your breasts with your hands pressed down on your hips.
- Inspect your breasts with your arms raised overhead and the palms of your hands pressed together.
- Lift your breasts to see if ridges along the bottom are symmetrical.
- Use the pads of your three middle fingers to feel your breasts. Imagine the face of a clock over your breast or the slices of a pie. Begin near your collarbone and examine that section, moving your fingers toward your nipple. Then move your fingers to the next section.

Don't panic if you find a change or lump in your breast. Breasts feel different in different places. Some changes in breasts may occur at various points in the menstrual cycle or with age. Talk to your provider if you have concerns about your breasts.

Bronchitis

WHAT IS IT? Bronchitis is an inflammation of the lining of the bronchial tubes. The condition may be acute or chronic.

Acute bronchitis typically develops from a cold or other respiratory infection. Chronic bronchitis is associated with constant irritation or inflammation of the bronchial tube lining, often due to smoking. Chronic bronchitis is one of the conditions included in chronic obstructive pulmonary disease (COPD).

Signs and symptoms of bronchitis include:

- Cough
- Production of clear or yellowish-green mucus (sputum)
- Fatigue
- Shortness of breath
- Slight fever and chills
- Chest discomfort

With acute bronchitis, a nagging cough may linger for several weeks after the inflammation resolves. With chronic bronchitis, a cough persists for months and recurs often.

TREATMENT Before making a diagnosis, your health care provider may order tests to rule out other conditions, such as pneumonia.

Most cases of acute bronchitis resolve without medical treatment in about two weeks. In some circumstances, a provider may prescribe an inhaler to help open narrowed passageways in your lungs or cough medicine to help you sleep at night. Because bronchitis typically results from a viral infection, antibiotics aren't effective. However, they may be prescribed if a bacterial infection is suspected.

If you have chronic bronchitis, you may benefit from a breathing exercise program to help you breathe more easily.

Other measures that may help include avoiding air irritants and using a humidifier to keep the air warm and moist. If cold air aggravates your cough and causes shortness of breath, wear a face mask before you go outside.

Bunions

WHAT IS IT? A bunion is a bony bump that forms on the joint at the base of your big toe. It occurs when your big toe pushes against your next toe, forcing the joint of your big toe to get bigger and stick out. Smaller bunions (bunionettes) also can develop on the joints of your little toes.

Bunions result when the pressures of bearing and shifting your weight fall unevenly on the joints and tendons in your feet. This imbalance makes your big toe joint unstable. Over time, the joint is molded into a knob that juts out. Factors that increase your risk of bunions include:

- **Heredity.** An inherited structural foot problem may increase the tendency to develop bunions.
- **A deformity or injury.** A deformity at birth or a foot injury that creates an imbalance in foot pressure may lead to a bunion.
- **Arthritis.** Bunions may be associated with certain types of arthritis, particularly inflammatory types such as rheumatoid arthritis. Pain from osteoarthritis that changes the way you walk also may make you more likely to get bunions.
- **High-heeled shoes.** Wearing high heels forces your toes into the front of your shoes, often crowding your toes.
- **Ill-fitting shoes.** People who wear shoes that are too tight, too narrow or too pointed are more prone to get bunions.

SYMPTOM CHECKER Signs and symptoms may include:

- A bulging bump on the outside of the base of the big toe
- Swelling, redness or soreness around the big toe joint
- Thickening of the skin at the base of the big toe
- Corns or calluses — these often develop where the first and second toes overlap
- Persistent or intermittent pain
- Restricted movement of the big toe

TREATMENT A doctor generally can identify a bunion fairly easily by examining your foot. Treatment options vary depending on the severity of the bunion and the amount of pain it causes.

Conservative treatment

Nonsurgical treatments to relieve the pain and pressure include:

Padding and taping or splinting. These methods can cushion and support your foot in a corrected position to reduce stress on the bunion.

Medications. Over-the-counter pain relievers may help control the pain of a bunion. Cortisone injections also may be helpful.

Shoe inserts. Padded shoe inserts may help distribute pressure more evenly when you walk. Inserts can reduce symptoms and prevent your bunion from getting worse. Over-the-counter arch supports may help some people; others may require prescription orthotics.

Applying ice. Icing may help relieve soreness and inflammation.

Surgery

If conservative treatment isn't helpful, you may need surgery to correct the position of your toe. Surgery for a bunion may involve one of the following procedures:

- Removing the swollen tissue from around your big toe joint
- Straightening your big toe by removing part of the bone
- Realigning the long bone between the back part of your foot and your big toe to straighten the irregular angle in your big toe joint
- Permanently joining (fusing) the bones of your affected joint

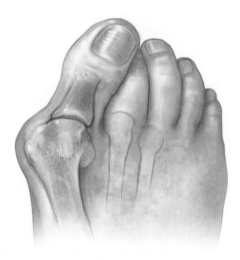

A bunion forms when the big toe joint becomes enlarged, causing the toe to crowd against the other toes.

Bursitis

WHAT IS IT? Bursitis is a painful condition that affects the small, fluid-filled sacs (bursae) that cushion bones, tendons and muscles near your joints. When one or more of the small sacs become inflamed, the result is bursitis.

The most common locations for bursitis are in the shoulder, elbow and hip. But you can also have bursitis by your knee, heel and the base of your big toe.

Bursitis often occurs near joints that perform frequent repetitive motion. Anyone can develop bursitis, but certain factors increase the risk:

- **Age.** Bursitis is more common with age.
- **Occupations or hobbies.** If work or a hobby requires repetitive motion or pressure on particular bursae, the risk of developing bursitis increases. Examples include carpet laying, tile setting, gardening, painting, throwing a baseball and playing a musical instrument.
- **Other medical conditions.** Certain diseases and conditions — such as rheumatoid arthritis, gout and diabetes — increase the risk of developing bursitis.

SYMPTOM CHECKER A joint affected by bursitis may:

- Feel achy or stiff
- Hurt more when you move it or press on it
- Look swollen and red

TREATMENT Bursitis is often diagnosed after a medical history and physical exam. Treatment typically involves resting the affected joint and protecting it from further trauma. In most cases, bursitis pain goes away within a few weeks with proper treatment, but recurrent flare-ups are common.

Types
Conservative measures, such as rest, ice and taking a pain reliever, are often effective in relieving symptoms. If conservative measures don't work, other options include:

Medication. An antibiotic may be prescribed if the inflammation is related to a bacterial infection.

Injections. A corticosteroid drug may be injected into a bursa in a shoulder or hip to relieve inflammation. This treatment often brings rapid pain relief. In many cases, only one injection is needed.

Therapy. Physical therapy to help strengthen the muscles in the affected area may ease the pain and prevent a recurrence.

Surgery. Sometimes an inflamed bursa must be surgically drained, but only rarely is removal of the affected bursa necessary.

LIFESTYLE You can reduce your risk of some forms of bursitis by changing how you perform certain tasks.

- **Use kneeling pads.** A pad reduces the pressure on your knees.
- **Lift properly.** Failing to bend your knees when you lift puts extra stress on the bursae in your hips.
- **Wheel heavy loads.** Carrying heavy loads puts stress on the bursae in your shoulders. Use a dolly or a wheeled cart instead.
- **Take frequent breaks.** Rest between repetitive tasks.
- **Maintain a healthy weight.** Being overweight places more stress on your joints.
- **Exercise.** Strengthening your muscles and tendons helps protect your joints.

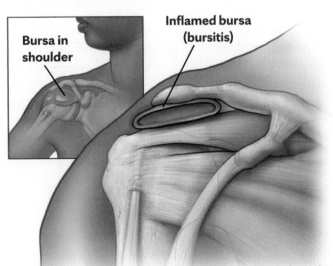

Bursae (shown in blue) are small, fluid-filled sacs that help cushion the moving parts in your joints.

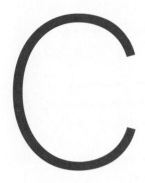

Cancer

WHAT IS IT? Cancer refers to any one of a large number of diseases characterized by the development of cells that divide uncontrollably and have the ability to infiltrate and destroy body tissue. Cancer that starts in one part of the body has the ability to spread throughout the body.

WHAT'S THE CAUSE? Cancer is caused by changes (mutations) to the DNA within cells. Each cell's DNA contains a set of instructions telling it how to grow and divide. Errors in these instructions can allow a cell to become cancerous.

Most commonly, a gene mutation may instruct a healthy cell to do one of the following:

- **Grow too fast.** The cell grows and divides more rapidly than it should. This creates many new cells that have the same mutation.
- **Forget to apply the brakes.** Healthy cells know when to stop growing. Cancer cells lose such control. They continue to grow and accumulate.
- **Overlook DNA errors.** Specialized genes called repair genes look for errors in a cell's DNA and make corrections. A mutation in a repair gene may prevent an error from being corrected.

Risk factors

Some gene mutations are inherited but most occur after you're born. A number of factors can produce gene mutations and lead to cancer. They include the following:

- **Age.** Because cancer can take decades to develop, it's most common in people age 65 and older. However, it can occur at any age.
- **Habits.** Certain lifestyle choices are known to increase the risk of cancer. Smoking, excessive alcohol use, excessive exposure to the sun, lack of exercise, and having unsafe sex can contribute to cancer. A diet rich in vegetables and fruits may help prevent it.
- **Weight management.** Carrying extra pounds may increase the risk of cancer, while losing weight may lower the risk.
- **Family history.** Only a small portion of cancers are inherited. Having an inherited genetic mutation increases your risk but doesn't necessarily mean you'll get cancer.
- **Health.** Some chronic conditions can markedly increase your risk of developing certain cancers. Ulcerative colitis, for example, significantly increases the risk of colon cancer.
- **Environment.** Harmful chemicals in the environment can increase the risk of cancer. Examples include secondhand smoke or chemicals such as asbestos and benzene.

SYMPTOM CHECKER Signs and symptoms associated with cancer vary depending on what part of the body is affected. Some general signs and symptoms include:

- Fatigue
- Lump or area of thickening that can be felt under the skin
- Weight changes, including unintended loss or gain
- Skin changes, such as yellowing, darkening or redness of the skin, sores that won't heal, or changes to existing moles
- Changes in bowel or bladder habits
- Persistent cough
- Difficulty swallowing or hoarseness
- Persistent indigestion or discomfort after eating
- Persistent, unexplained muscle or joint pain
- Persistent, unexplained fevers or night sweats

WHAT TESTS TO EXPECT Cancer is most often diagnosed using a combination of these approaches:

Physical exam
During a physical exam, your health care provider may feel areas of your body for lumps that may indicate a tumor. Your provider may also look for changes in skin color or enlargement of an organ.

Laboratory tests

Laboratory tests, such as urine and blood tests, may help your health care provider identify changes associated with cancer. For instance, in people with leukemia, a common blood test called a complete blood count (CBC) may reveal an unusual number of white blood cells.

Imaging tests

Imaging tests used in diagnosing cancer may include a computerized tomography (CT) scan, bone scan, magnetic resonance imaging (MRI), ultrasound and X-ray, among others. These tests can identify tumors and other changes associated with cancer.

Biopsy

In a biopsy, a sample of cells are collected for testing in a laboratory. There are several ways of doing this, depending on the type of cancer and its location. In most cases, a biopsy is the only way to definitively diagnose cancer. Under a microscope, cancer cells look less orderly than other cells, with varying sizes and shapes.

TREATMENT Health care providers have many tools when it comes to treating cancer. Treatment depends, in part, on the cancer itself.

Types

Treatment options include:

Surgery. The goal is to remove the cancer or as much of it as possible. Often, you'll have other treatments after surgery.

Chemotherapy. Chemotherapy uses medications to kill cancer cells. There are many chemotherapy drugs. Certain drugs are more effective for certain cancers.

Radiation therapy. Radiation therapy involves the use of high-powered energy beams, such as X-rays, to kill cancer cells.

Stem cell transplant. Also known as bone marrow transplant, this procedure involves transplanting your own stem cells or stem cells from a donor into your bone marrow. This is done to replenish the marrow and encourage the growth of healthy new blood cells after cancerous cells are destroyed by chemotherapy.

Immunotherapy. This treatment, also called biological therapy, uses the body's immune system to fight cancer. It helps your immune system "see" the cancer and attack it.

Hormone therapy. Some types of cancer, such as breast and prostate cancers, are fueled by hormones. Removing those hormones or blocking their effects may cause the cancer cells to stop growing.

Targeted drug therapy. Targeted drug treatments focus on specific characteristics within cancer cells. For example, one type of targeted therapy stops the formation of new blood vessels, cutting off blood supply to the tumor. Another type blocks an enzyme that plays a role in the growth of cancer cells.

Other treatments may be available, depending on the type of cancer.

LIFESTYLE There's no certain way to prevent cancer, but there are things you can do to reduce your risk:

- **Stop smoking.** Smoking is linked to several types of cancer — not just lung cancer.
- **Avoid excessive sun exposure.** Harmful ultraviolet (UV) rays from the sun can increase the risk of skin cancer. When outside, wear protective clothing or use sunscreen.
- **Eat a healthy diet.** Eat plenty of fruits and vegetables, which contain beneficial nutrients. Opt for whole grains and lean proteins.
- **Exercise.** Regular exercise is linked to a lower risk of cancer. Aim for at least 30 minutes of exercise most days of the week.
- **Maintain a healthy weight.** Obesity and being overweight can increase the risk of cancer. You can lose weight through a combination of a healthy diet and regular exercise.
- **Limit alcohol.** If you choose to drink alcohol, do it in moderation. For healthy adults, that's up to one drink a day for women and two drinks a day for men.
- **Get cancer screening exams.** Talk to your health care provider about what screening exams are best for you based on your risk factors.
- **Be up to date on your vaccinations.** Certain viruses increase your risk of cancer. Vaccinations may help prevent those viruses, including hepatitis B, which increases the risk of liver cancer, and human papillomavirus (HPV), which increases the risk of cervical cancer and other cancers.

Carpal tunnel syndrome

?

C

WHAT IS IT? Carpal tunnel syndrome is a hand and arm condition caused by a pinched nerve in the wrist that produces numbness, tingling and weakness.

The carpal tunnel is a narrow passageway located on the palm side of your wrist that's bound by bones and ligaments. This tunnel protects a main (median) nerve to your hand and the tendons that bend your fingers.

In general, anything that crowds, irritates or compresses the median nerve in the carpal tunnel space can lead to carpal tunnel syndrome. Factors that can increase your risk of carpal tunnel syndrome include:

- **Injury.** A wrist fracture or dislocation that alters the space within the carpal tunnel can create pressure on the median nerve.
- **Nerve-damaging conditions.** Some chronic illnesses, such as diabetes, increase your risk of nerve damage, including damage to the median nerve.
- **Inflammatory conditions.** Illnesses such as rheumatoid arthritis can affect the tendons in your wrist, exerting pressure on the median nerve.
- **Imbalance in body fluids.** Fluid retention, common during pregnancy or menopause, may increase the pressure within the carpal tunnel, irritating the median nerve.
- **Workplace factors.** The scientific evidence is conflicting, but it's possible that working with vibrating tools or performing a job that requires prolonged or repetitive flexing of the wrist may create pressure on or irritate the median nerve.

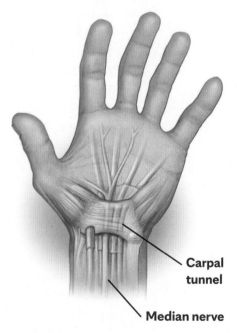

Carpal tunnel

Median nerve

Carpal tunnel syndrome occurs when the median nerve, which runs from your forearm to your hand, gets compressed or irritated.

SYMPTOM CHECKER Common symptoms of carpal tunnel syndrome include:

Tingling or numbness. You may experience tingling and numbness — especially in your thumb and index, middle or ring fingers, but not in your little finger. This sensation may occur while holding a steering wheel, newspaper or phone or while sleeping. It may extend from your wrist up your arm.

Weakness. You may experience weakness in your hand and find yourself frequently dropping objects. This may be due to weakening of the thumb's pinching muscles, which are controlled by the median nerve, or to numbness in the hand.

TREATMENT Your health care provider will ask about your symptoms and likely examine your wrist. Other tests may include those to evaluate the action of certain muscles and nerves.

Some people with mild symptoms can ease their discomfort by taking frequent breaks to rest their hands, avoiding activities that worsen symptoms and applying cold packs to reduce swelling.

Types
If self-care techniques don't offer relief, additional treatment options include wrist splinting, medications and surgery.

Wrist splinting. A splint that holds your wrist still while you sleep can help relieve nighttime symptoms of tingling and numbness.

Nonsteroidal anti-inflammatory drugs (NSAIDs). These medications may help relieve pain associated with carpal tunnel syndrome.

Corticosteroids. Your provider may inject your carpal tunnel with a corticosteroid such as cortisone. Corticosteroids decrease inflammation and swelling, which relieves pressure on the median nerve.

Surgery. The goal of carpal tunnel surgery is to relieve pressure on your median nerve by cutting the ligament that's pressing on it. During the healing process after the surgery, the ligament tissues gradually grow back together while allowing more room for the nerve than was there before.

Cataracts

WHAT IS IT? A cataract is a clouding of the clear lens of the eye. Seeing through a cloudy lens is a bit like looking through a frosty or fogged-up window.

Most cataracts are a result of aging. As you get older, the lenses in your eyes become less flexible, less transparent and thicker. Tissues within the lens may break down and clump together, clouding small areas. At first, the cloudiness may affect only a small part of the eye's lens. As the cataract grows, the blurring becomes more widespread.

Some cataracts are related to inherited genetic disorders. Cataracts may also stem from other eye disorders; medical conditions such as diabetes or high blood pressure; trauma; or past eye surgery.

Long-term use of corticosteroid medications also can increase the risk of cataracts. So can excessive exposure to sunlight.

SYMPTOM CHECKER Signs and symptoms may include:

- Clouded, blurred or dim vision
- Increasing difficulty with vision at night
- Sensitivity to light and glare
- Seeing "halos" around lights
- Frequent changes in eyeglass or contact lens prescription
- Fading or yellowing of colors
- Double vision in a single eye

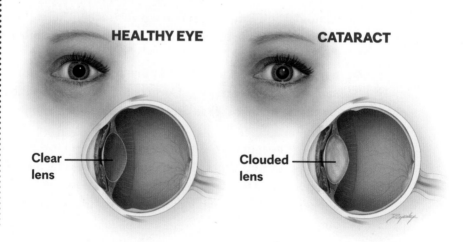

HEALTHY EYE   **CATARACT**

Clear lens   Clouded lens

WHAT TESTS TO EXPECT To determine whether you have a cataract, you'll have an eye examination that will likely include these basic tests.

- **Visual acuity test.** For this test you're asked to read an eye chart with progressively smaller letters.
- **Slit-lamp examination.** This test allows your eye doctor to see the structures at the front of your eye under magnification to look for any irregularities.
- **Retinal examination.** Before this test, dilating drops are placed in your eyes to open your pupils wide. This makes it easier to examine the back of your eyes (retina). Using a slit lamp or a device called an ophthalmoscope, your eye doctor can examine your lens for signs of a cataract.

TREATMENT The only effective treatment for cataracts is surgery. It's up to you and your health care provider to decide when cataract surgery is right for you. Surgery is recommended for most people when their cataracts begin to affect their quality of life or interfere with their ability to perform regular daily activities, such as reading or driving at night.

Cataract surgery involves removing the clouded lens and replacing it with a clear artificial lens. The artificial lens is positioned in the same place as your natural lens, and it remains a permanent part of your eye. The surgery is generally done under local anesthesia as an outpatient procedure.

For some people, other eye problems prohibit the use of an artificial lens. In these situations, once the cataract is removed, vision may be corrected with eyeglasses or contact lenses.

PREVENTION

No studies have proved that cataracts can be prevented, but eating plenty of colorful fruits and vegetables may help. Fruits and vegetables have many antioxidants thought to maintain eye health. A systematic review of research found that certain antioxidants do appear to protect against cataracts. More studies are needed to determine the doses required for protection or any adverse effects.

Celiac disease

WHAT IS IT? Celiac disease is an immune reaction to eating gluten, a protein found in wheat, barley and rye.

Among people who have the disease, their immune systems react to gluten similarly to how they respond to viruses or bacteria — they try to attack and destroy the protein. This reaction inflames and damages the lining of the small intestine and prevents the absorption of essential nutrients.

Celiac disease tends to run in families. Certain gene changes (mutations) are associated with the development of celiac disease. However, having one of these mutations doesn't mean you'll get the disease — just that you're at increased risk.

Similar to many immune disorders, celiac disease is thought to result from an interplay between genetics and something in the environment that triggers its development. It's possible that changes in gut bacteria could play a role. In some people, celiac disease becomes active for the first time after a serious viral infection or a major life event — such as surgery, pregnancy, childbirth or severe emotional stress.

SYMPTOM CHECKER The signs and symptoms of celiac disease vary greatly. Classic signs and symptoms include belly pain, bloating, excessive gas, and very odorous mushy stools or diarrhea.

Some people experience fatigue due to anemia or headaches. Some lose weight while others gain weight. Some are bothered by an itchy, blistering rash. And some people don't have any symptoms.

In children, the disease can affect growth and development.

WHAT TESTS TO EXPECT A diagnosis of celiac disease generally involves ruling out other possible causes of your symptoms and a few tests and procedures:

Blood tests. Elevated levels of certain substances in your blood (antibodies) indicate an immune reaction to gluten. In certain cases, a genetic test may be used to help rule out celiac disease.

Endoscopy. Your health care provider may order this procedure if blood tests suggest possible celiac disease. During endoscopy, a long tube with a tiny camera is put into your mouth and passed down your throat. Your provider can view the small intestine and take a sample of tissue (biopsy) to analyze for damage.

Capsule endoscopy. This procedure uses a tiny wireless camera to take pictures of the entire small intestine. Your provider may be able to see evidence of damage to the tissue.

TREATMENT The only way to treat celiac disease is to stop eating foods that contain gluten. That means all foods made from wheat, barley and rye. Oats are often harvested and processed in the same places as wheat, barley and rye, too, so they may have cross-contamination unless they are specifically labeled gluten-free.

Gluten-containing grains are pervasive in many foods, such as bread, pasta, baked goods and many processed products, such as chips, crackers and cookies. Gluten is present in most beers and in many salad dressings, sauces and seasonings. You can even find gluten in some luncheon meats and candies. Fortunately, more food processors are manufacturing gluten-free versions of their products.

If you have celiac disease, it's important to work with a dietitian to learn which foods are safe to eat and which are not. A dietitian can teach you how to read food labels and what ingredients to look for to alert you that the product contains gluten.

Once gluten is removed from the diet, inflammation of the small intestine begins to improve — often within days to weeks. However, complete healing may take several months to several years. Healing of the small intestine tends to occur more quickly in children than in adults.

In rare instances, the inflammation associated with celiac disease doesn't respond to a gluten-free diet. This is known as refractory celiac disease. Further testing is often necessary. Other treatments may be prescribed to manage symptoms.

Left untreated, the disease can lead to a number of serious conditions, including osteoporosis, anemia, infertility, vitamin deficiencies and cancer. That's why it's important for people with the disease — even those who don't experience symptoms — to follow a gluten-free diet.

Chronic fatigue syndrome

WHAT IS IT? Chronic fatigue syndrome is a complicated disorder characterized by extreme fatigue that lasts at least six months and can't be explained by any underlying medical condition. The fatigue may worsen with physical or mental activity, and it doesn't improve with rest.

This condition is also known as myalgic encephalomyelitis (ME). Sometimes it's abbreviated as ME/CFS. In addition, the disorder has been called systemic exertional intolerance disease (SEID).

The cause is unknown, although there are many theories — ranging from viral infections to psychological stress. Immune system problems and hormonal imbalances have been studied as well. Experts believe the condition may be related to a combination of factors.

These factors may increase your risk of chronic fatigue syndrome:

- **Age.** Chronic fatigue syndrome can occur at any age, but it most commonly affects young to middle-aged adults.
- **Sex.** The condition is diagnosed much more often in women than in men. However, it may be that women are simply more likely to report their symptoms to a health care provider.
- **Stress.** Difficulty managing stress may contribute to development of chronic fatigue syndrome.

SYMPTOM CHECKER For a diagnosis of chronic fatigue syndrome, symptoms must last for at least six months and be so severe that they limit your usual activities. Symptoms don't resolve with sleep and are worse after physical, mental or emotional exertion. The syndrome also involves at least one of these two symptoms: problems with memory and focus or dizziness that gets worse with moving from lying or sitting to standing (orthostatic intolerance).

Other signs and symptoms vary from person to person and may include:

- Loss of memory or concentration
- Sore throat
- Enlarged lymph nodes in the neck or armpits
- Unexplained muscle pain
- Headache of a new type, pattern or severity

- Joint pain without swelling or redness
- Chills and night sweats
- Nausea
- Light and sound sensitivity
- New allergies or sensitivities to food, chemicals or smells

WHAT TESTS TO EXPECT There's no single test to confirm a diagnosis of chronic fatigue syndrome. You may need to undergo medical tests to rule out other health problems with similar symptoms, such as a sleep disorder, a mental health issue, anemia, an underactive thyroid (hypothyroidism) or adrenal insufficiency.

TREATMENT The focus of treatment for chronic fatigue syndrome is on relieving symptoms.

Medications. Low doses of some antidepressants can help improve sleep and relieve pain, in addition to treating depression that may accompany the disease. Medications may also help with dizziness and pain.

Therapy. Many people with chronic fatigue syndrome benefit from an individualized therapy approach that combines psychological counseling with a gentle exercise program.

- **Psychological counseling.** A counselor can help build coping skills and find practical options for working around some of the limitations caused by the condition.
- **Paced activity.** Exercise often improves symptoms. A physical therapist can help determine what types of exercise are best. Inactive people often begin with range-of-motion and stretching exercises. As strength and endurance improve, you can increase the intensity.

Self-care. There are other steps you can take that may help relieve your symptoms and improve your quality of life. They include:

- **Find ways to relax.** Learn how to limit and respond to overexertion and emotional stress. And allow yourself time each day to relax. Relaxation therapies may be beneficial.
- **Avoid stimulants.** A good night's sleep is important. Caffeine, alcohol and nicotine can interfere with sleep.
- **Pace yourself.** Keep your activity at an even level. On days when you're feeling well, try not to overdo it.

Cold sore

WHAT IS IT? Cold sores — also called fever blisters — are tiny, fluid-filled lesions that occur on and around your lips. These blisters are often grouped together in patches.

Cold sores spread from person to person through close contact, such as kissing. Sharing eating utensils, razors and towels also can spread cold sores. The sores are caused by herpes simplex virus type 1 (HSV-1), which is closely related to the type that causes genital herpes (HSV-2). Both types can affect your mouth or genitals and can be spread by oral sex. Cold sores are contagious even if you don't see the sores.

SYMPTOM CHECKER A cold sore usually passes through several stages, which include:

- **Tingling and itching.** Many people feel an itching, burning or tingling sensation around their lips for a day or two before cold sore blisters erupt.
- **Blisters.** Small fluid-filled blisters typically break out along the border where the outside edge of the lips meets the skin of the face. Blisters can also occur around the nose or on the cheeks. Children younger than age 5 may have cold sores inside their mouths that are mistaken for canker sores.
- **Oozing and crusting.** The small blisters may merge and then burst, leaving shallow open sores that will ooze fluid and then crust over.

TREATMENT A cold sore generally clears up without treatment within about two weeks. Sometimes medications to speed the healing process may be prescribed. They include the drugs acyclovir (Zovirax), valacyclovir (Valtrex), famciclovir and penciclovir (Denavir).

If you develop cold sores frequently or if you're at high risk of serious complications, your health care provider may prescribe an antiviral medication to take on a regular basis.

A cream called docosanol (Abreva) may be used to treat cold sores and is available without a prescription. It must be applied frequently and may shorten an outbreak by a few hours or a day.

Colon cancer

WHAT IS IT? Colon cancer develops in the large intestine (colon). It is also sometimes called colorectal cancer.

The colon is part of the digestive system, which helps break down food to make energy.

ANATOMY O F THE LARGE INTESTINE (COLON)

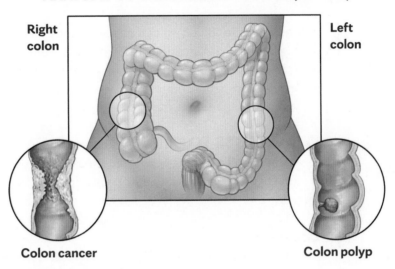

Right colon

Left colon

Colon cancer

Colon polyp

WHAT'S THE CAUSE? Colon cancer is one of the most common cancers in men and women. The cause of it isn't known. However, certain risk factors may make some people more likely to develop it, including:

- Being older. Colon cancer is diagnosed most often in people over age 40.
- Having small clumps of cells on the lining of the colon (colon polyps). Most polyps are harmless, but some can develop into colon cancer.
- Having a family history of colon polyps or cancer.
- Having more than three alcoholic drinks a week.
- Smoking.
- Being overweight and not exercising .
- Eating a diet high in red meat and low in vegetables.
- Having Crohn's disease or chronic ulcerative colitis.
- Being African American.

SYMPTOM CHECKER In the early stages of colon cancer, you may have no symptoms. The following symptoms may develop at later stages of the disease:

- Changes in bowel habits
- Blood in the stool, which may be bright red, maroon or black
- Diarrhea
- Constipation
- Narrow stools
- Inability to empty the bowel
- Unplanned weight loss

A large tumor in the colon can partially block your bowel. This may cause pain, nausea or vomiting. Polyps in the colon can bleed slowly over time, taking iron from the body. That may lead to iron deficiency anemia, resulting in tiredness and weakness.

WHAT TESTS TO EXPECT Routine screening for colon cancer is recommended beginning at age 45. There are several types of screening tests. Work with your health care provider to decide which test is best for you.

Colonoscopy

During this test, a thin, flexible tube is placed in the lower part of the colon (rectum). A tiny camera at the end of the tube lets your health care provider see inside your rectum and your entire colon.

People usually are given sedation for a colonoscopy. Your provider will tell you about changes in diet that you need to make and a colon cleansing routine you need to follow to prepare for the test.

A colonoscopy takes about 30 to 60 minutes. If polyps are found, they can be removed during the test. If the colonoscopy shows that you aren't at increased risk of colon cancer, you don't need to have another one for 10 years.

Virtual colonoscopy

This test takes about 10 minutes. It's done by using computerized tomography (CT) to make images of the colon and rectum. A small tube called a catheter is placed inside your rectum. It's used to fill your colon with air or carbon dioxide.

No sedation or colon cleansing is needed before a virtual colonoscopy. You do have to change your diet and drink a solution of contrast medium for the scan images.

This test can find most large polyps and some small ones. However, if anything of concern is found, you'll need a colonoscopy to remove it. If there's nothing unusual, you'll need to repeat the test every five years.

Stool DNA test

This test shows whether you have DNA changes in cells, which may mean you have colon cancer or precancerous clumps of cells (polyps). It can also find signs of blood in your stool.

To take a stool DNA test, you collect a stool sample at home and mail it to a lab. If the results show DNA changes or blood, you'll need to have a colonoscopy. Otherwise, you'll need to repeat the test every three years.

Fecal immunochemical test (FIT)

This test can show whether you have hidden blood in a sample of your stool. It doesn't require a change in diet, colon cleansing or sedation. You only need to collect a stool sample.

If the FIT shows blood in your stool, you need to have a colonoscopy. You'll need to repeat the test every year if it doesn't find anything out of the ordinary.

TREATMENT Most people with colon cancer have some type of surgery to remove the affected area (colectomy). Other therapies may be part of treatment as well.

Surgery

Several types of surgery may be recommended to treat colon cancer. The extent of the surgery depends on the stage of the disease. Stage 1 disease is only in the lining of the colon. Stage 2 cancer is in the colon wall but not nearby lymph nodes. Stage 3 cancer is in bowel wall and nearby lymph nodes. Stage 4 disease has spread to another organ, often the liver or lungs.

Surgical options for colon cancer may include:

Colon cancer screening tests

	Colonoscopy	
How often do I need to be screened if I don't have an increased risk of colon cancer?	10 years	
Does it require colon cleansing or diet changes?	Yes	
When can you return to work after the test?	The next day	
Is it recommended if there is a family history of colon cancer?	Yes	
Can it find polyps?	Can find most large and small polyps	
Can polyps be removed during the test?	Yes	
Is a colonoscopy needed if the test is positive?	N/A	

Source: Health Education & Content Services (Patient Education).

- **Local excision.** For early-stage disease, the cancer may be removed from the colon with a small border of healthy tissue.
- **Lower anterior resection.** For cancer in the upper rectum, part of the rectum can be removed. The remainder is reattached to the colon.
- **Proctectomy.** If cancer is in the lower to middle area of the rectum, part or all of the rectum may be removed. You may need a temporary attachment of the intestine to an opening created in your abdomen (ileostomy). This allows waste to leave your body through the opening (stoma). Later, a second surgery is needed to reverse the ileostomy.

Chemotherapy

Chemotherapy uses medications to kill cancer cells. It may be injected into a vein or taken in pill form. Sometimes, chemotherapy is combined with radiation therapy (chemoradiation).

	Virtual Colonoscopy	Stool DNA Test	Fecal Immunochemical Test (FIT)
	5 years	3 years	Every year
	Yes	No	No
	Immediately	Immediately	Immediately
	No	No	No
	Can find most large and some small polyps	Can find most large and some small polyps	Can find most large and a few small polyps
	No	No	No
	Yes	Yes	Yes

Colorectal cancer screening. Mayo Clinic; 2019.

Radiation therapy
This treatment uses high-energy beams, such as X-rays and protons, to destroy cancer cells. It can be used before and after surgery.

Biological therapy
These options use your body's immune system to attack cancer cells. There are many types of biological therapy. Some stop cancer cells from growing. Others stop cancer cells from getting nutrients.

LIFESTYLE You can reduce your risk of colon cancer with healthy daily habits: Eat a variety of fruits, vegetables and whole grains; exercise on most days; maintain a healthy weight; don't smoke; and limit alcohol.

Common cold

WHAT IS IT? The common cold is a viral infection of your upper respiratory tract — your nose and throat. A common cold is usually harmless, although it may not feel that way at the time.

What makes a cold different from other viral infections is that you generally won't have a high fever. You're also unlikely to experience significant fatigue from a common cold.

SYMPTOM CHECKER Because any one of more than 100 viruses can cause a cold, signs and symptoms can vary greatly and may include:

- Runny or stuffy nose
- Itchy or sore throat
- Cough
- Congestion
- Slight body aches or a mild headache
- Sneezing
- Watery eyes
- Low-grade fever
- Mild fatigue

TREATMENT There's no cure for the common cold. The goal of treatment is to relieve symptoms as much as possible.

Medications

Antibiotics are of no use against cold viruses, and over-the-counter cold medicine generally won't make a cold go away any sooner. Products that may help include:

Pain relievers. A pain reliever can help a fever, sore throat and headache feel better. All pain relievers can have potentially serious side effects in infants and children, so it's best to check with your health care provider before giving any medication to your child. With acetaminophen (Tylenol, others) and ibuprofen (Advil, Motrin IB, others), make sure to read and follow label directions carefully.

Aspirin is approved for use in children older than age 3, but it's been linked to Reye's syndrome, a rare but potentially life-threatening condition in children and teens. It's best to consult with a health care provider before giving aspirin to your child.

Decongestant nasal sprays. They may help relieve congestion, but adults shouldn't use them for more than a few days and children shouldn't use them at all. Prolonged use can cause rebound inflammation of the mucous membranes, which can worsen congestion.

Cough syrups. Cough and cold medicines shouldn't be given to children younger than age 6 because of potential side effects, including fatal overdoses in children younger than 2 years old. In fact, studies haven't proved that these medicines work in young children. And while cold medicines aim to relieve symptoms temporarily, they won't make a cold go away any sooner.

Self-care

Use these strategies to help ease symptoms:

Drink lots of fluids. Water, juice, clear broth and warm lemon water are good choices. They help replace fluids lost during mucus production or fever. Avoid alcohol and caffeine, which are dehydrating.

Try chicken soup. It temporarily speeds the movement of mucus through the nose, helping relieve congestion and limiting the time viruses are in contact with the nasal lining.

Soothe your throat. A saltwater gargle — a teaspoon salt dissolved in an 8-ounce glass of warm water — can temporarily relieve a sore or scratchy throat.

Use saline nasal drops. To help relieve nasal congestion, try saline nasal drops. You can buy them without a prescription, and they're effective, safe and nonirritating, even for children. In infants, place several saline drops into one nostril, then gently suction that nostril with a bulb syringe (insert the bulb syringe about ¼ to ½ inch).

Get some rest. Rest helps your body fight illness.

Adjust the temperature and humidity. Keep your home warm but not too hot. For dry air, use a cool-mist humidifier or vaporizer to moisten the air and help ease congestion and coughing. Keep the unit clean to prevent mold or bacteria growth.

Concussion

WHAT IS IT? A concussion is a traumatic brain injury that alters the way your brain functions. It often leads to headaches and problems with concentration, memory and balance.

The most common cause is a blow to the head, for example, in a fall or while playing a contact sport. A concussion can also occur when the head and upper body are violently shaken.

A concussion can cause you to lose consciousness, but most do not. Because of this, some people have concussions and don't realize it.

SYMPTOM CHECKER Signs and symptoms of a concussion can be subtle and not immediately apparent. Symptoms can last for days, weeks or even longer. Fortunately, most people usually recover fully.

Signs and symptoms of a concussion may include:

- Headache or a feeling of pressure in the head
- Temporary loss of consciousness
- Confusion or feeling as if in a fog
- Amnesia surrounding the traumatic event
- Dizziness or "seeing stars"
- Ringing in the ears
- Nausea and vomiting
- Slurred speech
- Delayed response to questions
- Appearing dazed
- Fatigue

Other symptoms that may not be immediately apparent include concentration and memory complaints, sensitivity to light and noise, and irritability and other personality changes.

In young children, indications of a concussion can include appearing dazed, irritability and crankiness, excessive crying, or listlessness.

WHAT TESTS TO EXPECT If you've had a head injury, it's important to get a medical evaluation, even if emergency care isn't required.

During evaluation, a health care provider may review your signs and symptoms and perform or recommended one or more of the following:

- **Neurological examination.** A neurological examination checks vision, hearing, strength and sensation, balance, coordination, and reflexes.
- **Cognitive testing.** Cognitive tests are used to evaluate your thinking (cognitive) skills, including your memory, concentration and ability to recall information.
- **Imaging tests.** In case of severe headaches, seizures, repeated vomiting or other worsening signs or symptoms, imaging tests may be performed to look for bleeding or swelling in your skull. This may involve a computerized tomography (CT) scan or magnetic resonance imaging (MRI).

TREATMENT Treatment generally involves rest and observation. If your health care provider agrees that you may be observed at home, someone should stay with you and check on you for at least 24 hours to ensure your symptoms aren't worsening.

Rest is the most appropriate way for your brain to recover from a concussion. This means avoiding general physical exertion, including sports or any vigorous activities, until you have no symptoms.

Rest also includes limiting activities that require thinking and mental concentration, such as playing video games, watching TV, schoolwork, reading, texting or using a computer.

Your health care provider may recommend shortened workdays or school days, taking breaks during the day, or reduced workloads or work assignments while you recover.

For a headache, take acetaminophen (Tylenol, others). Avoid ibuprofen (Advil, Motrin IB, others) and aspirin because of the possibility these medications may increase the risk of bleeding.

If you or your child sustained a concussion while playing sports, ask a health care provider when it's safe to return to play. Resuming sports too soon increases the risk of a second concussion and of a lasting, potentially fatal brain injury. Evidence is emerging that some people who've had multiple concussions during their lives are at greater risk of brain impairment that limits their ability to function.

Constipation

WHAT'S THE CAUSE? Constipation often results from too little fluids, too little fiber, too little activity and older age. It can also be a side effect of some medications.

Signs and symptoms of constipation may include:

- Less than three bowel movements a week
- Bowel movements that are hard, dry and difficult to pass
- Pain while having a bowel movement

TREATMENT Although it can be bothersome, the condition usually isn't serious. Simple changes in your diet and routine are often very effective:

- **Eat a high-fiber diet.** High-fiber foods soften and add bulk to stool. Foods high in fiber include beans, whole grains, and fresh fruits and vegetables. To reduce gas, increase fiber gradually.
- **Get adequate fluids.** Water and other fluids soften stool.
- **Be active.** Regular physical activity helps stimulate bowel function.
- **Don't rush or delay bowel movements.** Develop a bathroom routine. Don't ignore the urge to have a bowel movement and give yourself plenty of time to pass stool.
- **Check your medications.** If you take a drug that may be contributing to your constipation, talk to your health care provider.

Medications

Laxatives can relieve or prevent constipation. They shouldn't be given to children without a health care provider's instruction.

- **Fiber supplements.** Fiber supplements add bulk to stool. They include FiberCon, Metamucil and Citrucel. Make sure to drink plenty of water with these products.
- **Osmotics.** Products such as milk of magnesia, magnesium citrate and polyethylene glycol (MiraLax) help fluids move into the colon and stimulate bowel movements.
- **Stool softeners.** They help stool absorb more water from the intestines. Examples include docusate (Colace, others).

Coronary artery disease

WHAT IS IT? Coronary artery disease results when the major blood vessels that supply blood and oxygen to your heart (coronary arteries) become damaged or diseased. Inflammation and the accumulation of cholesterol-containing deposits (plaques) in the arteries are usually to blame for coronary artery disease.

The condition is thought to begin with damage or injury to the inner layer of a coronary artery, possibly as a result of smoking, high blood pressure, high cholesterol or diabetes.

Once the inner wall is damaged, plaques may accumulate at the injury site. If the plaques severely reduce the diameter of the artery, you may experience symptoms of chest pain. If the plaques break off or rupture, blood cells (platelets) will clump at the site to try to repair the artery. The clump can block the artery, causing heart attack symptoms.

SYMPTOM CHECKER Signs and symptoms may include:

- **Chest pain (angina).** You may feel pressure or tightness in your chest, as if someone were standing on it. This pain, called angina, is usually triggered by physical or emotional stress and typically goes away once the activity stops. In some people, the pain may be felt in the abdomen, back or arm.
- **Shortness of breath.** If your heart can't pump enough blood, you may develop shortness of breath or extreme fatigue with exertion.

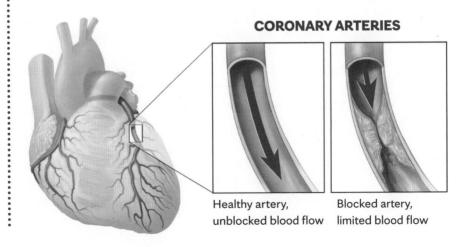

CORONARY ARTERIES

Healthy artery, unblocked blood flow

Blocked artery, limited blood flow

WHAT TESTS TO EXPECT Your health care provider will perform a physical exam and listen to your heart. In addition to routine bloodwork, tests you may have include:

- **Electrocardiogram (ECG).** This test records electrical signals as they travel through your heart. An ECG can often reveal evidence of a previous heart attack or one that's in progress. Certain results may indicate that you have inadequate blood flow to the heart.
- **Echocardiogram.** An echocardiogram uses ultrasound technology to produce images of your heart. It can reveal if parts of your heart have been damaged as a result of a heart attack or if they may be receiving too little oxygen.
- **Stress test.** During this test you walk on a treadmill or ride a stationary bike while being monitored with an ECG. There are several variations of this test. In some cases, medication to stimulate the heart may be used instead of exercise.
- **Heart-imaging tests.** During a coronary angiogram, a special dye is injected into your bloodstream. The dye outlines narrowed spots and blockages in the coronary arteries, which can be seen with various X-ray techniques. Computerized tomography (CT) or magnetic resonance imaging (MRI) procedures may be used to check for blockages or narrowed areas.

TREATMENT Treatment for coronary artery disease usually involves lifestyle changes, medications and, possibly, surgery.

Medications

Several different drugs may be used. They include:

- **Cholesterol-modifying medications.** These drugs decrease the amount of cholesterol in the blood, thereby reducing the amount of cholesterol to deposit within the coronary arteries.
- **Aspirin.** Aspirin reduces the tendency of your blood to clot.
- **Beta blockers.** They slow your heart rate and decrease your blood pressure, decreasing your heart's demand for oxygen.
- **Nitroglycerin.** Nitroglycerin may help reduce chest pain by opening up your coronary arteries and lessening your heart's demand for blood.
- **Angiotensin-converting enzyme (ACE) inhibitors and angiotensin 2 receptor blockers (ARBs).** These medications, which are similar, decrease blood pressure and may help prevent progression of the disease.

Surgical procedures

Sometimes more-aggressive treatment is needed, such as:

Angioplasty and stent placement. A long, thin tube (catheter) is inserted into the narrowed part of your artery. A wire with a deflated balloon is passed through the catheter to the narrowed area. The balloon is inflated, compressing the deposits against your artery walls.

A tiny device called a stent may be left in the artery to help keep it open. Some stents slowly release medication to help keep the artery open.

Coronary artery bypass surgery. A surgeon creates a graft to bypass a blocked coronary artery using a vessel from another part of your body. This allows blood to flow around the blockage. Because this requires open-heart surgery, it's most often reserved for cases of multiple narrowed coronary arteries.

LIFESTYLE Making healthy lifestyle changes is a key part of treatment for coronary artery disease. Your daily habits can go a long way in working toward healthier arteries.

Steps you can take include:

- **Stop smoking.** Nicotine constricts blood vessels and forces your heart to work harder. If you smoke, quitting is one of the best ways to reduce your risk of a heart attack.
- **Exercise.** Exercise helps you achieve and maintain a healthy weight and control diabetes, elevated cholesterol and high blood pressure — all risk factors for coronary artery disease.
- **Eat well.** A heart-healthy diet that emphasizes plant-based foods, such as fruits, vegetables, whole grains, legumes and nuts — and is low in saturated fat, cholesterol and sodium — can help you control your weight, blood pressure and cholesterol.
- **Maintain a healthy weight.** Being overweight increases your risk of coronary artery disease. Losing even just a few pounds is beneficial.
- **Manage stress.** Reduce stress as much as possible. Good techniques for managing stress include muscle relaxation, deep breathing and practices such as yoga and tai chi.
- **Control medical conditions.** If you have a chronic condition such as high blood pressure, high cholesterol or diabetes, keep it under control.

COVID-19

WHAT IS IT? Coronavirus disease 2019 (COVID-19) is an infectious disease caused by a virus. It's related to the common cold and often includes symptoms similar to those of a cold or flu. However, it can cause severe medical complications and can lead to death in some people.

WHAT'S THE CAUSE? COVID-19 is caused by the virus SARS-CoV-2. It's spread from person to person in droplets. When an infected person breathes, coughs or sneezes, the droplets come out. Someone nearby can breathe them in or they can land on their eyes, nose or mouth. Very small droplets can stay in the air for hours. Being closer than 6 feet from a person with COVID-19 increases your risk of getting infected.

There are different types (variants) of the virus that causes COVID-19. Certain variants spread more easily than others and some may cause more severe disease than others.

SYMPTOM CHECKER COVID-19 may cause mild to severe illness or no symptoms at all. Symptoms of COVID-19 may appear 2 to 14 days after exposure. Common symptoms include:

- Fever
- Cough
- Tiredness

In addition, losing your sense of taste or smell can be an early sign of COVID-19. Other symptoms include:

- Shortness of breath or difficulty breathing
- Muscle aches
- Chills
- Sore throat
- Runny nose
- Headache
- Chest pain
- Pink eye (conjunctivitis)
- Nausea or vomiting
- Diarrhea
- Rash

Some people with COVID-19 have no symptoms, but they can still transmit the virus to others. Children typically have similar symptoms to adults and generally have mild illness.

Risk of serious illness

Being older increases your risk of serious illness from COVID-19. So do certain medical conditions, including, but not limited to:

- Serious heart disease
- Cancer
- Chronic obstructive pulmonary disease (COPD)
- Diabetes
- Obesity
- High blood pressure
- Smoking
- Chronic kidney disease
- Weakened immune system
- Pregnancy
- Asthma

Long-term effects

Most people recover within a few weeks. For some, the symptoms last months or even longer. This condition has been called post-COVID-19 syndrome or long COVID-19. Ongoing symptoms may include:

- Fatigue
- Difficulty breathing
- Coughing
- Anxiety
- Headache
- Trouble thinking clearly
- Muscle weakness
- Loss of taste or smell

There is no test for long COVID-19 or quick fix for the symptoms. Recovery takes time. Your doctor can help you get on a path to feeling better.

Prevention

Vaccination, including booster shots, can help protect you and others around you from getting COVID-19. It also lowers the risk of serious symptoms if you become infected. Vaccination isn't 100% effective, but it's a safer way to build immunity than being infected with the virus.

COVID-19 vaccines available in the United States include Pfizer-BioNTech, Moderna and Johnson & Johnson/Janssen. The Pfizer and Moderna vaccines are authorized for use in people age 6 months and older. The Johnson & Johnson/Janssen vaccine is authorized for ages 18 and older. All of the vaccines are safe and have been studied rigorously. They don't cause the virus or treat it, and they won't alter your DNA.

The Pfizer-BioNTech and Moderna vaccines are messenger RNA (mRNA) vaccines. They contain mRNA created in a lab. The mRNA teaches your cells how to make a protein that will trigger your immune system to fight COVID-19. The Johnson & Johnson/Janssen vaccine is a viral vector vaccine. It contains a modified version of a different virus (vector virus) that triggers your immune system to fight COVID-19.

TESTS TO EXPECT There are two kinds of tests for diagnosing COVID-19 (viral tests).

- **PCR test.** This detects genetic material from the virus using a lab technique called reverse transcription polymerase chain reaction (PCR).
- **Antigen test.** This test detects certain proteins in the virus.

PCR tests are very accurate when done properly by a health care provider. Some give results in minutes. Others take longer because they have to be processed by a lab.

A positive antigen test result is considered accurate if you follow the instructions carefully. It's possible, however, to be infected with COVID-19 and have a negative antigen test. Depending on the situation, your provider may suggest a PCR test to confirm a negative antigen test result.

You can get an at-home viral test for COVID-19 from health centers and pharmacies. Some viral tests give results in 15 minutes. Others require that you mail a sample to a laboratory for special processing, so it takes longer to get results.

With either type of at-home test, you follow simple steps to collect a sample from your own nose or mouth. You should test for COVID-19 if you have symptoms, especially if you've been near someone with it.

If you test positive for COVID-19 or think you've been infected:

- Contact your health care provider or local health department for advice on testing and quarantine recommendations
- Stay home for five days after exposure to see if you develop symptoms
- Stay away from other people in your house and use a different bathroom, if possible
- Do not share personal items with other people in your house
- Carefully monitor your symptoms
- Rest and stay hydrated
- Cover your nose and mouth with a tissue or your elbow when you cough or sneeze
- Wash your hands often
- Clean surfaces that you touch often, such as counters and doorknobs

TREATMENT Get medical care immediately if you have emergency COVID-19 symptoms, including:

- Trouble breathing
- Persistent chest pain or pressure
- Inability to stay awake
- New confusion
- Pale, gray or blue-colored skin, lips or nail beds, depending on skin color

If you need to go to a hospital, call ahead so that health care providers can take steps to ensure that others aren't exposed.

For at-home treatment of mild to moderate COVID-19, you can help relieve symptoms by taking pain relievers to reduce fever and body aches. Options include ibuprofen (Advil, Motrin) or acetaminophen (Tylenol, others). You can also drink water to stay hydrated and get plenty of rest.

People who have a higher risk of severe symptoms may be prescribed monoclonal antibodies. These drugs are given through an IV in a clinic. They help a person's immune system recognize and respond better to the virus. For adults and older children who are hospitalized with COVID-19, the antiviral drug remdesivir may be prescribed. It is given through an IV to people who need supplemental oxygen or have a higher risk of serious illness.

Several medications taken as pills also are authorized for people who have a higher risk of severe disease. Treatments are changing throughout the COVID-19 pandemic. Talk with a health care provider about your options.

LIFESTYLE Wearing a mask when you're around others can help prevent you from getting COVID-19 or spreading the virus. Choose the most protective mask that fits well and is comfortable enough to keep on over your nose and mouth. For a mask to be effective, it should:

- Cover your nose, mouth and chin
- Be snug against the sides of your face
- Have more than one layer of tightly woven, breathable fabric
- Have a nose wire

N95 respirators, which are masks approved by the National Institute for Occupational Safety & Health (NIOSH), offer the most protection from COVID-19. Next in effectiveness are KN95 respirators, followed by disposable surgical masks. Cloth masks that fit well can provide some protection. Masks that have exhalation valves or vents aren't recommended because they allow virus particles to escape.

STEPS FOR PUTTING ON AND TAKING OFF A MASK

- Wash or sanitize your hands before and after putting on your mask.
- Place your mask over your mouth and nose and chin.
- Tie it behind your head or use ear loops. Make sure it's snug against your face.
- Don't touch your mask while wearing it.
- If you accidentally touch your mask, wash or sanitize your hands.
- If your mask becomes wet or dirty, switch to a clean one. Put the used mask in a sealable bag until you can get rid of it or wash it.
- Remove the mask by untying it or lifting off the ear loops without touching the front of the mask or your face. Fold the outside corners together.
- Regularly wash cloth masks in the washing machine or by hand. (They can be washed along with other laundry.) Dry them in the dryer or hang them outside in the sun.
- Throw away disposable masks after wearing them once. If using an N95 respirator, check the manufacturer's instructions for when to throw it away. Don't use a respirator once it becomes wet or dirty.

Croup

WHAT IS IT? Croup, which is most common in young children, is an infection of the upper airway that obstructs breathing and produces a barking cough. It's typically caused by a virus.

Inflammation around the vocal cords, windpipe and bronchial tubes is what produces the respiratory symptoms. When a cough forces air through this narrowed passage, the swollen vocal cords produce a noise similar to that of a seal barking. Likewise, taking a breath may produce a high-pitched whistling sound (stridor). Other signs may include fever and a hoarse voice.

Most cases of croup are mild and improve within a couple of days. In a small percentage of cases, the airway swells enough to interfere with breathing.

TREATMENT If the condition isn't severe, self-care measures at home are often all that's needed.

To reduce symptoms and manage croup, try these steps:

- **Keep your child calm.** Crying and agitation can make airway obstruction worse and make breathing more difficult, so try to comfort your child. Hold your child, sing lullabies or read quiet stories. Offer a favorite blanket or toy.
- **Moisten the air.** Humid air may help a child's breathing. You can use a humidifier or sit with your child in a bathroom filled with steam generated by running hot water from the shower.
- **Keep your child upright.** Sitting upright makes breathing easier. Hold your child on your lap, or place your child in a favorite chair.
- **Offer fluids.** For babies, water, breast milk or formula is fine. For older children, soup or frozen fruit pops may be soothing.
- **Encourage rest.** Sleep helps your child fight the infection.
- **Use an over-the-counter pain reliever.** If your child has a fever, acetaminophen (Tylenol, others) may help.

Your child's cough may improve during the day, but don't be surprised if it returns at night. You may want to sleep near your child or even in the same room so that you can take quick action if your child's symptoms become severe.

D

Depression

WHAT IS IT? Depression is a mood disorder that causes a persistent feeling of sadness and loss of interest.

Depression is more than just "the blues," and it isn't something that you can "snap out" of. It's a medical illness that affects how you feel, think and behave, and it can lead to a variety of emotional and physical problems.

WHAT'S THE CAUSE? It's not known exactly what causes depression. As with many mental disorders, a variety of factors may be involved, such as:

- **Biological differences.** People with depression appear to have physical changes in their brains. The significance of these changes is still uncertain, but may eventually help pinpoint causes.
- **Brain chemistry.** Neurotransmitters are naturally occurring brain chemicals that act as messengers. Changes in the function and effect of these chemicals may play a significant role in depression and treatment.
- **Hormones.** Changes in the body's balance of hormones may be involved in causing or triggering depression. Hormone changes can result from thyroid problems, menopause or other conditions.
- **Inherited traits.** Depression is more common in people whose biological (blood) relatives have the condition. Researchers are looking for genes that may be involved in causing depression.
- **Life events.** Traumatic events such as the death or loss of a loved one, financial problems, high stress, or childhood trauma can trigger depression in some people.

SYMPTOM CHECKER For some people, depression symptoms are so severe that it's obvious something isn't right. Other people feel miserable or unhappy without knowing why. Signs and symptoms of depression may include:

- Feelings of sadness, emptiness or unhappiness
- Angry outbursts, irritability or frustration, even over small matters
- Loss of interest or pleasure in usual activities
- Sleep disturbances, including insomnia or sleeping too much
- Tiredness and lack of energy
- Changes in appetite causing weight loss or weight gain
- Anxiety, agitation or restlessness
- Slowed thinking, speaking or body movements
- Feelings of worthlessness or guilt, fixating on past failures, or blaming yourself for things that aren't your responsibility
- Trouble thinking, concentrating, remembering and making decisions
- Unexplained physical problems, such as back pain or headaches
- Frequent thoughts of death, suicidal thoughts or suicide attempts

 TREATMENT Your primary care provider or psychiatrist can prescribe medications to treat depression. Most people feel better with medications, psychological counseling (psychotherapy) or both.

Medications

There are many types of antidepressant medications. You may need to try several medications before you find one that works. If a family member has responded well to an antidepressant, it may help you too.

Selective serotonin reuptake inhibitors (SSRIs). These medications are typically a first line of treatment. They're safer and generally cause fewer side effects than do other types of antidepressants. SSRIs include fluoxetine (Prozac), paroxetine (Paxil), sertraline (Zoloft), citalopram (Celexa) and escitalopram (Lexapro).

Serotonin and norepinephrine reuptake inhibitors (SNRIs). Examples of SNRI medications include duloxetine (Cymbalta), venlafaxine (Effexor XR), desvenlafaxine (Pristiq) and levomilnacipran (Fetzima).

Atypical antidepressants. These medications don't fit neatly into other antidepressant categories. They include trazodone and mirtazapine (Remeron), which are sedating, vortioxetine (Trintellix) and bupropion

(Wellbutrin XL, Aplenzin, others). Trazodone, mirtazapine and bupropion are some of the few antidepressants that aren't typically associated with sexual side effects.

Tricyclic antidepressants. These drugs — such as imipramine (Tofranil) and nortriptyline (Pamelor) — are used less often because they tend to cause more-severe side effects than newer antidepressants such as SSRIs.

Monoamine oxidase inhibitors (MAOIs). MAOIs — such as tranylcypromine (Parnate) and phenelzine (Nardil) — are typically prescribed when other medications haven't worked. Using MAOIs requires a strict diet because of dangerous interactions with foods and some medications. Selegiline (Emsam), a newer MAOI in the form of a skin patch, may cause fewer side effects than other MAOIs.

Psychotherapy

Psychotherapy involves treating depression by talking about your condition and related issues with a mental health provider. Psychotherapy can help you identify issues that may be contributing to your depression, adjust to a crisis or difficulty, replace negative thoughts with positive ones, find better ways to problem-solve, improve relationships, set realistic goals, and find healthy ways to deal with stress.

Newer alternatives to face-to-face office sessions may be an effective option for some people. Therapy can be provided as a computer program, by online sessions, or using videos or workbooks. Talk with your health care provider or therapist before trying one of these options.

Other treatments

For some, brain stimulation therapies may be suggested. These include:

Electroconvulsive therapy (ECT). With ECT, electrical currents are passed through the brain to impact the function of neurotransmitters. This therapy is generally used only in people who don't get better with medications, can't take antidepressants or are at high risk of suicide.

Transcranial magnetic stimulation (TMS). During TMS, a coil placed on your scalp sends magnetic pulses to stimulate brain cells involved in mood regulation. It's another option when other therapies don't work.

Diabetes

WHAT IS IT? Diabetes mellitus refers to a group of diseases that affect how your body uses blood sugar (glucose). Glucose is an important source of energy for the cells that make up your muscles and tissues. It's also your brain's main source of fuel.

If you have diabetes, it means you have too much glucose in your blood, which can lead to serious health problems.

Types
There are different types of diabetes. The most common are type 1 and type 2.

Type 1. With this type, which typically develops during childhood or adolescence, your pancreas is no longer able to produce the hormone insulin. This is critical because insulin is needed for glucose to enter your body's cells. It's like the key that unlocks the door.

Type 2. This type is more common in older adults, although it can occur in younger adults and children. With type 2 diabetes, your body either resists the effects of insulin or it doesn't produce enough insulin to maintain a healthy glucose level.

Gestational diabetes. This form of the disease develops during pregnancy and may resolve itself after the baby is born.

Prediabetes is a condition that often precedes diabetes, especially type 2. With prediabetes, your blood sugar levels are higher than a typical healthy range, but not high enough to be classified as diabetes.

WHAT'S THE CAUSE? The cause of diabetes is different for each type.

Type 1 diabetes. With type 1 diabetes, your immune system — which typically fights harmful bacteria or viruses — attacks and destroys insulin-producing cells in the pancreas. Type 1 is thought to result from a combination of genetic susceptibility and environmental factors, although what many of those factors are is still unclear. Your risk of type 1 diabetes is increased if a parent or sibling has it.

Type 2 diabetes. In type 2 diabetes, your cells become resistant to the action of insulin — making it more difficult for glucose to enter your cells and be used for energy. Exactly why this happens is uncertain. Genetics and environmental factors are thought to play a role. Being overweight is strongly linked to the development of type 2 diabetes. High blood pressure and high triglyceride levels are associated with an increased risk of diabetes as well.

Gestational diabetes. During pregnancy, the placenta produces hormones to sustain your pregnancy. These hormones make your cells more resistant to insulin. Typically, the pancreas responds by producing extra insulin. Sometimes it can't keep up and diabetes results.

SYMPTOM CHECKER Initially, some people don't experience any signs or symptoms. The most common signs and symptoms of type 1 and type 2 diabetes are:

- Increased thirst
- Frequent urination
- Extreme hunger
- Unexplained weight loss
- Ketones — a byproduct of the breakdown of muscle and fat — in the urine
- Fatigue
- Irritability
- Blurred vision
- Slow-healing sores
- Frequent infections, such as gum, skin and vaginal infections

WHAT TESTS TO EXPECT Depending on the type of diabetes you may have, you may receive one or more of the following tests.

- **Hemoglobin A1C test.** This blood test indicates your average blood sugar level for the past 2 to 3 months. It does this by measuring the percentage of blood sugar attached to hemoglobin, the oxygen-carrying protein in red blood cells. The higher your blood sugar levels, the more hemoglobin you'll have with sugar attached. A result of 6.5% or above indicates diabetes.
- **Random blood sugar test.** A blood sample is taken at a random time, regardless of when you last ate. A random blood sugar level of 200 milligrams per deciliter (mg/dL) or higher suggests diabetes.

- **Fasting blood sugar test.** A blood sample is taken after an overnight fast. A fasting blood sugar level less than 100 mg/dL is normal. A fasting blood sugar level from 100 to 125 mg/dL is considered prediabetes. If it's 126 mg/dL or higher on two separate tests, you have diabetes.
- **Oral glucose tolerance test.** You fast overnight, and your fasting blood sugar level is measured. Then you drink a sugary liquid, and your blood sugar level is tested periodically for the next two hours. A blood sugar level less than 140 mg/dL is normal. A reading of more than 200 mg/dL after two hours indicates diabetes. A reading between 140 and 199 mg/dL indicates prediabetes.
- **Urine test.** If type 1 diabetes is suspected, your urine may be tested for ketones.

TREATMENT Your treatment will depend on the type of diabetes you have. Managing your diabetes as needed with insulin and other therapies — along with monitoring blood sugar, eating a healthy diet and staying active — can help you avoid serious health problems.

Insulin. If you have type 1 diabetes, you need daily insulin to survive. Some people with type 2 diabetes also take insulin.

Insulin comes in many forms, including fast-acting and long-acting forms. Most often, the hormone is injected using a fine needle and syringe or an insulin pen — a device that looks like a large ink pen. An insulin pump also may be an option. Worn on the outside of your body, it dispenses the hormone as instructed.

Other medications. Other oral or injected medications may be prescribed for type 2 diabetes. Some stimulate your pancreas to produce more insulin. Others inhibit the production and release of glucose from your liver, so you need less insulin to transport sugar into your cells. Still others block stomach or intestinal enzymes that break down carbohydrates or make your tissues more sensitive to insulin. Another class of medication prevents the kidneys from reabsorbing sugar into the blood.

Transplantation. For some people with type 1 diabetes, a pancreas transplant may be an option. But transplants aren't always successful and they pose serious risks. Because the side effects can be more dangerous than the diabetes, transplants are usually reserved for people whose diabetes can't be controlled or people who also need a kidney transplant.

Bariatric surgery. Although not specifically a treatment for type 2 diabetes, people with a body mass index higher than 35 may benefit from this type of surgery. People who've undergone gastric bypass have seen significant improvements in their blood sugar levels.

LIFESTYLE Healthy daily habits are a key part of managing diabetes. These include:

Lose weight. Fat cells interfere with insulin's ability to work properly. Weight loss can help control blood sugar, especially among people with type 2 diabetes.

Eat a healthy diet. Follow a diet that's centered on fruits, vegetables and whole grains — foods high in nutrition and fiber and low in fat and calories — and that limits animal products, refined carbohydrates and sweets. A registered dietitian can help create a healthy meal plan. You'll also learn about carbohydrate counting, especially if you have type 1 diabetes.

Be physically active. Exercise increases your sensitivity to insulin, which means your body needs less insulin to transport sugar into your cells. Regular exercise can also prevent prediabetes from turning into diabetes.

Monitor your blood sugar. You may need to check your blood sugar level daily, perhaps even several times a day.

SIGNS OF TROUBLE

If your blood sugar is very high or drops very low, serious conditions can result.

High blood sugar (hyperglycemia). It can cause frequent urination, excessive thirst, blurred vision, fatigue and nausea. Insulin is needed to relieve symptoms.

Low blood sugar (hypoglycemia). People who take glucose-lowering medications or insulin are most at risk. Signs and symptoms include sweating, shakiness, dizziness, headache, blurred vision, heart palpitations, irritability, drowsiness, confusion, fainting and seizures. Low blood sugar is treated with glucose tablets or a food or beverage high in carbohydrates that's quickly absorbed.

Diarrhea

WHAT IS IT? Diarrhea occurs when food and fluids you ingest pass too quickly through your colon or in too large of an amount or both. Typically, the colon absorbs liquids from the food you eat, leaving a semisolid stool. If the liquids aren't absorbed, the result is a watery bowel movement.

D-E

If your diarrhea lasts longer than two days or is severe and accompanied by a high fever or bloody stools, see your health care provider. It may be a sign of a serious disorder or infection that needs further investigation. Prolonged or severe diarrhea can also lead to dehydration.

WHAT'S THE CAUSE? A number of diseases and conditions can cause diarrhea. Common causes include:

- **Viruses.** Viruses that can cause diarrhea include norovirus, cytomegalovirus and viral hepatitis. Rotavirus is a common cause of acute childhood diarrhea.
- **Bacteria and parasites.** Contaminated food or water can transmit bacteria and parasites to your body. Parasites such as *Giardia lamblia* and cryptosporidium can cause diarrhea. Common bacterial causes of diarrhea include campylobacter, salmonella, shigella and *Escherichia coli (E. coli)*.
- **Medications.** Many medications can cause diarrhea. The most common are antibiotics, which destroy good and bad bacteria, and can disturb the natural balance of bacteria in your intestines.
- **Lactose intolerance.** Lactose is a sugar found in milk and other dairy products. Many people have difficulty digesting lactose and experience diarrhea after eating dairy products.
- **Fructose.** Fructose, a sugar found naturally in fruits and honey and added as a sweetener to some beverages, can cause diarrhea in people who have trouble digesting it.
- **Artificial sweeteners.** Sorbitol and mannitol, artificial sweeteners found in chewing gum and other sugar-free products, can cause diarrhea in some people.
- **Surgery.** Some people may experience diarrhea after undergoing abdominal surgery or gallbladder removal surgery.
- **Other digestive disorders.** Several conditions may cause chronic diarrhea including Crohn's disease, ulcerative colitis, celiac disease, microscopic colitis and irritable bowel syndrome.

TREATMENT Diarrhea that isn't linked to a chronic condition often can be treated at home.

To help you cope until your diarrhea goes away:

- **Drink plenty of clear liquids.** This includes water, juice and broth. Avoid caffeine and alcohol. Prolonged or severe diarrhea can create an electrolyte imbalance. Fruit juice supplies needed potassium, and soup and broth provide sodium. Some sports drinks also contain electrolytes.
- **Avoid certain foods.** Dairy products, fatty foods, high-fiber foods or highly seasoned foods can worsen symptoms.
- **Consider anti-diarrheal medications.** Over-the-counter anti-diarrheal medications, such as loperamide (Imodium A-D) and bismuth subsalicylate (Pepto-Bismol), may reduce the number of watery bowel movements you experience. However, certain infections may worsen with the use of these medications because they prevent your body from getting rid of what's causing the diarrhea. Anti-diarrheals aren't always safe for children, so check with your health care provider before giving these medications to a child. (If you're traveling to a country with inadequate sanitation and contaminated food and water, some providers suggest taking Pepto-Bismol to help reduce the risk of experiencing diarrhea.)
- **Try probiotics.** Probiotics contain strains of living bacteria similar to the healthy bacteria typically found in the digestive system. Probiotics may boost the number of healthy bacteria present to fight germs in your digestive tract. Probiotics are found in some yogurts and cheese and are sold as supplements.
- **Add low-fiber foods gradually.** As your diarrhea improves, try soda crackers, toast, eggs, rice or chicken.

If self-care doesn't work, your health care provider may recommend:

- **Antibiotics.** Antibiotics may help treat diarrhea caused by bacteria or parasites. If a virus is causing your diarrhea, antibiotics won't help.
- **Fluid replacement.** For most people, replacing fluids means drinking water, juice or broth. If drinking liquids upsets your stomach or causes diarrhea, your health care provider may recommend getting fluids through a vein in your arm.
- **Medication adjustment.** If an antibiotic or another medication is causing your diarrhea, your provider may modify the dose or switch to a different medication.

Diverticulitis

WHAT IS IT? It's not uncommon for small, bulging pouches (diverticula) to form in the lining of your digestive tract. The pouches are most often found in the lower large intestine (colon). They develop when weak spots in the colon give way under pressure.

Seldom do the pouches cause problems. But sometimes one or more can become inflamed or infected, a condition called diverticulitis.

Several factors may increase your risk of developing diverticulitis, including being overweight, smoking, not getting enough exercise, and eating a diet high in animal fat and low in fiber.

SYMPTOM CHECKER Signs and symptoms include:

- Pain, which may be constant and persist for several days. The pain is usually in the lower left side of the abdomen, but may occur on the right.
- Nausea and vomiting.
- Fever.
- Abdominal tenderness.
- Constipation or, less commonly, diarrhea.

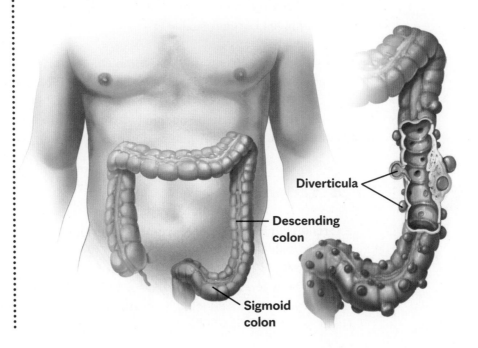

Diverticula

Descending colon

Sigmoid colon

About 10% to 15% of people with severe (acute) diverticulitis develop complications, which may include peritonitis, a condition in which an infected or inflamed pouch ruptures and spills intestinal contents into the abdominal cavity. Peritonitis is a medical emergency.

TREATMENT Treatment depends on the severity of your signs and symptoms.

If your symptoms are mild, you may be treated at home. This may include taking antibiotics to treat infection. You may also need to follow a liquid diet while your bowel heals. An over-the-counter pain reliever can treat the pain.

If you have a severe attack or you have other health problems, you may need to be hospitalized. You'll likely receive antibiotics intravenously. If a pocket of pus (abscess) has formed in one of the pouches, the abscess may need to be drained.

Surgery may be necessary in case of a serious complication, such as perforation, fistula, bowel obstruction or severe abscess. Surgery may also be needed if you don't respond to antibiotics or if you've had multiple diverticulitis attacks. The two most common surgeries are:

Primary bowel resection. A surgeon removes diseased segments of your intestine and then reconnects the healthy segments. This allows you to have bowel movements as usual.

Bowel resection with colostomy. Sometimes there's so much inflammation it's not possible to rejoin healthy segments and a colostomy is necessary. Your colon is connected to an opening (stoma) in the abdominal wall. Waste passes through the opening into a bag. Once the inflammation has eased, the colostomy may be reversed.

LIFESTYLE To help prevent future attacks:

- **Exercise regularly.** Exercise promotes bowel function and reduces pressure inside the colon.
- **Eat more fiber.** High-fiber foods, such as fresh fruits and vegetables and whole grains, soften stool and help it pass more easily through your colon, reducing pressure inside your digestive tract.
- **Drink plenty of fluids.** Fiber can be constipating.

Dizziness

WHAT IS IT? The term *dizziness* is used to describe everything from feeling faint or lightheaded to feeling weak or unsteady. Although an occasional dizzy spell or constant dizziness can be annoying and interrupt daily activities, dizziness rarely signals a serious, life-threatening condition.

D-E

Dizziness may be described as one of the following sensations:

- The false sense of motion or spinning (vertigo)
- Lightheadedness or the feeling of near fainting
- Loss of balance or unsteadiness (disequilibrium)
- Other sensations such as floating, swimming or heavy-headedness

A number of underlying health conditions can cause these problems. Often, dizziness stems from disruption or confusion in the signals your brain receives from your eyes, inner ear or sensory nerves.

WHAT'S THE CAUSE? The way dizziness makes you feel — such as the sensation of vertigo or the feeling that you've lost your balance — provides clues for possible causes. Treatment of the condition triggering the dizziness will often reduce or eliminate the problem.

Vertigo

Vertigo usually results from a sudden or temporary change in the activity of the balance structures in your inner ear or in their connections into the brain. These connections sense movement and changes in your head position. Sometimes vertigo is severe enough to cause nausea, vomiting and balance problems. The good news is, it generally doesn't last long. Within a couple of weeks, the body usually adapts to whatever is causing the dizziness.

Causes of vertigo may include:

Benign paroxysmal positional vertigo (BPPV). This condition causes intense, brief episodes of vertigo immediately following a change in the position of your head, such as when you turn over in bed or sit up in the morning. BPPV is the most common cause of vertigo. It's thought to result when tiny crystals in the inner ear that help maintain orientation and balance become dislodged. The crystals move into other parts of the ear, where they become sensitive to sudden head changes. A procedure in which a health care provider or therapist carefully maneuvers the position of your head to reposition the crystals is often effective.

Inflammation in the inner ear. Signs and symptoms of inflammation of the inner ear include the sudden onset of intense, constant vertigo that may persist for several days, along with nausea, vomiting and trouble with balance. The symptoms may be so severe that you have to stay in bed. When associated with sudden hearing loss, this condition is called labyrinthitis. The condition generally clears up on its own, but early medical treatment may speed recovery.

Meniere's disease. This condition involves the excessive buildup of fluid in your inner ear. It's characterized by sudden episodes of vertigo lasting as long as several hours, accompanied by fluctuating hearing loss, ringing in the ear and a feeling of fullness in the affected ear. Diuretic medications and a low-sodium diet to help reduce fluid retention may improve symptoms.

Vestibular migraine. Just as some people experience a visual "aura" with their migraines, others can get vertigo episodes and have other types of dizziness even when they're not having a severe headache. Such vertigo episodes can last hours to days and may be associated with headache as well as light and noise sensitivity. Certain medicines may help prevent attacks of vestibular migraine or make them less uncomfortable by providing relief of nausea and vomiting.

Acoustic neuroma. An acoustic neuroma is a noncancerous (benign) growth on the vestibular nerve, which connects the inner ear to your brain. Signs and symptoms of an acoustic neuroma generally include progressive hearing loss and tinnitus on one side accompanied by dizziness or imbalance. Surgery may be necessary to relieve the dizziness.

Other causes. Rarely, vertigo can be a symptom of a more serious condition such as a stroke, brain hemorrhage or multiple sclerosis. In such cases, other neurological signs and symptoms are usually present, such as double vision, slurred speech, facial weakness or numbness, or uncoordinated limb movements.

Feeling faint

Sometimes nausea, pale skin and clamminess accompany a feeling of faintness. Causes of this type of dizziness include:

Drop in blood pressure (orthostatic hypotension). A dramatic drop in your systolic blood pressure — the higher number in your blood pressure reading — may cause lightheadedness or a feeling of faintness. This can occur after sitting up or standing too quickly.

Inadequate blood flow from the heart. Certain conditions such as diseases of the heart muscle (cardiomyopathy), an irregular heart rhythm (arrhythmia) or a decrease in blood volume may cause inadequate blood output from the heart.

Loss of balance (disequilibrium)

Disequilibrium is the loss of balance or the feeling of unsteadiness when you walk. Causes may include:

Inner ear problems. Problems with your inner ear can cause you to feel like you're unsteady while walking.

Medications. Loss of balance can be a side effect of certain medications, such as anti-seizure drugs, sedatives and tranquilizers.

Nerve disorders. Nerve damage in your legs (peripheral neuropathy) may make it difficult to maintain balance.

Joint and muscle problems. Muscle weakness and osteoarthritis involving your weight-bearing joints can contribute to loss of balance.

Neurological conditions. Various neurological disorders can lead to progressive loss of balance, such as Parkinson's disease and cerebellar ataxia.

Other sensations

Sensations that are more difficult to describe, such as floating, swimming or heavy-headedness, are often referred to as nonspecific dizziness. Causes include:

Medications. Blood pressure lowering medications may cause unspecific dizziness if they lower your blood pressure too much. Many other medications can cause dizziness that resolves when you stop taking them.

Inner ear disorders. Some inner ear problems can cause persistent, non-vertigo-type dizziness.

Anxiety disorders. Certain anxiety disorders, such as panic attacks, may cause dizziness that's associated with hyperventilation.

Low iron levels (anemia). Other signs and symptoms that may occur along with dizziness include fatigue, weakness and pale skin.

Low blood sugar (hypoglycemia). This condition generally occurs in people with diabetes who use insulin. The dizziness may be accompanied by sweating and confusion.

Ear infections. Sometimes, ear infections can lead to dizziness. This type of dizziness will go away when the infection clears up.

WHAT TESTS TO EXPECT The types of tests you receive will depend on what your health care provider thinks may be the cause. Possible tests include:

- **Eye movement testing.** Your health care provider watches the path of your eyes when you track a moving object. You may also be given what's called a caloric test, in which the movement of your eyes is observed when cold and warm water are placed in your ear canal at different times.
- **Posturography testing.** This test tells your health care provider which parts of the balance system you rely on the most and which parts may be giving you problems. You stand in your bare feet on a platform and try to keep your balance under various conditions.
- **Rotary-chair testing.** During this test, you sit in a computer-controlled chair that moves very slowly in a full circle. At faster speeds, it moves back and forth in a very small arc.
- **Magnetic resonance imaging (MRI).** An MRI may be performed to rule out an acoustic neuroma or other concerns with the brain that may cause vertigo.
- **Blood tests and more.** You may have blood tests to check for infection. Other tests may check your heart and blood vessel health.

TREATMENT The treatment of dizziness is dependent on the cause of the condition. The best way to treat dizziness is to find out what's causing it and eliminate or control the cause.

Even if no cause is found, medications and other treatments may be able to make your symptoms more manageable.

Dry skin

WHAT'S THE CAUSE? Dry skin can occur for a variety of reasons. Most commonly, it's the result of dry air, cold weather, hot showers, harsh soaps and detergents, or too much sun.

Dry skin is often temporary — you get it only in winter, for example — but it may be a lifelong problem. Most cases of dry skin respond well to lifestyle and home remedies. See your health care provider if your skin doesn't improve in spite of your best efforts or you have large areas of scaling or peeling skin or open sores from scratching.

TREATMENT If you have a more serious skin disease, such as atopic dermatitis or psoriasis, your health care provider may prescribe prescription creams or other therapies to treat the condition. Otherwise, the following steps can help to keep your skin healthy.

- **Moisturize.** Moisturizers provide a seal over your skin to keep water from escaping. Apply them several times a day. Thicker moisturizers (brands such as Eucerin and Cetaphil) work best. If your skin is extremely dry, apply an oil, such as baby oil, while your skin is still moist. Oil has more staying power than do moisturizers and keeps water from evaporating from the surface of your skin. Ointments that contain petroleum jelly are helpful, but they may feel too greasy.
- **Apply moisturizers after bathing.** Gently pat your skin dry with a towel so that some moisture remains. Immediately moisturize your skin to help trap water in the surface cells.
- **Limit showers.** Long showers or baths and hot water remove oils from your skin. If possible, don't bathe daily (use a washcloth to cleanse key areas). Keep your shower time limited to 5 to 10 minutes and use warm, not hot, water.
- **Avoid harsh, drying soaps.** Choose mild soaps with added oils and fats.
- **Use a humidifier.** Dry indoor air can worsen itching and flaking. A portable humidifier or one attached to your furnace adds moisture to inside air. Be sure to keep the humidifier clean.
- **Choose skin-friendly fabrics.** Natural fibers, such as cotton and silk, allow your skin to breathe. Wool, though natural, can irritate your skin. Wash your clothes with detergents that don't contain dyes or perfumes, both of which can irritate your skin.

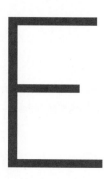

Ear infection

WHAT IS IT? An ear infection (acute otitis media) is a viral or bacterial infection that affects the middle ear — the area behind the eardrum that contains the tiny vibrating bones of the ear.

An ear infection often follows an upper respiratory infection that produces swelling, inflammation and mucus, blocking the tiny eustachian tubes that drain fluid from the ears. Fluid accumulates and serves as a breeding ground for viruses and bacteria.

Children ages 6 months to 2 years are most susceptible to ear infections because of the size and shape of their eustachian tubes and because their immune systems aren't fully developed.

SYMPTOM CHECKER Signs and symptoms of an ear infection may develop rapidly. In children, they include:

- Ear pain, especially when lying down
- Tugging or pulling at an ear
- Difficulty sleeping
- Crying or acting more irritable than usual
- Difficulty hearing or responding to sounds
- Fever of 100 F (37.8 C) or higher
- Loss of balance
- Drainage of fluid from the ear
- Loss of appetite

Common signs and symptoms in adults include ear pain, drainage of fluid from the ear and diminished hearing.

TREATMENT Most ear infections resolve on their own. In some instances antibiotics may be prescribed. Options include:

D-E

Wait-and-see approach. This may be recommended if your child is older than 6 months, appears to have mild symptoms, has had symptoms for less than 48 hours, and has a temperature of less than 102.2 F (39 C). To lessen the pain while the infection is healing, try:

- **A warm, moist compress.** Place it over the affected ear.
- **Pain medication.** Use acetaminophen (Tylenol, others) or ibuprofen (Advil, Motrin, others) and follow the directions on the label.
- **Eardrops.** Analgesic eardrops may relieve pain, but those that contain benzocaine aren't recommended for children younger than 2 years old. Benzocaine has been linked to a rare but potentially life-threatening condition that decreases oxygen in blood. If you use eardrops containing benzocaine, follow label instructions.

Antibiotics. Antibiotics are generally prescribed if:

- A child is 6 months of age or younger
- A child has severe symptoms
- Symptoms have persisted for more than 48 hours
- A child has an infection in both ears

Ear tubes. If your child has recurrent ear infections, a surgeon may create a tiny hole in the eardrum to suction fluids out of the middle ear. A tiny tube is placed in the opening to ventilate the middle ear and prevent the accumulation of fluids.

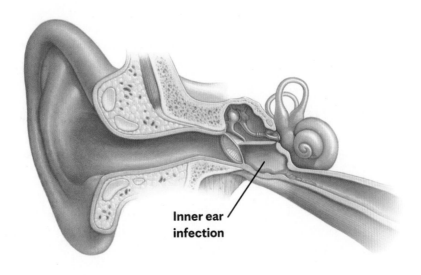

Inner ear infection

Eating disorders

WHAT ARE THEY? Eating disorders are serious conditions related to persistent, dangerous eating behaviors. People with an eating disorder are typically preoccupied with their weight, body shape and food. That leads them to adopt eating habits that can affect their ability to function and can be life-threatening.

D-E

The three most common eating disorders are:

- **Anorexia nervosa.** People with anorexia have a very low body weight and a distorted body image, and they make an extreme effort to control their weight and shape. They may eat very few calories, exercise excessively, use laxatives or diet aids, or vomit after eating.
- **Bulimia nervosa.** For someone with bulimia, self-image also is unduly influenced by body shape and weight. People with bulimia feel they can't control their eating. They typically eat a large amount of food in a short time. Then shame or fear of gaining weight leads to unhealthy actions such as vomiting to get rid of the extra calories. This is known as bingeing and purging. Someone with this illness may be at a healthy weight or may be even slightly overweight.
- **Binge-eating disorder.** People with this condition regularly binge — usually at least once a week. They also feel they can't control their eating. They don't purge but they do feel guilt, disgust or shame about their behavior. This often leads to hiding their eating habits. Someone who has binge-eating disorder may be at a healthy weight or be overweight.

Eating disorders are most common in teenagers and young adults, but anyone can be affected. These disorders can lead to serious problems with the heart, bones, digestive system, teeth and more.

WHAT'S THE CAUSE? No specific cause of eating disorders is known. Genes and biological factors, such as changes in brain chemicals, may play a role. Psychological and emotional problems also may contribute.

People with eating disorders tend to have low self-esteem, be perfectionists and impulsive, and have troubled relationships. Several things can increase a person's risk:

- History of an eating disorder in parents or siblings
- Personal history of an anxiety disorder, depression or obsessive-compulsive disorder
- Dieting and starvation
- Stress from a move, a new job or a family or relationship issue

SYMPTOM CHECKER Many people with eating disorders don't think they have one. Red flags include:

- Skipping meals or making excuses for not eating
- Avoiding family meals
- Focusing excessively on healthy eating
- Constantly worrying or complaining about being fat
- Talking about losing weight
- Checking in the mirror frequently for perceived flaws
- Using dietary supplements, laxatives or herbal products for weight loss
- Exercising to an extreme
- Eating in secret or hoarding food
- Leaving during meals to use the bathroom
- Eating much more food in a meal or snack than is considered healthy
- Expressing depression, disgust, shame or guilt about eating

Sores, scars or calluses on the knuckles and loss of tooth enamel may be signs of bulimia nervosa in people who repeatedly make themselves vomit. They may also have damaged gums, mouth sores and throat sores.

Getting help for an eating disorder at an early stage is important. Extreme weight loss or starvation can cause serious health problems, including:

- Tiredness or fatigue
- Headaches
- Dizziness, lightheadedness or problems concentrating
- Muscle cramps and muscle loss
- Loss of menstrual periods
- Dehydration
- Irregular heart rate
- Thinning hair or dry skin
- Low blood pressure

- Changes in bone density
- Depression

TREATMENT If you have an eating disorder, food is the main medicine and refeeding — restoring necessary nutrition — is the most important goal. A health care provider may do a physical examination and refer you to a special clinic for care. Recovery typically involves nutrition education, therapy and, sometimes, medications.

Therapy

Two types of therapy are commonly used with an eating disorder:

Family-based treatment (FBT). There are three phases to FBT, which typically is used for teenagers. In phase one, the parents are encouraged to support their child in creating healthy eating patterns. This includes supervising meals and periods of time after meals to prevent purging. In phase two, the teenager has to be able to keep up the healthy eating behaviors alone. In phase three, the therapist and family work to restore good family communication.

Cognitive behavior therapy (CBT). This type of therapy is used for teenagers and adults. The first goal is to get the person back to eating regular meals. After that, they learn to identify, judge and challenge the thoughts they have about weight, body shape and food.

CBT may work well for people with bulimia. The distress caused by bingeing and purging and their desire to control their eating habits may motivate them to change.

Medication

Some people with eating disorders also may have medication prescribed to help them recover.

People who have bulimia nervosa often take fluoxetine, a selective serotonin reuptake inhibitor. This medication can be effective when used with CBT.

A medication called lisdexamfetamine dimesylate (Vyvanse) is approved to treat adults who have moderate to severe binge-eating disorder.

There are no medications for anorexia nervosa. Some people are given antidepressants and anti-anxiety medications for depression and anxiety.

Eczema (atopic dermatitis)

WHAT IS IT? Eczema is a condition that makes white skin red and itchy and may cause dark spots on brown and Black skin. It's common in children but can occur at any age. Eczema is associated with allergies, and it may be accompanied by asthma or hay fever.

Other signs and symptoms include patches of thickened, cracked and scaly skin, and small, raised bumps that may leak fluid and crust over. In some people, eczema flares periodically and then clears up for a time.

TREATMENT Medications used to treat eczema include:

- **Creams that control itching and inflammation.** A corticosteroid cream or ointment may be used for a limited time.
- **Creams that repair the skin.** Drugs called calcineurin inhibitors, such as tacrolimus (Protopic) and pimecrolimus (Elidel), help maintain healthy skin, control itching and reduce flares.
- **Drugs to fight infection.** Antibiotics treat and prevent bacterial skin infection from an open sore or caused by scratching.
- **Drugs to control severe inflammation.** Oral corticosteroids such as prednisone or an injected corticosteroid may be used.
- **Injectable biologic (monoclonal antibody).** Dupilumab (Dupixent) is a newer medication that's used to treat people with severe disease who do not respond well to other treatment options.

Other treatments include:

- **Wet dressings.** Wrapping the area with topical corticosteroids and wet bandages can help severe eczema. This is labor intensive and requires medical expertise, but you can learn to do it at home.
- **Light therapy.** Phototherapy involves exposing your skin to controlled amounts of natural sunlight. Other forms use artificial ultraviolet (UV) A and narrow band UVB alone or with medications. Though effective, long-term light therapy has harmful effects, including increased risk of skin cancer.

Other measures that may help include adding oatmeal or baking soda to bath water and using a humidifier to moisturize dry indoor air. Among infants, treatment generally includes avoiding skin irritations and lubricating baby's skin with bath oils, lotions, creams or ointments.

Emphysema

WHAT IS IT? Emphysema gradually damages the air sacs in your lungs, making you progressively more short of breath. It's one of several diseases known collectively as chronic obstructive pulmonary disease (COPD).

The main symptom of emphysema is shortness of breath, which usually begins gradually. You may start avoiding activities that cause you to be short of breath. Eventually, the condition causes shortness of breath even while resting.

WHAT'S THE CAUSE? Emphysema often results from long-term exposure to airborne irritants. Rarely, it stems from an inherited disorder called alpha-1-antitrypsin deficiency emphysema.

Factors that increase your risk of developing emphysema include:

- **Smoking.** Smoking is the leading cause of emphysema. The condition is most likely to develop in cigarette smokers, but cigar and pipe smokers also are susceptible.
- **Exposure to secondhand smoke.** Regular exposure to secondhand smoke increases emphysema risk.
- **Occupational exposure to fumes or dust.** If you breathe fumes from certain chemicals or dust from grain, cotton, wood or mining products, you're more likely to develop emphysema.
- **Exposure to indoor and outdoor pollution.** Breathing indoor pollutants, such as fumes from heating fuel, as well as outdoor pollutants, such as car exhaust, increases your risk.

People who have emphysema, especially severe emphysema, are at increased risk of developing other health conditions including a collapsed lung, large holes in the lungs and heart problems.

TREATMENT To determine if you have emphysema, you may undergo lung function tests to measure how much air your lungs can hold and how well they deliver oxygen to your bloodstream.

Emphysema can't be cured, but treatments can relieve symptoms and slow its progression.

D-E

Medications

Medications used to treat emphysema include:

Bronchodilators. These drugs help relieve coughing, shortness of breath and breathing problems by relaxing constricted airways. They're not as effective in treating emphysema as they are in treating asthma or chronic bronchitis.

Inhaled steroids. Corticosteroids inhaled as aerosol sprays may help relieve shortness of breath. Prolonged use may increase your risk of side effects.

Therapy

Other treatments include:

Pulmonary rehabilitation. It includes breathing exercises and other techniques to reduce breathlessness and improve your activity level.

Nutrition therapy. In the early stages of emphysema, many people need to lose weight, while people with late-stage emphysema often need to gain weight.

Supplemental oxygen. It increases blood oxygen levels. The oxygen typically is administered via tubing that fits into your nostrils.

Surgery

In certain situations, surgery may be performed to remove small wedges of damaged tissue. This may help remaining lung tissue expand and work more efficiently, improving breathing.

LIFESTYLE To control symptoms and avoid complications:

- **Stop smoking.** This is the most important measure you can take.
- **Avoid other respiratory irritants.** This includes secondhand smoke, paint or chemical fumes, and automobile exhaust.
- **Exercise regularly.** Exercise increases your lung capacity.
- **Avoid cold air.** In cold weather, wear a cold-air mask or scarf over your mouth and nose before going outside.
- **Prevent respiratory infections.** Get annual flu shots and pneumonia vaccinations as advised by your health care provider.

Endometriosis

WHAT IS IT? Endometriosis is an often painful disorder in which tissue that lines the inside of the uterus (endometrium) spreads and grows outside the uterus. Rarely, endometrial tissue may spread beyond the pelvic region.

The displaced endometrial tissue continues to act as if it were inside the uterus — it thickens, breaks down and bleeds with each menstrual cycle. Because the tissue has no way to exit your body, it becomes trapped. Surrounding tissue can become irritated, eventually developing scar tissue and adhesions.

SYMPTOM CHECKER Signs and symptoms include:

- **Painful periods.** Pelvic pain and cramping may begin before and extend several days into your period.
- **Pain with intercourse.** Pain during or after sex is common.
- **Pain with bowel movements or urination.** These symptoms are most common during your period.
- **Excessive bleeding.** You may experience occasional heavy periods or bleeding between periods.
- **Other symptoms.** You may also experience fatigue, diarrhea, constipation or nausea, especially during menstrual periods.

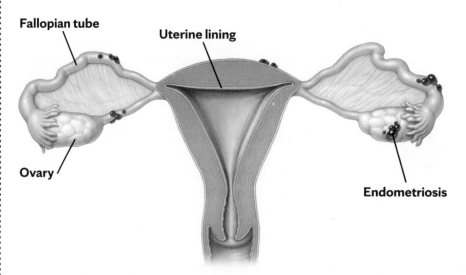

In endometriosis, tissue that normally lines the uterus may spread to the ovaries, fallopian tubes, bowel and pelvic lining.

The main complication of endometriosis is impaired fertility. Approximately one-third to one-half of people with endometriosis have difficulty getting pregnant. Ovarian cancer also occurs at higher than expected rates in people with endometriosis.

TREATMENT In making a diagnosis of endometriosis, your health care provider will likely perform a pelvic exam. An ultrasound exam may reveal cysts associated with endometriosis. Sometimes minimally invasive laparoscopic surgery is performed to look for endometrial tissue outside the uterus.

The type of treatment you may receive depends on the severity of your symptoms and whether you hope to become pregnant.

Hormone therapy. Hormone medication may slow the growth of endometrial tissue outside the uterus and prevent new growths from forming. Therapies used to treat endometriosis include:

- **Hormonal contraceptives.** Birth control pills, patches and vaginal rings help control those hormones responsible for the buildup of endometrial tissue each month.
- **Gonadotropin-releasing hormone (Gn-RH) agonists and antagonists.** They block the production of ovarian-stimulating hormones, lowering estrogen levels, preventing menstruation and causing endometrial tissue to shrink. The drugs can force endometriosis into remission, sometimes lasting for months to years. Because the drugs create an artificial menopause, other medications may be required to decrease menopausal side effects.
- **Progestin therapy.** A variety of progestin therapies, including an intrauterine device with levonorgestrel (Mirena, Skyla, others), contraceptive implant (Nexplanon), contraceptive injection (Depo-Provera) or progestin pill (Camila), can halt menstrual periods and the growth of endometrial tissue outside the uterus.

Conservative surgery. If you're trying to become pregnant, surgery to remove as much displaced tissue as possible while preserving your uterus and ovaries may increase your chances of success.

Hysterectomy. In severe cases of endometriosis, surgery to remove the uterus and cervix as well as both ovaries (total hysterectomy) may be the best treatment. This is typically considered a last resort because it ends the possibility of future pregnancies.

Epilepsy

WHAT IS IT? Epilepsy is a neurological disorder in which nerve cell activity in your brain is disturbed, producing a seizure. Generally, at least two unprovoked seizures are required to be diagnosed with epilepsy.

Seizure symptoms vary. Some people with epilepsy simply stare blankly for a few seconds during a seizure, while others repeatedly jerk their arms or legs. Other signs and symptoms may include temporary confusion and loss of consciousness.

WHAT'S THE CAUSE? In about half the people with epilepsy, the condition may be traced to various factors.

- **Genetic influence.** Some types of epilepsy run in families, and researchers have linked some types to specific genes. For most people, genes are thought to be only part of the cause. They may make a person more sensitive to environmental conditions that trigger seizures.
- **Head trauma.** Head trauma that occurs due to a car accident or other traumatic injury can cause epilepsy.
- **Brain conditions.** Conditions that damage the brain, such as tumors or strokes, can cause epilepsy. Stroke is a leading cause of epilepsy in adults older than age 35.
- **Infectious diseases.** Diseases, such as meningitis, AIDS and viral encephalitis, may trigger epilepsy.
- **Prenatal injury.** Before birth, several factors, such as an infection in the mother, poor nutrition or oxygen deficiencies, may cause brain damage that produces seizures.
- **Developmental disorders.** Epilepsy may be associated with developmental disorders, such as autism and neurofibromatosis.

WHAT TESTS TO EXPECT To diagnose your condition, your health care provider may order several tests. In addition to blood tests and an evaluation of your thinking, memory and speech skills, these may include:

- **Electroencephalogram (EEG).** Electrodes that record the electrical activity of your brain are attached to your scalp. If you have epilepsy, it's common to have changes in your normal pattern of brain waves, even when you're not having a seizure.

- **Computerized tomography (CT) or magnetic resonance imaging (MRI).** They can reveal brain changes that might be causing your seizures, such as tumors, bleeding or cysts.
- **Positron emission tomography (PET).** A small amount of low-dose radioactive material is injected into a vein to help visualize active areas of the brain and detect problems.
- **Single-photon emission computerized tomography (SPECT).** It creates a map of blood flow activity in your brain during seizures.

 TREATMENT Treatment generally begins with medication.

Medication

Many people with epilepsy can become seizure-free by taking anti-seizure medication, called anti-epileptic medication. Others may be able to decrease the frequency and intensity of their seizures with medication. Your health care provider will consider the frequency and severity of your seizures, your age, and other factors when selecting a drug to prescribe.

Surgery

Surgery is most often done when tests show that your seizures originate in a small, well-defined area of your brain that doesn't interfere with vital functions such as speech, language, motor function, vision or hearing. During surgery, the area of your brain causing the seizures is removed. You may be awake during part of the surgery.

Other therapies

Additional treatments include:

Vagus nerve stimulation. In this procedure a stimulator is placed underneath the skin of your chest, and wires from the stimulator are connected to the vagus nerve in your neck. The stimulator sends bursts of electrical energy through the vagus nerve to the brain. The device may reduce seizures by 20% to 40%.

Ketogenic diet. Some children with epilepsy have been able to reduce their seizures by following a strict diet that's high in fats and low in carbohydrates.

Erectile dysfunction

WHAT IS IT? Erectile dysfunction (impotence) is the inability to get or keep an erection firm enough for sexual intercourse. Occasional trouble with erectile dysfunction isn't a cause for concern, but if the problem is ongoing you should seek treatment.

Problems getting or keeping an erection can be a sign of an underlying health condition, and treating the problem may be enough to reverse your erectile dysfunction. Stress and mental health problems also can cause or worsen erectile dysfunction. Often, the condition results from a combination of physical and psychological issues.

Factors that can contribute to erectile dysfunction include:

- Medical conditions, particularly diabetes or heart problems
- Tobacco use, which restricts blood flow to veins and arteries
- Being overweight
- Certain medical treatments, such as prostate surgery or radiation treatment for cancer
- Damage to the nerves that control erections
- Medications, including antidepressants, antihistamines, and medications to treat high blood pressure, pain or prostate cancer
- Drug and alcohol use, especially long-term use or heavy drinking
- Prolonged bicycling, which may compress nerves and affect blood flow to the penis, causing temporary erectile dysfunction

TREATMENT See your primary care provider if you have erectile problems. A physical exam and a medical history often are all that's needed to make a diagnosis. If your provider suspects an underlying problem, you may need further tests. A variety of treatment options exist. They include:

Oral medications
Oral medications such as sildenafil (Viagra), tadalafil (Cialis, others) and vardenafil (Levitra, Staxyn) can successfully treat erectile dysfunction. These drugs enhance the effects of nitric oxide, a natural chemical your body produces that relaxes muscles in the penis. This increases blood flow and allows you to get an erection in response to sexual stimulation. They don't automatically cause an erection.

Before taking any medication for erectile dysfunction (including supplements or herbal remedies), get your health care provider's OK. The drugs may be dangerous if taken with certain medications or if you have heart disease or uncontrolled high blood pressure.

Other medications

Other medications for erectile dysfunction include:

- **Self-injection.** With this method, you use a fine needle to inject medication into the base or side of your penis. Because the needle used is very fine, pain from the injection is usually minor.
- **Penile suppository.** You use a special applicator to insert a tiny suppository containing medication into the penile urethra.
- **Testosterone replacement.** If erectile dysfunction is caused by low levels of the hormone testosterone, testosterone replacement therapy may be prescribed.

Other options

If medications don't work or aren't an option, other choices include:

- **Pumps.** A tube is placed over your penis, and a pump sucks out the air inside the tube. This creates a vacuum that pulls blood into your penis, creating an erection. To keep the penis firm, you slip a tension ring around its base.
- **Penile implants.** It involves surgically placing inflatable or semi-rigid rods into the two sides of the penis. This treatment usually isn't recommended until other methods have been tried.

HERBAL VIAGRA

Some alternative products that claim to treat erectile dysfunction can be dangerous. The Food and Drug Administration has issued warnings about several types of "herbal viagra" that contain potentially harmful drugs not listed on the label. Some can interact with prescription drugs and cause dangerously low blood pressure. These products are especially dangerous when taken with nitrates.

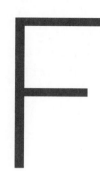

Fatty liver disease

WHAT IS IT? Fatty liver disease is the storage of too much fat in the cells of the liver. This can lead to inflammation and liver damage.

There are two forms of fatty liver disease: alcoholic and nonalcoholic (NAFLD). Alcoholic fatty liver disease typically develops in people who drink heavily over many years. NAFLD refers to a range of fatty liver conditions affecting people who drink little to no alcohol.

WHAT'S THE CAUSE? Different forms of the disease have different causes. Alcoholic fatty liver disease results from drinking too much alcohol. As the liver breaks down alcohol to remove it from the body, it produces harmful substances that can damage liver cells.

It's unclear why some people get NAFLD, but the causes may include:

- Being overweight
- Insulin resistance, in which cells don't take in sugar from the bloodstream in response to the hormone insulin
- High blood sugar (hyperglycemia)
- High levels of fats, particularly triglycerides, in the blood

Diseases and conditions that can increase the risk of NAFLD include:

- Metabolic syndrome
- Polycystic ovary syndrome
- Sleep apnea
- Type 2 diabetes
- Underactive thyroid (hypothyroidism)

- Underactive pituitary gland (hypopituitarism)
- Family history of fatty liver disease

Some people develop an aggressive form of NAFLD called nonalcoholic steatohepatitis (NASH). The liver inflammation seen with NASH can lead to advanced scarring (cirrhosis) and liver failure. This is similar to damage caused by heavy alcohol use. The risk of NASH is higher in people who are older, who have diabetes or whose body fat is concentrated in the abdomen.

SYMPTOM CHECKER Fatty liver disease often causes no signs or symptoms. When it does, they may include fatigue and pain or discomfort in the upper right abdomen.

In people with alcoholic fatty liver disease, yellowing of the skin and eyes (jaundice), weight loss, and fever are common. If you have cirrhosis — advanced scarring of the liver — signs may include:

- Abdominal swelling (ascites)
- Enlarged blood vessels just beneath the surface of the skin
- Enlarged spleen
- Red palms

Taking care of your liver is important because if you have too much fat in it, the organ can become inflamed. That can lead to areas of scarring (fibrosis). If the fat build-up continues, the fibrosis can spread to more liver tissue (cirrhosis) and result in:

- Swelling of veins in the esophagus (esophageal varices), which can rupture and bleed
- Liver cancer
- End-stage liver failure, in which the liver has stopped functioning.

WHAT TESTS TO EXPECT Some people are diagnosed with fatty liver disease when their livers look unusual on an ultrasound or after an enzyme test.

The following tests also may help identify an issue:

Blood tests. Your health care provider may look at bloodwork to diagnose fatty liver disease and see how severe it is, including:

- Complete blood count
- Liver enzyme and liver function tests
- Tests for chronic viral hepatitis
- Celiac disease screening
- Fasting blood sugar
- Hemoglobin A1C, to see how stable your blood sugar is
- Lipid profile to measure the fat in your blood

Imaging. You may also have imaging tests, such as:

- Abdominal ultrasound
- Computerized tomography scanning or magnetic resonance imaging
- Transient elastography, a form of ultrasound to measure the stiffness of the liver
- Magnetic resonance elastography, which creates a visual map that shows stiffness of body tissues

If testing is inconclusive, your provider may recommend taking a sample (biopsy) of your liver to look for signs of inflammation and scarring.

TREATMENT Eliminating alcohol is the first line of treatment for alcoholic fatty liver disease. For NAFLD, your health care provider may recommend losing weight through a combination of healthy diet and exercise. That can help improve the risk factors for NASH.

Losing 10% of your body weight may be ideal, but even losing 3% to 5% of your starting weight can help. Weight-loss surgery may be an option if you need to lose a lot of weight. Liver transplantation may be an option if you have cirrhosis.

LIFESTYLE You can make daily choices and changes to reduce your risk of fatty liver disease. They include:

- Protecting your liver by avoiding alcohol and following instructions on all medications and over-the-counter drugs
- Eating a plant-based diet rich in fruits, vegetables, whole grains and healthy fats
- Maintaining a healthy weight
- Exercising most days of the week
- Controlling your diabetes
- Lowering your cholesterol

Fever

WHAT IS IT? A fever is a temporary rise in your body temperature, often due to an illness. Having a fever is a sign that something out of the ordinary is going on in your body.

The average normal body temperature is 98.6 F (37 C). However, normal body temperature can vary by a degree or more — from about 97 F (36.1 C) to 99 F (37.2 C). A temperature over 100.4 F (38 C) that's taken using a mouth (oral) thermometer is considered a fever.

Fevers generally go away within a few days. Over-the-counter medications can treat a fever, but sometimes it's better left untreated. A fever plays a key role in helping the body fight off infection.

Sometimes the cause of a fever can't be identified. Often, a fever is related to the following:

- A viral or bacterial infection
- Heat exhaustion or extreme sunburn
- Heavy exercise
- The menstrual cycle
- Certain inflammatory conditions, such as rheumatoid arthritis
- Some medications, such as antibiotics and high blood pressure and seizure medications
- Some immunizations

When to see a health care provider

A fever is greater cause for concern in infants and young children than in older children and adults. It's generally recommended to get medical care if your child is:

- **Younger than age 3 months** and has a rectal temperature of 100.4 F (38 C) or higher.
- **3 to 6 months old** and has a temperature higher than 102 F (38.9 C), or has a temperature up to 102 F (38.9 C) and seems unusually irritable, lethargic or uncomfortable.
- **Ages 6 months to 24 months** and has a temperature higher than 102 F (38.9 C) that lasts longer than a day but shows no other symptoms. If your child has other signs and symptoms, such as a cough or diarrhea, you might call your child's doctor sooner.

- **A newborn** and has a lower than normal temperature — less than 97 F (36.1 C). Very young babies may not regulate body temperature well when they're ill and may become cold rather than hot.

In older children, call a health care provider if your child has a fever of 102 F (38.9 C) or higher that lasts longer than three days or is accompanied by other symptoms, including severe headache; stomachache; throat swelling; skin rash; irritability; listlessness; confusion or vomiting.

Ask your child's health care provider for guidance in special circumstances, such as a child with a weakened immune system or with a preexisting illness.

It's generally recommended that adults seek medical care if they have a temperature of 103 F (39.4 C) or higher, a fever that lasts more than three days, or a fever along with other symptoms that are worrisome.

TREATMENT As long as your temperature and other symptoms aren't severe, self-care is often all that's needed to treat a fever. Steps you can take at home include:

- **Drinking plenty of fluids.** A fever can cause fluid loss and dehydration, so drink water, juice or broth. For a baby less than 1 year old, use an oral rehydration solution such as Pedialyte. These solutions contain water and salts proportioned to replenish fluids and electrolytes.
- **Resting.** You need rest to recover, and activity can raise your body temperature.
- **Staying cool.** Dress in light clothing, keep the room temperature cool, and sleep with only a sheet or light blanket.

Medication

In the case of a high fever, your health care provider may recommend an over-the-counter medication. If you have a medical condition, check with your provider before taking nonprescription drugs.

Acetaminophen or ibuprofen. Use these medications according to the label instructions or as recommended by your provider. Be careful to avoid taking too much. High doses or long-term use of acetaminophen or ibuprofen may cause liver or kidney damage, and acute overdoses can be fatal. If your child's fever remains high after a dose, don't give more medication; call your health care provider instead.

Aspirin. Aspirin is generally not recommended for children because it may trigger a rare, but potentially fatal, disorder called Reye's syndrome. Don't give your child aspirin unless your health care provider has specifically prescribed it.

LIFESTYLE Often, fevers develop as part of the body's response to an infectious disease. You can take the following steps to reduce your exposure to germs that cause illness:

- **Wash your hands often.** Washing hands is especially important before eating, after using the toilet and after being around someone who's sick. Teach your children to do the same.
- **Try to avoid touching your nose, mouth or eyes.** These are the main ways that viruses and bacteria can enter the body.
- **Cover up.** Cover your mouth when you cough and your nose when you sneeze. Teach children to do the same.
- **Avoid sharing.** This applies to cups, water bottles and utensils.

FEBRILE SEIZURES

A febrile seizure is a convulsion in a young child generally caused by a spike in body temperature from an infection. Febrile seizures represent a unique response of a young child's brain to an increase in body temperature. Although alarming for parents, the vast majority of febrile seizures cause no lasting effects. If a seizure occurs:

- Lay the child on his or her side or stomach on the floor or ground
- Remove any sharp objects that are near the child
- Loosen tight clothing
- Hold the child to prevent injury
- Don't place anything in the child's mouth or try to stop the seizure

Most febrile seizures stop on their own. Get medical care as soon as possible afterward to determine the cause of the fever. If the seizure lasts more than 5 minutes or if your child has repeated seizures, call for emergency help.

Fibrocystic breasts

WHAT IS IT? Fibrocystic breasts refers to breasts that are composed of tissue that feels lumpy or ropelike in texture. The condition is common. More than half of women — mainly those in their 20s to 50s — experience fibrocystic breast changes at some point in their lives.

Fibrocystic breasts can cause breast pain, tenderness and lumpiness — especially in the upper, outer area of the breasts. Symptoms tend to be most bothersome just before menstruation. Signs and symptoms may include:

- Breast lumps or areas of thickening that tend to blend into the surrounding breast tissue
- Generalized breast pain or tenderness
- Breast lumps that fluctuate in size
- Monthly increase in breast pain or lumpiness from midcycle to just before your period
- Changes that occur in both breasts, rather than just one
- Green or dark brown nonbloody nipple discharge that may leak without pressure or squeezing

TYPICAL BREAST

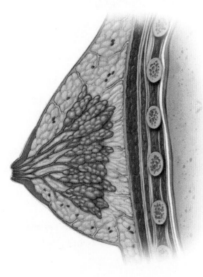

FIBROCYSTIC BREAST

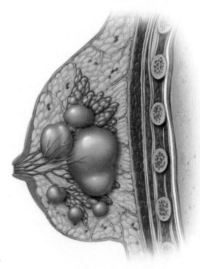

Fibrocystic breasts are composed of fluid-filled sacs (cysts) and more-prominent scar-like (fibrous) tissue that make breasts feel tender and lumpy or "ropy."

The exact cause of fibrocystic breast changes isn't known, but experts suspect that reproductive hormones — especially estrogen — play a role. Hormone fluctuations may cause your breasts to develop lumpy areas that feel tender, sore and swollen. The pain and lumpiness tend to clear up once your period begins.

WHAT TESTS TO EXPECT To evaluate your condition, your health care provider will likely perform a breast exam, checking your breast for areas of thickening, lumps and cysts associated with fibrocystic breasts. You may undergo additional tests to rule out other possible causes, including:

- **Mammogram.** If your provider detects a breast lump or unusual thickening in your breast tissue, you may have a mammogram to evaluate the area and rule out a cancerous tumor.
- **Ultrasound.** Women younger than age 30 might have an ultrasound exam instead of, or in addition to, a mammogram. Ultrasound can better evaluate dense breast tissue, which is more common in younger women than older women. Ultrasound can also help distinguish between fluid-filled breast cysts and solid masses. Other imaging procedures also may be performed.
- **Fine-needle aspiration.** If your health care provider thinks the lump detected on the clinical exam has the consistency of a cyst, you may have an ultrasound to confirm the presence of a cyst. Then a very fine needle may be used to attempt to draw fluid from the cyst.
- **Breast biopsy.** A small sample of breast tissue is removed from the suspicious area for microscopic analysis. A breast biopsy is generally performed when it's unclear if a lump or area of thickening seen during an imaging exam is benign or cancerous.

TREATMENT If you don't experience symptoms or if your symptoms are mild, no treatment may be needed. Severe pain or large, painful cysts associated with fibrocystic breasts may warrant treatment.

Breast cysts

Options for treating painful cysts include:

Fine-needle aspiration. A hair-thin needle is used to drain the fluid from the cyst. Removing the fluid confirms that the lump is a breast cyst, not a solid mass. Removal of fluid also relieves the discomfort caused by the cyst.

Surgical excision. Rarely, surgery is needed to remove a persistent cyst-like lump that doesn't resolve after other treatments.

Breast pain

To treat breast pain your health care provider may recommend:

- **Over-the-counter pain relievers.** These include acetaminophen (Tylenol, others) or nonsteroidal anti-inflammatory drugs (NSAIDs), such as ibuprofen (Advil, Motrin IB, others).
- **Oral contraceptives.** They lower the levels of cycle-related hormones linked to fibrocystic breast changes.

LIFESTYLE Other strategies to relieve symptoms include:

- **Wear a firm support bra.** Try to buy one fitted by a professional. Wear a sports bra when exercising and even when sleeping.
- **Limit or avoid caffeine.** Studies of caffeine's effect on breast pain are inconclusive, but some women find limiting caffeine helpful.
- **Decrease the fat in your diet.** Reduced fat may decrease breast pain or discomfort associated with fibrocystic breasts.
- **Use a heating pad or warm water bottle.** Apply it to painful areas to relieve your discomfort.

BREAST LUMPS

If you find a breast lump or other change in your breast, you may worry that it's breast cancer. That's understandable, but remember that breast lumps are common and not necessarily cancerous. Consult your health care provider if:

- You find a breast lump that's new or unusual
- A new breast lump doesn't go away after your next period
- An existing breast lump seems to have changed — it gets bigger, for instance
- You notice breast skin changes, such as redness, crusting, dimpling or puckering
- You notice changes in your nipple — it turns inward or appears flatter, for example
- You notice nipple discharge that's clear, yellow, green, brown or red

---

Fibromyalgia

WHAT IS IT? Fibromyalgia is a disorder characterized by widespread musculoskeletal pain that's often accompanied by other symptoms, including fatigue or sleep difficulties.

Researchers believe that among people with fibromyalgia the way that the brain processes pain signals is amplified. In addition, the brain's pain receptors become more sensitive than normal, causing them to overreact to pain signals.

Because fibromyalgia tends to run in families, there may be certain genetic mutations that may make individuals more susceptible to the disorder. Symptoms may begin after a physical trauma, surgery, infection or significant psychological stress. Women are much more likely to develop fibromyalgia than are men.

SYMPTOM CHECKER Symptoms of fibromyalgia include:

- **Widespread pain.** The pain associated with fibromyalgia often is described as a constant dull ache that has lasted for at least three months. To be considered widespread, the pain must occur on both sides of the body and above and below the waist.
- **Fatigue.** People with fibromyalgia often awaken tired, even though they report sleeping for long periods. Some people have sleep disorders such as restless legs syndrome and sleep apnea.
- **Cognitive difficulties.** A symptom commonly referred to as "fibro fog" impairs the ability to focus, pay attention and concentrate on mental tasks.
- **Other problems.** Some people experience depression, headaches, and pain or cramping in the lower abdomen.

TREATMENT Because many of the signs and symptoms of fibromyalgia are similar to other disorders, it may take a while to receive a diagnosis.

In the past, health care providers would check 18 specific points on a person's body to see how many of them were painful when firmly pressed. Newer guidelines don't require a tender point exam. Instead, a diagnosis can be made if a person has had widespread pain for more than three months — with no other medical condition that could cause the pain.

Treatments for fibromyalgia include both medication and therapy, with an emphasis on minimizing symptoms.

Medications

Medications are used to reduce pain and improve sleep.

Antidepressants. Duloxetine (Cymbalta) and milnacipran (Savella) may be prescribed to treat pain and fatigue. Amitriptyline or cyclobenzaprine are sometimes prescribed to help promote sleep.

Anti-seizure drugs. Medications to treat epilepsy may reduce certain fibromyalgia pain. Pregabalin (Lyrica) was the first drug approved by the Food and Drug Administration to treat fibromyalgia. Gabapentin (Neurontin) also may relieve symptoms.

Pain relievers. Over-the-counter pain relievers may help. If over-the-counter products and other medications don't work, your health care provider might suggest a prescription pain reliever such as tramadol (Ultram, others). Other opioids aren't advised. They can lead to dependence and worsen chronic pain.

Cognitive behavioral therapy

Some people find talking with a counselor and learning strategies for dealing with fibromyalgia to be helpful in reducing symptoms.

LIFESTYLE To help manage fibromyalgia symptoms:

- **Reduce stress.** Try to avoid or limit overexertion and emotional stress. Allow yourself time each day to relax, but remain active.
- **Get enough sleep.** Adequate sleep is essential. Practice good habits, such as following a sleep schedule and limiting napping.
- **Exercise regularly.** At first, exercise may increase your pain. But doing it regularly often decreases symptoms.
- **Pace yourself.** Moderation means not overdoing it on your good days, and not doing too little on the days when symptoms flare.
- **Maintain a healthy lifestyle.** Eat a balanced diet, limit your caffeine and don't smoke. Do something enjoyable every day.

Flu (influenza)

WHAT IS IT? Influenza is a viral infection that attacks the respiratory system — the nose, throat and lungs. Commonly called "the flu," influenza isn't the same as stomach "flu" viruses that cause diarrhea and vomiting.

Flu viruses travel through the air in droplets when an infected person coughs, sneezes or talks. You can inhale the droplets or you can pick up the germs by touching an object and then transfer them to your eyes, nose or mouth. People with the flu are generally contagious from the day before symptoms first appear until 5 to 10 days after they begin.

If you're young and healthy, the flu usually isn't serious. Although you may feel miserable, it usually goes away with no lasting effects. Children and adults at high risk may develop complications such as pneumonia, bronchitis, asthma flare-ups, and sinus and ear infections. For older adults and people with chronic illnesses, pneumonia can be deadly.

People at higher risk of developing flu complications include young children, adults older than age 65, pregnant women, people with weakened immune systems and people who have chronic illnesses.

SYMPTOM CHECKER Initially, the flu may seem like a common cold. But colds usually develop slowly, whereas the flu tends to come on suddenly, and symptoms are often worse than a cold. Common signs and symptoms of the flu include:

- Fever over 100 F (38 C)
- Aching muscles, especially in your back, arms and legs
- Chills and sweats
- Headache
- Dry cough
- Fatigue and weakness
- Nasal congestion

TREATMENT Most people who get the flu can treat themselves at home and often don't need medical care.

Self-care

If you come down with the flu:

- **Drink plenty of liquids.** Choose water, juice and warm soups to prevent dehydration.
- **Rest.** Sleep helps your immune system fight the infection.
- **Use pain relievers as needed.** An over-the-counter pain reliever, such as acetaminophen (Tylenol, others) or ibuprofen (Advil, Motrin IB, others), can combat the achiness associated with influenza. Don't give aspirin to children or teens because of the risk of Reye's syndrome, a rare, but potentially fatal, disease.

Medications

Your provider may prescribe an antiviral medication, such as oseltamivir (Tamiflu), zanamivir (Relenza), peramivir (Rapivab) or baloxavir (Xofluza). If taken soon after symptoms begin, these drugs may shorten the duration of the flu by a day or so and help prevent serious complications.

Oseltamivir is an oral medication. Zanamivir is inhaled through a device similar to an asthma inhaler. It shouldn't be used by anyone with respiratory problems, such as asthma and lung disease. Side effects of the medications may include nausea and vomiting. Oseltamivir has also been associated with delirium and abnormal behaviors in teenagers.

LIFESTYLE To help reduce the spread of infection:

- **Wash your hands.** Thorough and frequent hand-washing is the best way to prevent many common infections.
- **Contain your coughs and sneezes.** Cover your mouth and nose.
- **Avoid crowds.** Flu spreads easily wherever people congregate.

PREVENTION

The Centers for Disease Control and Prevention recommends an annual flu vaccination for all Americans over the age of 6 months. Each year's vaccine contains protection from viruses expected to be the most common during the upcoming flu season. The vaccine may be given as an injection or a nasal spray.

Food poisoning

 WHAT'S THE CAUSE? Food poisoning, also known as foodborne illness, is caused by eating contaminated food. Infectious organisms — including bacteria, viruses and parasites, or their toxins — are the most common causes of food poisoning.

Contamination can happen at any point during food production: growing, harvesting, processing, storing, shipping or preparing. The organism responsible, the amount of exposure, your age and your health generally determine the severity of the illness.

 SYMPTOM CHECKER Signs and symptoms, which can start within hours of eating contaminated food, vary with the source of contamination. They generally include:

- Nausea
- Vomiting
- Watery diarrhea
- Abdominal pain and cramps
- Fever

Seek immediate treatment for severe signs and symptoms, which may include an inability to keep liquids down, frequent vomiting, blood in vomit or stool, severe abdominal cramping, diarrhea that lasts more than three days, a temperature higher than 100.4 F (38 C), and neurological symptoms such as blurry vision or muscle weakness.

You should also seek medical care for symptoms of dehydration — the severe loss of water and essential salts and minerals. Signs or symptoms include excessive thirst, little or no urination, severe weakness, dizziness, or lightheadedness. Severe dehydration may require hospitalization.

 TREATMENT Depending on your symptoms and their severity, your health care provider may conduct tests, such as a blood test or stool culture to identify the microorganism responsible and confirm the diagnosis.

For most people, the illness resolves on its own within a few days, though some types of food poisoning may last longer.

Replacement of lost fluids. Fluids and minerals such as sodium, potassium and calcium that maintain the balance of fluids in your body need to be replaced. Drink water, clear soda or noncaffeinated sports drinks, such as Gatorade. Oral rehydration fluid (Pedialyte, Enfalyte, others) is often recommended for children.

Antibiotics. Your health care provider may prescribe antibiotics if you have certain kinds of bacterial food poisoning and your symptoms are severe. Generally, the sooner treatment begins, the better. During pregnancy, prompt antibiotic treatment may keep the infection from affecting the baby.

Anti-diarrheals. Adults with diarrhea that isn't bloody and who don't have a fever may get relief from taking the over-the-counter medication loperamide (Imodium A-D) or bismuth subsalicylate (Pepto-Bismol). Ask your provider about these options.

Self-care. To keep yourself comfortable and prevent dehydration:

- **Let your stomach settle.** Don't eat and drink for a few hours. Suck on ice chips.
- **Rest.** The illness can weaken and tire you.
- **Ease back into eating.** Eat bland, easy-to-digest foods, such as soda crackers, toast and gelatin. Until you feel better, avoid dairy products, caffeine, and fatty or highly seasoned foods.

DANGEROUS INFECTIONS

Food poisoning can cause potentially serious complications in some people.

Listeria monocytogenes

Early in pregnancy, a listeria infection may lead to miscarriage. Later on, it may lead to stillbirth, premature birth, a potentially fatal infant infection after birth, or long-term neurological damage and delayed development. Listeria may be found in hot dogs, luncheon meats, unpasteurized milk and cheeses, and unwashed raw produce.

Escherichia coli (E. coli)

Certain E. coli strains can cause hemolytic uremic syndrome, which damages the kidneys. Older adults, children under age 5 and people with weakened immune systems are at increased risk. E. coli is spread mainly through undercooked ground beef.

Frostbite

WHAT IS IT? Frostbite is an injury caused by freezing of the skin and underlying tissues. It's most common on the fingers, toes, nose, ears, cheeks and chin. Exposed skin in cold, windy weather is most vulnerable to frostbite.

F-G

Frostnip, the first stage of frostbite, doesn't cause permanent skin damage and can be treated with first-aid measures. All other frostbite requires medical attention because it can damage skin and underlying tissues.

Signs and symptoms of frostbite include:

- Cold skin and a prickling feeling
- Numbness
- Red, white, bluish-white or grayish-yellow skin
- Hard or waxy-looking skin
- Clumsiness due to joint and muscle stiffness
- Blistering after rewarming, in severe cases

TREATMENT Treatment for frostbite depends on its severity.

To care for your skin after mild frostbite:

- **Gently rewarm frostbitten areas.** Soak hands or feet in warm, not hot, water for 15 to 30 minutes. Don't rewarm frostbitten skin with direct heat, such as a heat lamp or heating pad.
- **Take pain medicine.** Ibuprofen (Advil, Motrin IB, others) will help reduce pain and inflammation.
- **Apply aloe.** After the affected skin has been rewarmed, apply aloe vera gel or lotion several times a day.

For more severe frostbite, your health care provider may loosely wrap the area with sterile dressings to protect the skin. You may need to elevate the affected area to reduce swelling. To heal properly, frostbitten skin needs to be free of damaged or infected tissue. Because of this, some tissue may need to be removed. Soaking in a whirlpool bath can aid in healing. Antibiotics may be prescribed to protect against infection. Medications that help restore blood flow to damaged tissue also may be prescribed.

Fungal infections

WHAT IS IT? Fungi are microscopic organisms that live in warm, moist environments. Some fungi have beneficial uses; others can cause illness and infection.

Fungal infections most commonly occur on the nails, especially the toenails; on the feet, especially between the toes (athlete's foot); and in the groin area in men (jock itch).

SYMPTOM CHECKER Signs and symptoms of a fungal infection generally appear as follows:

- **Nail infection.** Infected nails may be thickened, brittle, crumbly or ragged, and distorted in shape. They may be yellowish or dull in color, or darkened from debris building up under the nail. Sometimes the infected nail separates from the nail bed.
- **Athlete's foot.** Athlete's foot generally causes a scaly, itchy rash that may also sting or burn.
- **Jock itch.** Jock itch typically produces an itchy, red rash that's often ring-shaped.

TREATMENT Treatment for a fungal infection depends on its location and severity.

Nail infections
Treatment options include:

Oral antifungal drugs. The most effective treatments are the prescription drugs terbinafine and itraconazole (Sporanox). They help a new nail grow free of infection. However, it may take four months or longer to eliminate the infection and grow the nail back.

Success seems to improve when combining oral and topical antifungal therapies.

Medicated nail polish. You paint an antifungal nail polish called ciclopirox (Penlac) on the infected nails and surrounding skin once daily. After seven days, you wipe the piled-on layers clean and begin fresh applications. You may need to use the polish daily for a year.

Medicated nail cream. The cream is rubbed into the infected nails after soaking them. These creams may work better if you first thin the nails so that the medications get through the hard nail surface.

Nail removal. If a nail infection is severe or extremely painful, your health care provider may suggest removing the nail. A new nail will usually grow in its place, but it may take up to a year to grow back.

Athlete's foot

If athlete's foot is mild, an over-the-counter antifungal ointment, lotion, powder or spray may be effective. If the rash doesn't improve, you may need a prescription-strength medication. Severe infections may require an oral antifungal medication.

Jock itch

For a mild case of jock itch, use an over-the-counter antifungal ointment, lotion, powder or spray. If the jock itch is severe or doesn't respond to over-the-counter products, a prescription-strength cream or ointment, or even antifungal pills, may be necessary.

LIFESTYLE To reduce jock itch, dry your genital area and inner thighs thoroughly after showering or exercising. Use powder around the groin area to prevent excess moisture. If you sweat a lot, change underwear often. Make sure your athletic supporter fits correctly.

To prevent toenail infection and athlete's foot, keep your feet dry, especially between the toes. Wear well-ventilated shoes and change socks often. In public showers or pools, wear waterproof sandals.

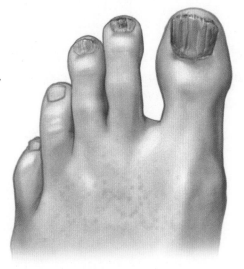

Nail fungus can cause the nail to become thick or ragged and appear yellow, brown or black.

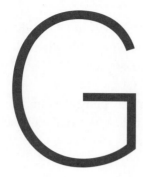

Gallstones

WHAT IS IT? Gallstones are hardened deposits of digestive fluid (bile) that can form in the gallbladder. The stones may be as small as grains of sand or as large as golf balls. Some people develop just one gallstone, while others develop many.

It's not clear what causes gallstones to form. Some may result if the digestive fluid (bile) produced by the gallbladder contains too much cholesterol or too much bilirubin. Bilirubin is a chemical that's produced when the body breaks down red blood cells. Gallstones may also result if the gallbladder doesn't empty properly.

Factors that may increase the risk of gallstones include being overweight, eating a high-fat or high-cholesterol diet, losing weight very rapidly, pregnancy, and a family history of gallstones. In the United States, the risk is also higher for American Indians and Mexican Americans.

SYMPTOM CHECKER Some gallstones don't cause any symptoms. If a stone lodges in a passageway (duct) and creates a blockage, symptoms may occur and include:

- Sudden, rapidly intensifying pain in the upper right part of the abdomen
- Sudden and rapidly intensifying pain in the center of the abdomen, just below the breastbone
- Back pain between the shoulder blades
- Pain in the right shoulder

Gallstone pain may last several minutes to a few hours.

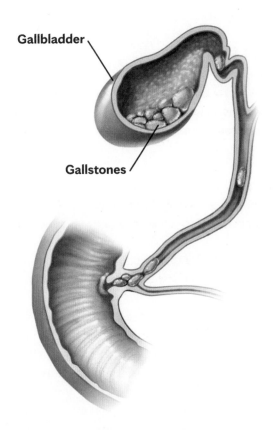

Gallbladder

Gallstones

TREATMENT Gallstones that don't cause signs and symptoms typically don't require treatment. If gallstones are causing pain or other symptoms, treatment options include:

Surgery to remove the gallbladder. Once the gallbladder is removed, bile flows directly from the liver into the small intestine, rather than being stored in the gallbladder. You don't need your gallbladder to live, and its removal doesn't affect your ability to digest food. You may experience diarrhea temporarily.

Medications to dissolve gallstones. It may take months or years to dissolve gallstones using medications, and sometimes the treatments don't work. This approach is generally reserved for people who can't undergo surgery.

LIFESTYLE To reduce your risk of gallstones:

- **Don't skip meals or fast.** It increases the risk of gallstones.
- **Lose weight slowly.** If you need to lose weight, aim to lose 1 or 2 pounds a week. Try to maintain a healthy weight.

Ganglion cyst

WHAT IS IT? Ganglion cysts are noncancerous lumps that most often develop along the tendons or joints of the wrists or hands. The cysts are typically round or oval and are filled with a jellylike lubricating fluid.

TREATMENT Ganglion cysts that are painless and don't affect joint movement generally don't require any treatment. If a cyst is bothersome, your health care provider may recommend:

Immobilization. Activity can cause a ganglion cyst to enlarge. One option is to wear a wrist brace or splint to immobilize the area.

Aspiration. A needle is inserted into the cyst to drain the fluid from it. Before the aspiration, an enzyme may be injected into the cyst to make the jellylike contents easier to remove. Afterward, a steroid may be injected into the cyst to reduce the chances of recurrence.

Surgery. If other treatments haven't worked, surgery may be necessary to remove the stalk that attaches the cyst to a joint or tendon. However, in some cases a cyst may recur after surgery.

An old home remedy for a ganglion cyst consisted of "thumping" the cyst with a heavy object. This isn't a good solution because the force of the blow can damage surrounding structures. Also, don't try to "pop" the cyst yourself by puncturing it with a needle. This is unlikely to be effective and can lead to infection.

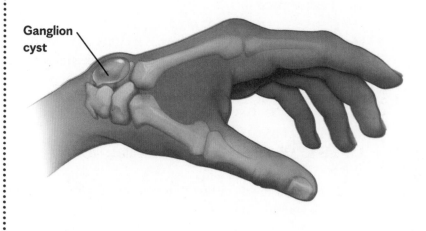

Ganglion cyst

GERD (gastroesophageal reflux disease)

WHAT IS IT? When you swallow, the lower esophageal sphincter — a circular band of muscle around the bottom part of your esophagus — relaxes to allow food and liquid to flow down into your stomach. Then it closes again. If this valve relaxes at other times or it weakens, stomach acid can flow back up (reflux) into your esophagus.

Acid reflux is common. Most people experience the condition on occasion, often due to overeating. When it occurs frequently — at least twice each week — or it interferes with your daily life, you may have gastroesophageal reflux disease (GERD).

GERD is a chronic digestive disease caused by frequent acid reflux that irritates and inflames the lining of the esophagus. Over time, the inflammation can erode the lining, causing complications such as bleeding, esophageal narrowing or a precancerous condition called Barrett esophagus.

Conditions that can increase your risk of GERD include a hiatal hernia, obesity, pregnancy, smoking, asthma, diabetes and delayed stomach emptying.

SYMPTOM CHECKER Signs and symptoms include:

- A burning sensation in your chest (heartburn), sometimes spreading to your throat, along with a sour taste in your mouth
- Regurgitation of food or sour liquid (acid reflux)
- Chest pain
- Difficulty swallowing
- Dry cough
- Hoarseness or sore throat
- Sensation of a lump in your throat

WHAT TESTS TO EXPECT A diagnosis of GERD can sometimes be made based on the common symptoms of heartburn and acid reflux. Other times, certain tests may be needed before a diagnosis is made.

Types

Tests used to diagnose GERD include the following:

- **Acid tests.** Ambulatory acid (pH) probe tests use a device placed in your esophagus to measure acid for 24 to 48 hours. They identify when, and for how long, stomach acid is regurgitated.
- **Upper digestive system X-ray.** Sometimes called a barium swallow or upper GI series, this test involves drinking a chalky liquid that coats the inside lining of your digestive tract before X-rays are taken. The coating allows your health care provider to see a silhouette of your esophagus, stomach and upper intestine.
- **Endoscopy.** During this procedure, a catheter equipped with a light and camera (endoscope) is inserted down your throat to view your esophagus and esophageal sphincter. A sample of tissue (biopsy) may be taken for further testing.
- **Esophageal manometry.** This test measures movement and pressure in the esophagus. For the test, a catheter is threaded through your nose and into your esophagus.

TREATMENT Treatment of GERD usually begins with nonprescription products that control acid. If you don't experience relief within a few weeks, your health care provider may recommend other treatments, including medications or surgery.

Nonprescription medications

Products that may help treat GERD include:

Antacids. Antacids, such as Maalox, Mylanta, Gaviscon, Rolaids and Tums, may provide quick relief. But they won't heal an inflamed esophagus damaged by stomach acid. Overusing these medications may cause side effects such as diarrhea.

Medications to reduce acid production. Called H-2-receptor blockers, they include cimetidine (Tagamet HB), famotidine (Pepcid AC) and nizatidine (Axid AR). H-2-receptor blockers don't act as quickly as antacids do, but they provide longer relief and may decrease acid production for up to 12 hours.

Medications that block acid production. Proton pump inhibitors are stronger acid blockers that provide time for damaged esophageal tissue to heal. Over-the-counter proton pump inhibitors include lansoprazole (Prevacid 24 HR) and omeprazole (Prilosec OTC, Zegerid OTC).

Prescription-strength medications

If GERD persists, your health care provider may recommend:

H-2-receptor blockers. They include higher dose prescription-strength cimetidine, famotidine, nizatidine and ranitidine.

Proton pump inhibitors. Prescription-strength proton pump inhibitors include esomeprazole (Nexium), lansoprazole (Prevacid), omeprazole (Prilosec), pantoprazole (Protonix), rabeprazole (Aciphex) and dexlansoprazole (Dexilant).

Baclofen. This medication may decrease acid reflux by reducing how often the lower esophageal sphincter relaxes. It's not as effective as proton pump inhibitors, but may help with severe reflux.

Surgery

Surgical options are rarely needed because medication is so effective. They include:

Nissen fundoplication. It involves tightening the lower esophageal sphincter to prevent reflux by wrapping the top of the stomach around the outside of the lower esophagus.

LINX Reflux Management System. This device is a ring made of tiny magnetic titanium beads that's wrapped around the junction of the stomach and esophagus. The magnetic pull between the beads is strong enough to prevent acid reflux but weak enough that food can pass through.

LIFESTYLE To help reduce symptoms of GERD:

- **Maintain a healthy weight.** Excess pounds put pressure on the abdomen, pushing on the stomach and causing acid to back up into the esophagus. If you're overweight, try to lose weight.
- **Avoid foods and drinks that trigger heartburn.** Common triggers include fatty or fried foods, tomato sauce, alcohol, chocolate, mint, garlic, onion, and caffeine.
- **Eat smaller meals.** Overeating can trigger symptoms.
- **Don't lie down after a meal.** Wait at least three hours after eating.
- **Adjust your bed.** Elevate your head by placing blocks under the top legs of your bed. Or insert a wedge pillow between your mattress and box spring.

Glaucoma

WHAT IS IT? Glaucoma isn't one eye disease but is a group of eye conditions that can damage the optic nerve and lead to vision loss. High pressure inside the eye is often the cause. This can happen when drainage channels become blocked and fluid builds up in the eye.

Factors that can increase your risk of glaucoma include age and a family history of glaucoma. Black people older than 40 have a much higher risk of developing glaucoma than white people do. People of Asian descent also are at increased risk of some forms of glaucoma.

Several conditions may increase your risk of developing glaucoma, including diabetes, heart disease, high blood pressure and an underactive thyroid gland (hypothyroidism).

SYMPTOM CHECKER Signs and symptoms of the most common forms of glaucoma include:

- Gradual loss of peripheral vision, usually in both eyes
- Tunnel vision in the advanced stages

Other signs and symptoms may include eye pain, blurred vision, halos around lights and reddening of the eye.

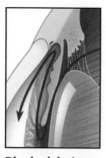

Blocked drainage channel

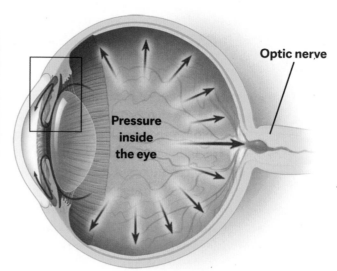

Optic nerve

Pressure inside the eye

TREATMENT The goal of treatment is to reduce the amount of pressure in your eye.

Eye drops

Treatment often starts with medicated eye drops. They increase the flow of fluid from the eye, decrease the production of fluid or both. These changes help reduce eye pressure. Prescription eye drops include:

- **Prostaglandins.** Examples include latanoprost (Xalatan, Xelpros) and bimatoprost (Lumigan). A new form of bimatoprost (Durysta) is available as an implant that dissolves in the eye.
- **Beta blockers.** Examples include timolol (Betimol, Timoptic, others) and betaxolol (Betoptic).
- **Alpha-adrenergic agonists.** Examples include apraclonidine (Iopidine) and brimonidine (Alphagan P, Qoliana).
- **Carbonic anhydrase inhibitors.** Examples include dorzolamide and brinzolamide (Azopt).
- **Rho kinase inhibitor.** This medication is available as netarsudil (Rhopressa).
- **Combined medications.** Sometimes doctors may prescribe a combined medication, such as a beta blocker and an alpha-adrenergic agonist, or a beta blocker and a carbonic anhydrase inhibitor.

If eye drops alone don't reduce eye pressure to a desired level, your health care provider may also prescribe an oral medication.

Surgery

Surgical procedures include:

Laser surgery. A high-energy laser beam is used to open clogged drainage canals and help fluid drain more easily from your eye.

Filtering surgery. An opening is made in the white of your eye (sclera) and a small piece of eye tissue is removed at the base of your cornea, allowing fluid to leave the eye through this opening.

Drainage implants. A surgeon inserts a small tube in your eye to facilitate drainage of fluid from the eye.

Some types of glaucoma are medical emergencies, requiring urgent treatment to reduce eye pressure. A laser may be used to create a small hole in your iris, allowing fluid to exit your eye.

Gout

WHAT IS IT? Gout is a complex form of arthritis characterized by sudden, severe attacks of pain, redness and tenderness in joints — often the joint at the base of the big toe. Gout can also occur in the feet, ankles, knees, hands and wrists.

Gout occurs when urate crystals accumulate in a joint, causing inflammation and intense pain. These crystals can form when you have high levels of uric acid in your blood.

Your body produces uric acid when it breaks down purines — substances found naturally in your body, as well as in certain foods, such as steak, organ meats and seafood. Alcoholic beverages, especially beer, and drinks sweetened with fruit sugar (fructose) also may promote increased uric acid.

Uric acid typically dissolves in your blood and passes through your kidneys into your urine. But sometimes your body produces too much or your kidneys excrete too little of it, and the acid can accumulate and form sharp, needlelike crystals in a joint or surrounding tissue. An attack of gout can occur suddenly, even waking you up in the middle of the night.

SYMPTOM CHECKER Signs and symptoms almost always occur without warning. They may include:

- **Intense joint pain.** The pain is likely to be most severe within the first 4 to 12 hours after it begins.
- **Lingering discomfort.** After the most severe pain subsides, joint discomfort may last from a few days to a few weeks.
- **Inflammation and redness.** The affected joint or joints become swollen, tender, warm and red.
- **Limited range of motion.** As gout progresses, you may notice that you have decreased mobility in your joints.

Your risk of gout is increased if you're overweight, your diet is high in meat and seafood, or you drink a lot of beverages sweetened with fructose. Drinking a lot of alcohol, especially beer, increases your risk too. If other members of your family have had gout, you're also more likely to develop it.

TREATMENT Medications are the main form of treatment for gout.

Medications to treat gout attacks
Drugs used to relieve gout flares include:

Nonsteroidal anti-inflammatory drugs (NSAIDs). NSAIDs include nonprescription products such as ibuprofen (Advil, Motrin IB, others) and naproxen sodium (Aleve), as well as more-powerful prescription NSAIDs such as indomethacin (Indocin) or celecoxib (Celebrex).

Colchicine. Colchicine (Colcrys, Gloperba, Mitigare) effectively reduces gout pain, but it can cause nausea, vomiting and diarrhea.

Corticosteroids. Corticosteroid medications, such as the drug prednisone, may control gout inflammation and pain. They're generally reserved for people who can't take NSAIDs or colchicine because of potential serious side effects.

Medications to prevent complications
If you experience several gout attacks each year or if your attacks are particularly painful, your doctor may recommend one of the following:

Xanthine oxidase inhibitors. The drugs allopurinol (Aloprim, Lopurin, Zyloprim) and febuxostat (Uloric) limit the amount of uric acid your body makes.

Probenecid (Probalan). This medication improves your kidneys' ability to remove uric acid from your body.

LIFESTYLE Certain lifestyle changes can help prevent or reduce gout attacks. Here are some tips that you can try:

- Limit alcoholic beverages and drinks sweetened with fructose.
- Limit foods that are high in purines, such as red meat, organ meats and seafood.
- Keep your body at a healthy weight.

Certain foods and beverages may have potential to lower uric acid levels. For example, there is some evidence of a possible benefit from coffee, cherries and foods high in vitamin C. But no study has found enough evidence to encourage consuming them as a treatment.

Graves' disease

WHAT IS IT? Graves' disease is an immune system disorder that results in the overproduction of thyroid hormones (hyperthyroidism). Although a number of disorders are associated with hyperthyroidism, Graves' disease is a common cause.

Factors that may increase your risk include having a family history of the disorder and having another autoimmune disorder, such as rheumatoid arthritis or type 1 diabetes. There's some indication that stressful life events or illness may act as a trigger for the onset of Graves' disease in people who are genetically susceptible.

SYMPTOM CHECKER Because thyroid hormones affect a number of different body systems, signs and symptoms associated with Graves' disease can be wide ranging and include:

- Anxiety and irritability
- A fine tremor of the hands or fingers
- Heat sensitivity, an increase in perspiration, or warm, moist skin
- Weight loss, despite usual eating habits
- Enlargement of the thyroid gland (goiter)
- Change in menstrual cycle
- Erectile dysfunction or reduced libido
- Bulging eyes (Graves' ophthalmopathy)
- Thick, red skin, usually on the shins or tops of the feet (Graves' dermopathy)
- Rapid or irregular heartbeat

About 25% to 40% of people with the disease experience Graves' ophthalmopathy. Inflammation and other changes to the muscles and tissues around your eyes can cause them to bulge. They may also feel gritty and appear red or inflamed.

TREATMENT Several tests may be performed in making a diagnosis. In one test, you're given a small amount of radioactive iodine and the rate at which your thyroid gland takes up the iodine is measured. (Iodine is needed to make thyroid hormones.) The goals of treatment are to inhibit the production of thyroid hormones and to block the hormones' effects on your body.

Radioactive iodine therapy. For this common treatment, you take radioactive iodine (radioiodine) by mouth. The radioiodine is absorbed by the thyroid cells, gradually destroying overactive cells. This causes your thyroid gland to shrink and symptoms to lessen. Because the radioiodine causes thyroid activity to decline, you'll likely need treatment later on to supply your body with thyroid hormones.

Because radioiodine therapy may cause or worsen Graves' ophthalmopathy, this treatment may not be recommended if you already have moderate to severe eye problems. And it's not used in those who are pregnant or breastfeeding.

Anti-thyroid medications. The medications propylthiouracil and methimazole interfere with the thyroid's use of iodine to produce hormones. These two drugs may be used alone or before or after radioiodine therapy.

Beta blockers. They block the effect of thyroid hormones and may provide fairly rapid relief of irregular heartbeats, tremors, anxiety and irritability, heat intolerance, sweating, diarrhea, and muscle weakness. Beta blockers include the drugs propranolol (Inderal, Innopran XL), atenolol (Tenormin), metoprolol (Lopressor, Toprol-XL) and nadolol (Corgard).

Surgery. Surgery to remove all or part of your thyroid gland is a last resort. After surgery, you'll need to take supplemental thyroid hormones.

Graves' ophthalmopathy

To treat this condition, your health care provider may recommend:

- **Corticosteroids.** Prescription corticosteroids, such as prednisone, may diminish swelling behind your eyeballs. However, corticosteroids have several side effects.
- **Orbital decompression surgery.** The bone between your eye socket and your sinuses is removed, giving your eyes room to move back to their original positions. This treatment may be used if pressure on the optic nerve threatens your vision.
- **Orbital radiotherapy.** This uses targeted X-rays over the course of several days to destroy some of the tissue behind your eyes. It may be considered if your eye problems are worsening and other treatments aren't an option.
- **Prisms.** If you have double vision, special lenses in your eyeglasses may help.

Gut microbiome imbalance

WHAT IS IT? Your gut microbiome is the "community" of microbes in your stomach and intestines. An imbalance or change in the composition of bacteria, fungi, parasites and viruses may make you more susceptible to health problems.

Your gut microbiome has trillions of bacteria in it. They work together to help your body digest food and synthesize vitamins. Scientists are just beginning to understand what these microbes do beyond digestion.

Studies have shown that the microbes in your gut can affect your metabolism and determine whether you are likely to become obese. A microbe imbalance caused by medication or diet can lead to diarrhea or constipation. The balance of microbes in your gut may be linked to your risk of having ulcerative colitis, Crohn's disease, celiac disease, stomach cancer or colorectal cancer.

Recent research suggests that the gut microbiome may play a role in many other processes too, including regulating brain chemistry and behavior. Studies of the gut microbiome are underway to learn:

- How exactly it affects human health and disease
- Why each person's gut microbiome is unique
- How the gut microbiome varies in pregnancy and childhood
- How gut microbiomes are different in healthy people and people with health conditions such as diabetes and depression
- Whether it's possible to alter people's gut microbiomes to help them stay well or get healthy

WHAT'S THE CAUSE? Each person's gut microbiome is different and determined in part by DNA. Scientists are studying what causes the gut microbiome to get out of balance.

One possibility is that "good" bacteria decrease if you eat a diet high in fat and processed foods and low in fiber and don't get enough exercise. A lack of diversity in your microbiome may change how your immune system reacts to challenges, and it may affect how you gain or lose weight.

Researchers continue to study how your diet and other factors, such as your genes and the environment you live in, play important roles in maintaining a healthy gut ecosystem. Things that are known to disturb the balance of gut bacteria include:

- Having an infection
- Taking antibiotics for a long time
- Using other medications that destroy the good bacteria
- Changes in diet

Scientists are also exploring the relationship of the gut microbiome to disease. One area of focus is probiotics, live microorganisms contained in certain foods. Eating probiotics may be helpful to the balance of bacteria in the body. However, the benefits haven't been conclusively proved.

F-G

 LIFESTYLE Diet, and especially intake of fat and fiber, dramatically impacts the makeup of your microbiome. The following steps are part of a healthy lifestyle and may have benefits for your gut health:

- Eating a diet rich in plant foods and fiber
- Choosing protein from a variety of animal and plant-based sources
- Exercising regularly
- Getting adequate sleep
- Managing stress

UNDERSTANDING PROBIOTICS

Some fermented foods, such as yogurt and sauerkraut, and dietary supplements contain probiotics. Probiotics are live organisms that are the same as or similar to the bacteria in your gut microbiome. Two of the most common are lactobacillus and bifidobacterium bacteria.

The theory behind taking probiotics is that they may help the gut microbiome regain balance after it's been disturbed. For example, some research shows that probiotics may prevent diarrhea associated with antibiotics.

However, dietary supplements that contain probiotics aren't regulated by the U.S. Food and Drug Administration (FDA). So there is no way to confirm that a probiotic contains live and active bacteria or verify any health claims on the label. If you're considering taking supplements, check with your doctor to be sure they're right for you.

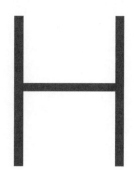

Headache

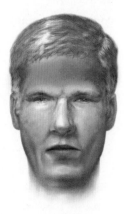

WHAT IS IT? Headache is pain in any region of the head.

Headaches may occur on one or both sides of the head, be isolated to a certain location, or radiate across the head. Headaches may appear gradually or come on suddenly. They may last less than an hour or for several days. There are many different types.

Tension headache

Tension headache refers to diffuse, mild to moderate head pain that's often accompanied by tightness or pressure across the forehead. Other symptoms may include tenderness in the scalp, neck and shoulders.

What causes tension headaches isn't known. Some experts theorize that people with tension headaches may have a heightened sensitivity to pain and possibly a heightened sensitivity to stress.

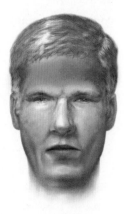

Tension

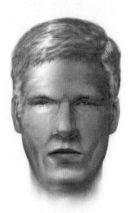

Migraine

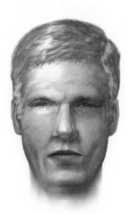

Cluster

Migraine

A migraine typically causes an intense throbbing or a pulsing sensation in one area of the head that may last for hours to days. The pain is often accompanied by nausea, vomiting, and sensitivity to light and sound. Some migraines are preceded by warning symptoms (auras), such as flashes of light, blind spots, or tingling in an arm or leg.

What causes migraines isn't well understood. They may be associated with brain chemical imbalances, changes in the brainstem and interactions with the trigeminal nerve, a major pain pathway. They are more common among women and people who have a family member with a history of migraines.

A number of things may trigger a migraine attack, including hormonal changes in women; salty or processed foods; some sweeteners or preservatives; alcohol; stress; a change of weather; and sensory stimuli, such as bright lights, unusual smells or loud sounds.

Cluster headache

Cluster headaches occur in cyclical patterns (clusters). The pain is very severe and often located in or around one eye on one side of the head. People say it feels like a hot poker being stuck in the eye. Other symptoms include redness or excessive tearing in the eye, a stuffy or runny nostril on one side of the face, and pain that radiates to other areas of the face or neck and shoulders.

Cluster headaches may occur frequently for weeks to months, usually followed by a remission period. Changes in an area of the brain called the hypothalamus may play a role.

TREATMENT It depends on the type of headache you have.

Tension headache

A variety of medications may be prescribed.

Pain-relieving medications. These medications are generally taken as soon as symptoms begin.

Nonprescription pain relievers, including aspirin and ibuprofen (Advil, Motrin IB, others), are usually the first line of treatment. Sometimes a health care provider will recommend a prescription pain reliever.

Preventive medications. These medications are prescribed to help reduce the frequency of tension headaches.

Tricyclic antidepressants, including amitriptyline and nortriptyline, are the most commonly used medications to prevent tension headaches. Other antidepressants may be beneficial in some people.

Migraine

Some medications are intended to stop symptoms, and others are intended to reduce the frequency of migraines. Some are not safe during pregnancy, so if you're pregnant or trying to get pregnant, talk with your health care provider before using any of these.

Pain-relieving medications. These medications should be taken as soon as symptoms begin.

- **Pain relievers.** Aspirin and ibuprofen (Advil, Motrin IB, others) may relieve mild migraines. Medicine that combines caffeine, aspirin and acetaminophen (Excedrin Migraine) may treat mild symptoms.
- **Triptans.** These are migraine-specific medications. They work by narrowing blood vessels and blocking pain pathways in the brain. These drugs are available as pills, nasal sprays and shots.
- **Dihydroergotamine (D.H.E. 45, Migranal).** This drug may be most helpful for people whose pain tends to last for more than 24 hours. It's available as a shot or a nasal spray.
- **Lasmiditan (Reyvow).** This newer oral tablet significantly improved headache pain in drug trials. It's approved to treat migraines with or without aura. Lasmiditan can cause dizziness and sedation, so you shouldn't drive or operate machinery for eight hours after taking it.
- **Calcitonin gene-related peptide receptor (CGRP) antagonists.** Ubrogepant (Ubrelvy) and rimegepant (Nurtec ODT) are oral CGRP antagonists recently approved for the treatment of acute migraine with or without aura in adults.
- **Opioid (narcotic) medications.** A narcotic may be prescribed for people with severe migraines who can't take other drugs. Opioids are habit-forming and used only as a last resort.

Preventive medications. These are taken on a regular basis by people with frequent migraines or when a predictable trigger, such as menstruation, is approaching.

- **Cardiovascular drugs.** Some medications used to treat high blood pressure and coronary artery disease, such as beta blockers and calcium channel blockers, may help prevent migraines.
- **Antidepressants.** Tricyclic antidepressants may help prevent migraines in some people.
- **Anti-seizure drugs.** The drugs valproate and topiramate (Topamax, Qudexy XR, others) seem to reduce the frequency of migraines.
- **OnabotulinumtoxinA (Botox).** For some adults with migraines, Botox injections in the forehead and neck every 12 weeks are helpful.
- **CGRP monoclonal antibodies.** Several newer drugs in this class are approved to treat migraines, given as monthly or quarterly shots.

Cluster headache

The goal is to relieve symptoms and reduce the frequency of cluster headache attacks. Rarely, if medication isn't effective, surgery may be an option.

Acute therapies. Treatments used to relieve symptoms include:

- **Oxygen.** Briefly inhaling 100% oxygen through a mask often provides dramatic relief.
- **Triptans.** The injectable form of sumatriptan (Imitrex) and the nasal spray zolmitriptan (Zomig), commonly used to treat migraines, may be effective treatments for acute cluster headaches.
- **Octreotide (Sandostatin).** This drug is an injectable synthetic version of the brain hormone somatostatin.
- **Local anesthetics.** The numbing effect of local anesthetics given through the nose may relieve cluster headache pain.
- **Dihydroergotamine.** The injected form may help cluster headaches.

Preventive medications. Medications to suppress attacks include:

- **Calcium channel blockers.** The medication verapamil (Calan SR, Verelan) is often a first choice of treatment.
- **Corticosteroids.** Your health care provider may prescribe corticosteroids if your cluster headaches only recently started or if you have a pattern of brief cluster periods and long remissions.
- **Lithium.** Used to treat bipolar disorder, this medication may be effective in preventing chronic cluster headaches.
- **Nerve block.** A numbing agent (anesthetic) and corticosteroid are injected near the occipital nerve, at the back of your head.
- **Melatonin.** Studies show a modest effect in treating attacks at night.

H

Heart arrhythmias

WHAT IS IT? Your heart is made up of four chambers — two upper chambers (atria) and two lower chambers (ventricles). The rhythm of your heart is controlled by a natural pacemaker (sinoatrial, or SA, node) located in the right atrium. The SA node produces electrical impulses that cause the chambers of your heart to contract and relax in a controlled manner.

Heart rhythm problems (heart arrhythmias) occur when the electrical impulses that coordinate your heartbeats don't work properly, causing your heart to beat too fast, too slow or irregularly.

Heart arrhythmia may result from a condition you're born with; it may be associated with a disease or disorder that occurs later in life, such as high blood pressure or coronary artery disease; or it may be related to factors such as smoking, stress, or excessive alcohol or caffeine.

Types

Arrhythmias are classified not only by where they originate (atria or ventricles) but also by the speed of heart rate they cause.

Tachycardia. Tachycardia refers to a fast heartbeat — a resting heart rate greater than 100 beats a minute. Forms of tachycardia include:

- **Atrial fibrillation.** Atrial fibrillation is a rapid heart rate caused by chaotic electrical impulses in the atria that produce an irregular, rapid rhythm of the ventricles. Atrial fibrillation may be temporary, but some episodes won't end unless treated.
- **Atrial flutter.** It's similar to atrial fibrillation, but the heartbeats tend to be more organized and the electrical impulses are more rhythmic.
- **Supraventricular tachycardia.** It includes many forms of arrhythmia originating above the ventricles (supraventricular).
- **Wolff-Parkinson-White syndrome.** This is a type of supraventricular tachycardia in which there's an extra electrical pathway between the atria and the ventricles at birth.
- **Ventricular tachycardia.** This is a rapid, regular heart rate that originates with irregular electrical signals in the ventricles.
- **Ventricular fibrillation.** It occurs when rapid, chaotic electrical impulses cause the ventricles to quiver and pump ineffectively. It's often fatal if not treated within minutes.

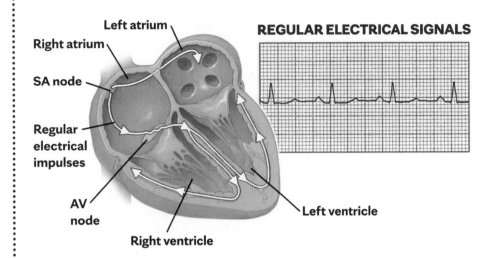

REGULAR ELECTRICAL SIGNALS

Left atrium

Right atrium

SA node

Regular electrical impulses

AV node

Right ventricle

Left ventricle

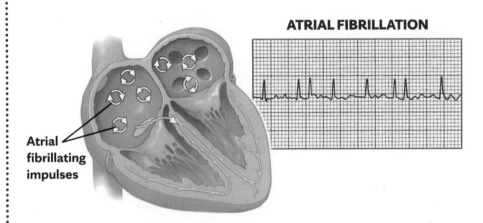

ATRIAL FIBRILLATION

Atrial fibrillating impulses

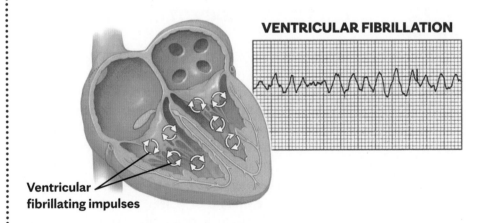

VENTRICULAR FIBRILLATION

Ventricular fibrillating impulses

In atrial fibrillation, electrical signals fire from multiple locations in the atria, causing the atria to beat chaotically and the loss of typical heart rhythm. In ventricular fibrillation, erratic electrical impulses in the ventricles cause the heart to quiver uselessly.

H

- **Long QT syndrome.** This condition can cause fast, chaotic heartbeats that may lead to fainting. It can be life-threatening. Some people are born with a genetic mutation that puts them at risk.

Bradycardia. Bradycardia refers to a slow heartbeat — a resting heart rate less than 60 beats a minute. Forms of bradycardia include:

- **Sick sinus syndrome.** In this condition your sinus node isn't sending impulses properly and your heart rate may be too slow. Your heart rate may speed up and slow down intermittently.
- **Conduction block.** The heart's electrical pathways become blocked in or near the AV node. Impulses between the upper and lower halves of your heart may slow, reducing your heart rate.

SYMPTOM CHECKER Some arrhythmias don't cause any signs or symptoms. Noticeable symptoms may include:

- A fluttering in your chest
- A racing heartbeat (tachycardia)
- A slow heartbeat (bradycardia)
- Chest pain
- Shortness of breath
- Lightheadedness
- Dizziness
- Fainting (syncope) or near fainting

WHAT TESTS TO EXPECT Heart-monitoring tests include:

- **Electrocardiogram (ECG).** An ECG measures the timing and duration of each electrical phase in your heartbeat.
- **Holter monitor.** This is a portable ECG device that records your heart's activity for 24 hours as you go about your daily routine.
- **Event monitor.** You activate this device when you have symptoms.
- **Echocardiogram.** This noninvasive test produces images of your heart's size, structure and motion.
- **Stress test.** During a stress test, you exercise on a treadmill or stationary bicycle while your heart activity is monitored.
- **Tilt table test.** You lie flat on a table. As it's tilted, you're monitored to evaluate how your heart and nervous system respond.
- **Electrophysiological mapping.** This invasive test maps out the spread of electrical impulses within your heart.

TREATMENT Treatment is generally required if the arrhythmia is causing significant symptoms or putting you at risk of a more serious condition.

Bradycardia

There aren't any medications that can reliably speed up your heart. Often, bradycardia is treated with a pacemaker. The device is implanted near your collarbone, and its wires run through your blood vessels to your inner heart. If your heart rate becomes too slow or it stops, the pacemaker sends out electrical impulses that stimulate your heart to beat at a steady rate.

Tachycardia

Treatment for a fast or chaotic heartbeat may include:

- **Medications.** Medication to restore regular heart rhythm is the primary treatment for many types of tachycardia. If you have atrial fibrillation, your health care provider may also prescribe a blood-thinning drug to help keep blood clots from forming.
- **Cardioversion.** For certain types of arrhythmia, such as atrial fibrillation, your provider may perform a procedure called cardioversion. A shock is delivered to your heart through paddles or patches on your chest. The shock affects the electrical impulses in your heart and can restore a regular rhythm.
- **Catheter ablation.** One or more catheters are threaded through your blood vessels to your heart. Electrodes on the catheter tips use heat, extreme cold or radiofrequency energy to damage (ablate) a small area of heart tissue, preventing transmission of the electrical signal that's causing the arrhythmia.
- **Pacemaker.** Similar to bradycardia, a pacemaker may be used to stimulate your heart to beat at a regular rate.
- **Implantable cardioverter-defibrillator** (**ICD**). This device works similar to a pacemaker. It continuously monitors your heart rhythm and sends out shocks to reset the heart to a regular rhythm, if needed.

Surgery

In the maze procedure, a series of surgical incisions are made in heart tissue in the upper half of the heart. This creates a maze of scar tissue. Because scar tissue doesn't conduct electricity, it interferes with stray electrical impulses that cause some types of arrhythmia.

Heart attack

WHAT IS IT? A heart attack occurs when the flow of blood to the heart is blocked, most often by a buildup of fat, cholesterol and other substances that form a hard deposit called plaque in a heart (coronary) artery. The interrupted blood flow can damage or destroy part of the heart muscle.

Another cause of a heart attack is a spasm in a coronary artery that shuts down blood flow to the heart. A heart attack can also result from a tear in a coronary artery.

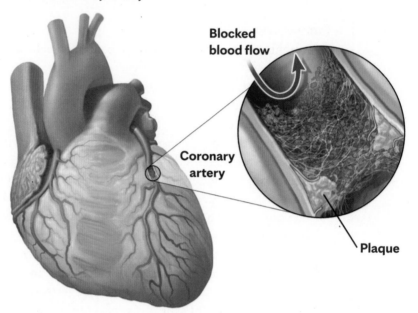

A heart attack results when deposits (plaques) form in a coronary artery, limiting blood flow. Some plaques become unstable and rupture. A blood clot forms at the rupture site, blocking blood flow through the artery and to the heart muscle.

Factors that can increase your risk of a heart attack include:

- **Age.** Men age 45 or older and women age 55 or older are at higher risk of a heart attack.
- **Tobacco.** Smoking and long-term exposure to secondhand smoke increase the risk of a heart attack.
- **High blood pressure.** Over time, high blood pressure can damage the arteries that feed your heart.
- **High blood cholesterol or triglyceride levels.** A high level of low-density lipoprotein (LDL, or "bad") cholesterol is most likely to

narrow arteries. A high level of triglycerides, a type of blood fat related to your diet, also raises your risk of heart attack.

- **Diabetes.** Having diabetes, especially uncontrolled diabetes, increases your risk of a heart attack.
- **Family history.** If your siblings, parents or grandparents had early heart attacks (by age 55 for male relatives and age 65 for female relatives), you may be at increased risk.
- **Inactivity.** An inactive lifestyle can increase your risk.
- **Obesity.** Obesity is associated with high blood cholesterol levels, high triglyceride levels, high blood pressure and diabetes.
- **Stress.** How you respond to stress can increase your risk.
- **Illegal drug use.** Using stimulant drugs can trigger a spasm of your coronary arteries that can cause a heart attack.

SYMPTOM CHECKER Common heart attack signs and symptoms include:

- Pressure, tightness, pain, or a squeezing or aching sensation in your chest or arms that may spread to your neck, jaw or back
- Nausea, indigestion, heartburn or abdominal pain
- Shortness of breath
- Cold sweat
- Fatigue
- Lightheadedness or sudden dizziness

Some heart attacks strike suddenly, but many people have warning signs and symptoms in advance. The earliest warning may be recurrent chest pain (angina) that's triggered by exertion and relieved by rest. It's caused by a temporary decrease in blood flow to the heart.

WHAT TESTS TO EXPECT You'll likely be asked about your symptoms and have your blood pressure, pulse and temperature checked. Tests that may be performed include:

- **Electrocardiogram (ECG).** It records the electrical activity of your heart via electrodes attached to your skin. Because injured heart muscle doesn't conduct electrical impulses well, the ECG may show that a heart attack has occurred or is in progress.
- **Blood tests.** Certain heart enzymes slowly leak into your blood if your heart has been damaged by a heart attack. Samples of your blood may be taken to test for the presence of these enzymes.

- **Chest X-ray.** It allows your health care provider to check the size of your heart and its blood vessels and to look for fluid in your lungs.
- **Echocardiogram.** It can help identify whether an area of your heart has been damaged by a heart attack and isn't pumping as usual or at peak capacity.
- **Coronary catheterization (angiogram).** A liquid dye is injected into the arteries of your heart through a long, thin tube (catheter) that's fed through an artery. The dye makes the arteries visible on X-ray, revealing areas of blockage.
- **Stress test.** After a heart attack, a stress test may be performed to measure how your heart and blood vessels respond to exertion. You may walk on a treadmill or pedal a stationary bike while attached to a monitoring device. Or you may receive a drug that stimulates your heart similar to exercise.
- **CT scan or MRI.** A computerized tomography (CT) scan or magnetic resonance imaging (MRI) may be used to diagnose heart problems, including the extent of damage from a heart attack.

TREATMENT With each passing minute after a heart attack, more heart tissue loses oxygen and other vital nutrients and the tissue deteriorates. The main way to prevent heart damage is to restore blood flow quickly.

Medications

Medications given to treat a heart attack include:

- **Aspirin.** Take aspirin immediately. It reduces blood clotting, helping maintain blood flow through a narrowed artery. If you have a regular tablet (not coated), chew it before swallowing.
- **Thrombolytics.** Also called clotbusters, they help dissolve a blood clot that's blocking blood flow to your heart.
- **Anti-platelet agents.** These drugs help prevent new clots and keep existing clots from getting larger.
- **Other blood-thinning medications.** Medications such as heparin make your blood less "sticky" and less likely to form clots.
- **Nitroglycerin.** This medication can help improve blood flow to the heart by widening (dilating) the blood vessels.
- **Beta blockers.** These drugs help relax your heart muscle, slow your heart rate and decrease blood pressure, making your heart's job easier.
- **Angiotensin-converting enzyme (ACE) inhibitors.** They lower blood pressure and help reduce stress on the heart.

Medical procedures

In addition to medications, you may undergo one of the following:

Coronary angioplasty and stenting. A long, thin tube (catheter) is threaded through an artery to the blocked artery in your heart. Once in position, a special balloon is briefly inflated to open the artery. A metal mesh stent may be inserted into the artery to keep it open long term. Some stents are coated with a slow-releasing medication to help prevent another blockage.

Coronary artery bypass surgery. Occasionally, doctors may perform emergency surgery at the time of a heart attack. Or you may undergo bypass surgery after your heart has had time to recover from a heart attack. Bypass surgery involves sewing veins or arteries in place around a blocked or narrowed coronary artery, allowing blood to bypass the narrowed section as it flows to the heart.

H

CHEST PAIN

People typically equate chest pain with a heart attack, but other problems can trigger chest pain. Often, the underlying cause has nothing to do with your heart.

- *Heartburn.* When stomach acid washes up from your stomach into the esophagus, it can produce a painful, burning sensation behind your breastbone.
- *Gallbladder or pancreas problems.* Gallstones or inflammation of your gallbladder or pancreas can cause abdominal pain that radiates to your chest.
- *Costochondritis.* In this condition, the cartilage that joins your ribs to your breastbone becomes inflamed and painful.
- *Injured ribs.* A bruised or broken rib can cause chest pain.
- *Pulmonary embolism.* When a blood clot becomes lodged in a lung (pulmonary) artery, blocking blood flow to lung tissue, pain can result in the chest.
- *Pleurisy.* If the membrane that covers your lungs becomes inflamed, it can cause chest pain that's worse when you inhale or cough.
- *Collapsed lung.* The pain typically comes on suddenly and can last for hours.
- *Panic attack.* Chest pain is a symptom of a panic attack. It may be accompanied by a rapid heartbeat, rapid breathing, sweating and shortness of breath.

Because it can be difficult to distinguish chest pain due to a heart problem from other types of chest pain, it's important to get any chest pain checked out.

Heart failure

WHAT IS IT? Heart failure, also called congestive heart failure, occurs when your heart muscle doesn't pump blood as well as it should, often because it's too weak or too stiff.

Heart failure typically develops after other conditions have damaged or weakened your heart. Diseases and conditions that most often lead to heart failure include high blood pressure, coronary artery disease, heart attack and diabetes.

The term *congestive heart failure* refers to the condition that causes blood to back up into (congest) the liver, abdomen, lower extremities and lungs. Not all heart failure is congestive.

SYMPTOM CHECKER Signs and symptoms of heart failure may include:

- Shortness of breath
- Fatigue and weakness
- Swelling (edema) in your legs, ankles and feet
- Rapid or irregular heartbeat
- Reduced ability to exercise
- Persistent cough or wheezing with white or pink phlegm
- Sudden weight gain from fluid retention
- Lack of appetite and nausea
- Elevated blood pressure

TREATMENT With treatment, symptoms of heart failure can improve and the heart sometimes becomes stronger.

Medications
Health care providers usually treat heart failure with a combination of medications. You may be prescribed one or more of the following drugs:

Angiotensin-converting enzyme (ACE) inhibitors. ACE inhibitors widen blood vessels to lower blood pressure, improve blood flow and decrease the workload on the heart. Examples include enalapril (Vasotec, Epaned), lisinopril (Qbrelis, Zestril) and captopril.

Angiotensin II receptor blockers. These drugs, which include losartan (Cozaar) and valsartan (Diovan), may be an alternative for people who can't tolerate ACE inhibitors.

Digoxin (Lanoxin). This drug, also referred to as digitalis, increases the strength of the heart muscle contractions. It also tends to slow the heartbeat.

Beta blockers. This class of drugs slows your heart rate, reduces blood pressure, and may limit or reverse some of the damage to your heart. Examples include carvedilol (Coreg), metoprolol (Lopressor) and bisoprolol.

Diuretics. Often called water pills, diuretics make you urinate more frequently, keeping fluid from collecting in your body.

Aldosterone antagonists. Drugs such as spironolactone (Aldactone, Carospir) and eplerenone (Inspra) may decrease mortality in severe cases.

Inotropes. These medications are used in people with severe heart failure to improve heart function and maintain blood pressure.

Surgery and medical devices

In some cases, surgery or another procedure is recommended to treat the underlying problem that led to heart failure. If severely blocked arteries are contributing to your heart failure, you may need coronary artery bypass surgery. If a faulty heart valve is causing your heart failure, you may need surgery to repair or replace the valve. If a heart rhythm problem is at fault, you may need an implantable device to help coordinate your heart rhythm.

Heart pumps. These devices are implanted into the abdomen or chest and attached to a weakened heart to help it pump. Doctors first used heart pumps to keep heart transplant candidates alive while they waited for a donor heart. They're now sometimes used as an alternative to transplantation. Heart pumps can extend and improve the lives of people who aren't eligible for transplants or who are waiting for new hearts.

Heart transplant. A transplant can dramatically improve survival and quality of life for people with severe heart failure. Candidates often have to wait a long time before a suitable donor heart is found.

Heart valve disease

WHAT IS IT? Your heart has four valves that keep blood flowing in the correct direction. The valves open and close once during each heartbeat. Sometimes the valves don't open or close properly, disrupting the flow of blood through the heart to the body.

In a condition called stenosis, a valve isn't able to open properly. In a condition called regurgitation, it doesn't close properly and can leak.

Heart valve disease includes the following four conditions:

Aortic valve disease

The valve between the main pumping chamber of your heart (left ventricle) and the main artery to your body (aorta) doesn't work properly. Aortic valve disease may be present at birth, or it may result from other causes. Types of aortic valve disease include:

- **Aortic valve stenosis.** The aortic valve opening is narrowed, preventing the valve from opening fully. This obstructs blood flow from your heart into your aorta.
- **Aortic valve regurgitation.** The aortic valve doesn't close properly, causing blood to flow backward into the left ventricle.

Mitral valve disease

The mitral valve located between your left atrium and left ventricle doesn't work properly. Types of mitral valve disease include:

- **Mitral valve regurgitation.** The flaps (leaflets) of the mitral valve don't close tightly, causing blood to leak backward into the left atrium of your heart. The most common cause of leakage is mitral valve prolapse, in which the leaflets bulge back into the left atrium as your heart contracts.
- **Mitral valve stenosis.** The flaps of the mitral valve become thick or stiff, and they may fuse together, narrowing the valve opening and reducing blood flow from the left atrium to the left ventricle.

Tricuspid valve disease

With this form of disease, the valve between the right ventricle and right atrium doesn't function properly. Several types of tricuspid valve disease exist, including stenosis and regurgitation. Some tricuspid valve disorders are present at birth.

Pulmonary valve disease

Pulmonary valve disease refers to any disorder of your heart's pulmonary valve, which is responsible for keeping blood flowing from your heart to your lungs. This may include a leaky valve (pulmonary valve regurgitation) or a narrowed valve (pulmonary valve stenosis).

SYMPTOM CHECKER Signs and symptoms may include:

- Chest pain or tightness
- Feeling faint or fainting with exertion
- Shortness of breath, especially with exertion
- Fatigue, especially during times of increased activity
- Heart palpitations — sensations of a rapid, fluttering heartbeat
- Heart murmur

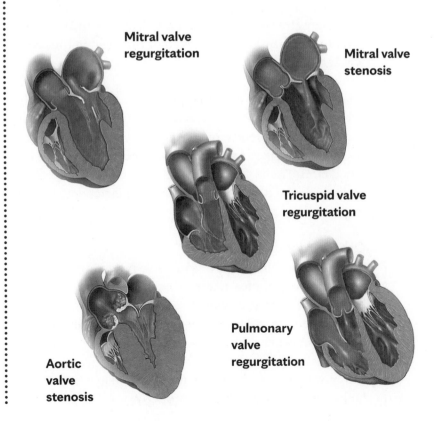

Mitral valve regurgitation

Mitral valve stenosis

Tricuspid valve regurgitation

Pulmonary valve regurgitation

Aortic valve stenosis

TREATMENT If your health care provider suspects that you may have a heart valve disorder, you may need to undergo tests that monitor the flow of blood through your heart and assess how well the valves are functioning. An echocardiogram is typically the primary test to diagnose heart valve disease.

Medications can't correct a heart valve disorder. However, your provider may prescribe certain medications to ease your symptoms. These may include medications that reduce fluid accumulation, slow your heart rate or control heart rhythm changes.

Surgery

Often, the only way to treat a heart valve condition is surgery to repair or replace the valve and open up the passageway. Surgery isn't always needed right away. If tests reveal that you have mild valve disease and you aren't experiencing any symptoms, your provider may suggest a wait-and-see approach and carefully monitor the valve so that surgery can be performed at the appropriate time.

Surgery is usually necessary when the stenosis or regurgitation becomes more severe and symptoms begin to develop. Your provider may also recommend surgery even if you aren't experiencing symptoms. If the valve isn't fixed or replaced in time, your heart may weaken permanently.

Sometimes it's necessary to replace a damaged valve with a mechanical or tissue valve. Mechanical valves, made from metal, are durable but carry the risk of blood clots forming. If you receive a mechanical valve, you'll need to take an anticoagulant medication for life to prevent blood clots. Tissue valves — which may come from a pig, a cow or a human deceased donor — may need replacement at some point.

Other procedures

If surgery isn't an option, less invasive procedures may be used. A thin, flexible tube (catheter) may be threaded through an artery into the heart. In case of valve stenosis, a balloon at the tip of the catheter is inflated and the balloon pushes open the valve and stretches the valve opening, improving blood flow.

Less invasive procedures also may be used in an attempt to repair a faulty valve that doesn't close properly.

Heatstroke

WHAT IS IT? Heatstroke is a condition that results when your body overheats — usually from spending too much time in hot, humid weather or from prolonged intense physical activity, especially in hot weather. When your temperature rises to 104 F (40 C), heatstroke may develop.

Heatstroke requires emergency treatment. Untreated heatstroke can quickly damage your brain, heart, kidneys and muscles. The damage worsens the longer treatment is delayed.

Factors that may increase your risk of heatstroke include being unaccustomed to hot weather, wearing clothing that prevents sweat from evaporating easily and cooling your body, drinking alcohol, and not getting enough fluids.

Some medications also can make you more susceptible to heatstroke, including medications that narrow your blood vessels (vasoconstrictors), regulate your blood pressure by blocking adrenaline (beta blockers), rid your body of sodium and water (diuretics), or reduce psychiatric symptoms (antidepressants or antipsychotics). Stimulants for attention-deficit/hyperactivity disorder (ADHD) also make you more vulnerable to heatstroke.

SYMPTOM CHECKER Signs and symptoms of heatstroke may include:

- **High body temperature.** A temperature of 104 F (40 C) or higher.
- **Altered mental state or behavior.** Confusion, agitation, slurred speech, irritability, delirium, seizures and coma may occur.
- **Alteration in sweating.** In heatstroke brought on by hot weather, your skin will feel hot and dry to the touch. In heatstroke brought on by strenuous exercise, your skin may feel moist.
- **Nausea and vomiting.** You may feel sick to your stomach or vomit.
- **Flushed skin.** As body temperature increases, skin may turn red, especially in people with white skin.
- **Racing heart rate.** Your pulse may significantly increase because heat stress places a tremendous burden on your heart to help cool your body.
- **Rapid breathing.** Your breathing may become rapid and shallow.
- **Headache.** Your head may throb.

TREATMENT While waiting for emergency treatment to arrive, take immediate action to cool the overheated person:

- Get the person into shade or indoors.
- Remove excess clothing.
- Cool the person with whatever means available — use a cool tub of water or a cool shower; spray with a garden hose; sponge with cool water; fan while misting with cool water; or place ice packs or cold, wet towels on the person's head, neck, armpits and groin.

At a hospital, the focus of treatment continues to be on lowering the internal body temperature. Methods of doing this include immersing the person in cold water, using evaporation cooling techniques and wrapping the person in a specialized cooling blanket.

HEAT EXHAUSTION AND HEAT CRAMPS

With a less serious heat emergency, such as heat exhaustion or heat cramps, the following steps may lower your body temperature and ease symptoms. With heat exhaustion, your internal body temperature doesn't rise as high. Other symptoms may include cool, moist skin with goose bumps while in the heat; heavy sweating; faintness and dizziness; a weak, rapid pulse; and muscle cramps.

- **Get to a shady or air-conditioned place.** If you don't have air conditioning at home, go someplace with air conditioning.
- **Cool off with damp sheets and a fan.** Cover yourself with damp sheets or spray yourself with cool water and direct the air from a fan onto yourself.
- **Take a cool shower or bath.** If you're outdoors, soaking in a cool pond or stream can help bring your temperature down.
- **Rehydrate.** Drink lots of fluids. Because you lose salt through sweating, consume sports drinks to replenish salt and water. If your fluid or salt intake is restricted, check to see how much you should drink and if you should replace salt.
- **Don't drink alcoholic or sugary beverages.** They can interfere with your body's ability to control your temperature.
- **Rest.** Don't resume strenuous activity for several hours after symptoms go away.

Heel pain (plantar fasciitis)

WHAT IS IT? Plantar fasciitis is a common cause of heel pain. It results from pain and inflammation in the thick band of tissue (plantar fascia) that runs across the bottom of your foot and connects your heel bone to your toes.

Under usual circumstances, your plantar fascia acts like a shock-absorbing bowstring, supporting the arch in your foot. If tension on that bowstring becomes too great, it can create small tears in the band of tissue. Repetitive stretching and tearing can cause the fascia to become irritated or inflamed.

Plantar fasciitis commonly causes stabbing pain that usually occurs with your very first steps in the morning. Once your foot limbers up, the pain typically lessens or disappears, but it may return after long periods of standing or after getting up from a seated position.

Plantar fasciitis is particularly common in runners. People who are overweight, who wear shoes with inadequate support, who have flat feet, or who spend a lot of time on their feet also are at higher risk.

TREATMENT Most people recover in a few months with conservative treatments. They include:

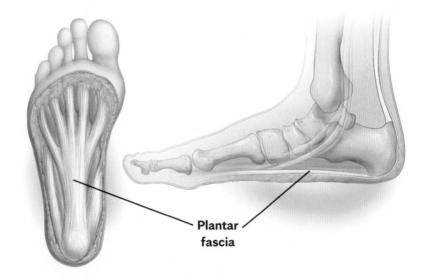

Plantar fascia

This is where the pain associated with plantar fasciitis is often felt.

Pain relievers. Medications such as ibuprofen (Advil, Motrin IB, others) and naproxen sodium (Aleve) may ease the pain and inflammation.

Exercises. A physical therapist can teach you exercises to stretch the plantar fascia and Achilles tendon and to strengthen lower leg muscles, which stabilize your ankle and heel. The therapist may also show you how to apply athletic tape to support the bottom of your foot.

Night splints. Wearing a splint holds the plantar fascia and Achilles tendon in a lengthened position overnight and facilitates stretching to help prevent morning symptoms.

Orthotics. Over-the-counter or custom-fitted arch supports (orthotics) can help distribute pressure to your feet more evenly.

Steroid shots. Injecting a steroid medication into the tender area of the foot can provide temporary pain relief.

Extracorporeal shock wave therapy. Sound waves are directed at the area of pain to stimulate healing. This treatment is generally used for chronic plantar fasciitis that doesn't respond to other treatments.

Surgery. Rarely, surgery is performed to detach the plantar fascia from the heel bone. It's an option only when the pain is severe and all else fails.

LIFESTYLE To reduce the pain and inflammation of plantar fasciitis or prevent it from occurring, try these tips:

- **Maintain a healthy weight.** It reduces stress on the plantar fascia.
- **Wear supportive shoes.** Avoid high heels. Buy shoes with low to moderate heels and good arch support. Don't go barefoot.
- **Replace worn-out athletic shoes.** If you're a runner, buy new shoes after about 500 miles of use.
- **Vary your sport.** Alternate swimming or bicycling with jogging or walking.
- **Apply ice.** Hold a cloth-covered ice pack over the painful area for 15 to 20 minutes three or four times a day or after an activity. Or freeze a water-filled paper cup and roll it over the site of discomfort for about 5 to 7 minutes.
- **Stretch your arches.** Do simple exercises that stretch your plantar fascia, Achilles tendon and calf muscles.

Hemorrhoids

WHAT IS IT? Hemorrhoids are swollen and inflamed veins in your anus and lower rectum. Hemorrhoids may result for a variety of reasons, including straining during bowel movements or increased pressure on the veins during pregnancy.

Hemorrhoids may be located inside the rectum (internal hemorrhoids), or they may develop under the skin around the anus (external hemorrhoids). The veins around your anus tend to stretch under pressure and may bulge or swell.

Factors that might cause increased pressure include straining during bowel movements, sitting for long periods of time on the toilet, chronic diarrhea or constipation, obesity, pregnancy, anal intercourse, and a low-fiber diet.

Hemorrhoids are common and more likely to occur as you get older because the tissues that support the veins in your rectum and anus can weaken and stretch with aging.

SYMPTOM CHECKER Signs and symptoms may include:

- Painless bleeding during bowel movements — small amounts of bright red blood on your toilet tissue or in the toilet bowl
- Itching or irritation in your anal region
- Pain or discomfort
- Swelling around your anus
- A lump near your anus, which may be sensitive or painful
- Leakage of feces

Symptoms usually depend on the location. You usually can't see or feel internal hemorrhoids, and they generally don't cause discomfort. But straining or irritation when passing stool can damage their delicate surfaces and cause bleeding. Occasionally, straining can push an internal hemorrhoid through the anal opening, which is known as a protruding or prolapsed hemorrhoid.

When external hemorrhoids around your anus can get irritated, they itch or bleed. Sometimes blood may pool in an external hemorrhoid and form a clot, causing severe pain, swelling and inflammation.

TREATMENT Most of the time, you can treat hemorrhoids on your own, but sometimes medical treatment is necessary.

Medications

If your hemorrhoids produce only mild discomfort, your health care provider may suggest creams, ointments, suppositories or pads that you can get without a prescription. These contain ingredients such as witch hazel or hydrocortisone that can temporarily help relieve pain and itching.

Don't use a nonprescription steroid cream for more than a week unless directed by your provider because it can thin your skin.

Minimally invasive procedures

If a blood clot has formed within an external hemorrhoid, your health care provider can remove the clot with a simple incision, which may provide prompt relief. For persistent bleeding or painful hemorrhoids, you may need another procedure.

Rubber band ligation. One or two tiny rubber bands are placed around the base of an internal hemorrhoid to cut off its circulation. The hemorrhoid withers and falls off within a week. This procedure is effective for many people.

Injection (sclerotherapy). A chemical solution is injected into the hemorrhoid tissue to shrink it.

Coagulation. Coagulation techniques use laser or infrared light or heat. They cause small, bleeding, internal hemorrhoids to harden and shrivel.

Surgical procedures

If other procedures haven't been successful or the hemorrhoids are large, your provider may recommend more-invasive options.

Hemorrhoid removal. A surgeon removes the excessive tissue causing the bleeding. Various techniques may be used. It's the most effective way to treat severe or recurring hemorrhoids.

Hemorrhoid stapling. This procedure blocks blood flow to hemorrhoidal tissue. Hemorrhoid stapling generally involves less pain, and recovery is quicker than with hemorrhoid removal, but it has a greater risk of recurrence.

Hepatitis

WHAT IS IT? Hepatitis is an inflammation of the liver, most commonly caused by a viral infection. The most common types of viral hepatitis are A, B and C. Hepatitis can result for a number of other reasons, including consuming alcohol.

Hepatitis A

You're most likely to contract hepatitis A from contaminated food or water or from close contact with someone who's infected. The hepatitis A virus usually is spread when a person ingests even tiny amounts of contaminated fecal matter — often when eating food handled by someone with the virus who doesn't thoroughly wash his or her hands after using the toilet. Another method of transmission is drinking contaminated water. You may have a mild illness that lasts a few weeks or a severe illness that lasts several months. Unlike other types of viral hepatitis, hepatitis A doesn't cause long-term liver damage, and it doesn't become chronic.

Hepatitis B

The hepatitis B virus is passed from person to person through blood, semen or other body fluids. For some people, hepatitis B infection becomes chronic. Having chronic hepatitis B increases your risk of liver failure, liver cancer or scarring of the liver (cirrhosis). Most adults with hepatitis B recover fully, even if their signs and symptoms are severe. Infants and children are more likely to develop a chronic infection.

Hepatitis C

Many people infected with the hepatitis C virus have no symptoms, and may not know they have hepatitis until liver damage occurs decades later. Hepatitis C is considered among the most serious of the hepatitis viruses. It's passed through contact with contaminated blood — most commonly through needles shared during illegal drug use.

Alcoholic hepatitis

Alcoholic hepatitis is most common in people who drink heavily over many years, but the relationship between alcohol and hepatitis is complex. Not all heavy drinkers develop alcoholic hepatitis, and the disease can occur in people who drink only moderately. If you're diagnosed with alcoholic hepatitis, you must stop drinking alcohol. People who continue to drink alcohol face a high risk of serious liver damage and death.

SYMPTOM CHECKER Signs and symptoms may include:

- Fatigue
- Nausea and vomiting
- Abdominal pain or discomfort, especially on your right side
- Clay-colored bowel movements
- Loss of appetite
- Low-grade fever
- Dark urine
- Joint pain
- Yellowing of the skin and eyes (jaundice)

TREATMENT If your hepatitis infection will likely improve on its own, you may not need treatment. Rest, good nutrition and fluids are important while your body fights the infection.

- **Rest.** Many people with hepatitis infection feel tired and sick and have less energy. Rest will help combat that.
- **Manage nausea.** Nausea can make it difficult to eat. Try snacking throughout the day rather than eating full meals. To get enough calories, consume high-calorie foods and beverages.
- **Rest your liver.** Your liver may have difficulty processing medications and alcohol. Review all your medications with your health care provider and don't drink alcohol.

Medications

If you have chronic hepatitis or severe symptoms, you may need treatment to reduce the risk of liver disease and to prevent passing the infection to others. Treatments include:

Antiviral medications. Several antiviral medications — including lamivudine (Epivir), adefovir (Hepsera), telbivudine and entecavir (Baraclude) — can help fight the virus and slow its ability to damage your liver. A combination of medications may be prescribed.

Interferon alfa-2b (Intron A). This injectable drug, a synthetic version of interferon-alpha produced by your body, is prescribed mainly for young people with hepatitis B who don't want to undergo long-term treatment or who might want to get pregnant in a few years.

Corticosteroid drugs. They've shown some short-term benefit among some people with alcoholic hepatitis. Steroids have significant side effects and aren't recommended if you have failing kidneys, gastrointestinal bleeding or an infection.

Liver transplant

If your liver has been severely damaged, a liver transplant is an option. For people with hepatitis C infection, a liver transplant isn't a cure. Antiviral medications are usually necessary after a transplant because the infection is likely to recur in the new liver.

For severe alcoholic hepatitis, a liver transplant is the only hope to avoid death. But medical centers may be reluctant to perform liver transplants for fear the individuals will resume drinking after surgery.

 LIFESTYLE To reduce the risk of passing viral hepatitis to others, avoid sexual activity during infection. If you're sexually active, tell your partner you have hepatitis and discuss the risk of transmission. Use a new latex condom every time you have sex, but remember that condoms don't absolutely eliminate the risk.

In the case of hepatitis A, wash your hands thoroughly after using the toilet, scrubbing vigorously for at least 20 seconds. Don't prepare food for others while you're actively infected.

Don't share razor blades or toothbrushes, which may carry traces of infected blood. If you use IV drugs, never share needles and syringes.

PREVENTION

Hepatitis A and B can be prevented through vaccination. There is no vaccine for hepatitis C. The hepatitis A vaccine is typically given in two doses. The hepatitis B vaccine is given as three or four injections.

Hernia

WHAT IS IT? A hernia occurs when soft tissue or part of an organ squeezes through a weak spot in a muscle wall or band of tissue. There are different types of hernias. The most common are hiatal, inguinal and umbilical.

Hiatal hernia

With a hiatal hernia, part of your stomach pushes upward through the large dome-shaped muscle that separates your chest cavity from your abdomen (diaphragm). Your esophagus passes into your stomach through an opening in the diaphragm called the hiatus. In a hiatal hernia, the muscle tissue surrounding this opening becomes weak, and the upper part of your stomach bulges through the diaphragm into your chest cavity.

A hiatal hernia may result from injury to the area, being born with an unusually large hiatus, persistent coughing or vomiting, or intense pressure on the surrounding muscles. Obesity, heavy lifting or straining during a bowel movement may produce intense pressure.

A small hiatal hernia generally doesn't cause problems. You may have one and not know it. A large hiatal hernia can allow food and acid to back up into your esophagus, producing heartburn. Symptoms of a hiatal hernia include heartburn, belching and difficulty swallowing.

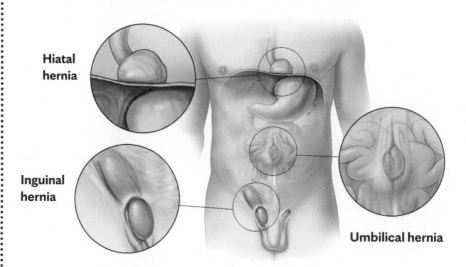

Hiatal hernia

Inguinal hernia

Umbilical hernia

A hernia occurs when an organ pushes through an opening in the muscle or tissue that holds the organ in place. Types of hernias include hiatal, umbilical and inguinal.

Inguinal hernia

An inguinal hernia occurs when soft tissue — usually the membrane lining the abdominal cavity (omentum) or part of the intestine — protrudes through a weak point in the abdominal muscles.

Often, weakness in the abdominal wall that leads to an inguinal hernia occurs at birth when the abdominal lining doesn't close properly. Men are more likely to have this type of muscle weakness due to how the male anatomy forms during gestation. Other inguinal hernias occur later in life when muscles weaken or deteriorate due to aging, strenuous physical activity or a chronic cough.

Some inguinal hernias don't cause symptoms. Often, though, you can see and feel the protrusion. It's usually more obvious when you stand upright, especially if you cough or strain.

Signs and symptoms of an inguinal hernia include:

- A bulge in the area on either side of your pubic bone
- A burning, gurgling or aching sensation at the bulge
- Groin pain or discomfort when bending over, coughing or lifting
- A heavy or dragging sensation in your groin
- Weakness or pressure in your groin
- Pain and swelling around the testicles if the protruding intestine descends into the scrotum

Umbilical hernia

An umbilical hernia occurs when part of the intestine protrudes through an opening in the abdominal muscles. It's most common in infants, but it can affect adults as well.

In an infant, an umbilical hernia may be especially evident when the infant cries, causing the baby's bellybutton to protrude. Many umbilical hernias close on their own by age 1; some take longer to heal. Among adults, being overweight or having multiple pregnancies may increase the risk of developing an umbilical hernia.

Umbilical hernias often aren't painful, but they can cause discomfort in some people. Complications can occur if the protruding tissue becomes trapped and can no longer be pushed back into the abdominal cavity. Blood flow to the section of trapped intestine is reduced, which can lead to pain and tissue damage.

TREATMENT Treatment is dependent on the type of hernia and its severity. If the hernia is small and it isn't causing problems, no treatment may be necessary. If the hernia is larger or you're bothered by symptoms, you may need medication or surgery.

Medications

For a hiatal hernia that causes heartburn and acid reflux, your health care provider may recommend:

- **Antacids that neutralize stomach acid.** These include products such as Maalox, Mylanta, Rolaids and Tums.
- **Medications to reduce acid production.** These include medications such as cimetidine (Tagamet HB), famotidine (Pepcid AC) and nizatidine (Axid AR).
- **Medications that block acid production and heal the esophagus.** These include medications such as lansoprazole (Prevacid) and omeprazole (Prilosec).

Surgery

Surgery is the most common treatment for inguinal and umbilical hernias that are causing symptoms.

Hiatal hernia. Surgery is generally reserved for emergency situations and for people who aren't helped by medications. It may involve pulling your stomach back down into your abdomen and making the opening in your diaphragm smaller; reconstructing a weak esophageal sphincter; or removing the hernia sac.

Inguinal hernia. Enlarged or painful inguinal hernias usually require surgery to relieve discomfort and prevent serious complications. This may be done using open surgery or minimally invasive hernia repair, in which a surgeon operates through several small incisions. During surgery, the protruding omentum or intestine is placed back into your abdomen and the weakened or torn muscle is sewn together. The weakened area may be reinforced with a synthetic mesh.

Umbilical hernia. In children, surgery is typically reserved for umbilical hernias that are painful, become trapped or block the intestines, are large, or don't disappear. In adults, surgery may be performed if the hernia is painful or to avoid possible complications. The protruding tissue is returned to the abdominal cavity, and the opening in the abdominal wall is closed and reinforced.

Hiccups

WHAT IS IT? Hiccups are involuntary muscle contractions of the diaphragm, which separates your chest and abdomen. The hiccup sound happens when the muscle contraction briefly closes your vocal cords.

Along with the sound, sometimes hiccups are accompanied by a slight tightening sensation in your chest, belly or throat.

WHAT'S THE CAUSE? Almost everyone gets hiccups. They usually seem to come on for no reason and end quickly. A large meal, an alcoholic or carbonated drink, and sudden excitement all could cause you to hiccup. A quick change in temperature or swallowing air while you're chewing gum or sucking on candy also may trigger a short bout of hiccups.

In most instances, hiccups resolve on their own within a few minutes. In rare cases, they may last longer than 48 hours. If you have hiccups for more than 48 hours, the cause may be serious, such as:

- Damage to the phrenic nerve, which serves your diaphragm
- A tumor or infection in your central nervous system
- A disorder that affects metabolism, such as diabetes or kidney disease
- Alcoholism
- Anesthesia
- Drugs such as barbiturates, steroids and tranquilizers
- An imbalance in electrolytes (salts and minerals that control your body's electrical impulses)

Long-term hiccups are more common in men than in women. Other risk factors for hiccups include mental health or emotional health issues. In addition, some people develop hiccups after undergoing general anesthesia or after surgical procedures that involve abdominal organs.

TREATMENT Most cases of hiccups go away on their own without medical treatment. See your health care provider if your hiccups last more than 48 hours or if they're so severe that they cause problems with eating, sleeping or breathing.

A physical is the first step in identifying the source of chronic hiccups. If your health care provider suspects that an underlying medical condition is the cause of prolonged hiccups, you may have tests such as:

- A check of your blood for signs of diabetes, infection and kidney disease
- A chest X-ray
- A CT scan
- Magnetic resonance imaging
- Endoscopy, in which a thin, flexible tube that contains a camera is passed down your throat to check for problems in your esophagus or windpipe

Medications

Drugs that may be used to treat long-term hiccups when the cause isn't an underlying medical condition include:

- Baclofen
- Chlorpromazine
- Metoclopramide

If medication doesn't cure your hiccups, your health care provider may recommend an injection of anesthetic to block your phrenic nerve. Surgery to implant a battery-operated device to deliver mild electrical stimulation to your vagus nerve also may help.

HOME REMEDIES

Home remedies for hiccups haven't been proved to be effective, but some people find them helpful. The following are generally safe to try:

- Breathing into a paper bag
- Gargling with ice water
- Holding your breath for 5 to 10 seconds
- Sipping cold water

If you have repeated bouts of hiccups, it may be helpful to eat smaller meals and avoid carbonated beverages and foods that make you gassy.

High blood pressure (hypertension)

 WHAT IS IT? High blood pressure is a condition in which the force of the blood against the artery walls elevates to the point that it can cause health problems.

Blood pressure is determined by the amount of blood your heart pumps and the amount of resistance to blood flow in your arteries. The more blood your heart pumps and the narrower your arteries, the higher your blood pressure.

Most people with high blood pressure have no symptoms, even when blood pressure readings reach quite high levels. Symptoms such as dull headaches, dizzy spells or a few more nosebleeds than usual often don't occur until the condition has reached a severe or life-threatening stage.

 WHAT'S THE CAUSE? There are two types of high blood pressure, and they develop in different ways.

- **Primary hypertension.** For most adults, there's no identifiable cause of their high blood pressure. This type, called primary (essential) hypertension, tends to develop gradually over many years.
- **Secondary hypertension.** In some people, high blood pressure results from an underlying condition. This is known as secondary hypertension. Conditions that can lead to secondary hypertension include kidney problems, adrenal gland tumors, thyroid problems, certain blood vessel defects and obstructive sleep apnea, as well as some medications, alcohol misuse and illegal drugs.

Many factors can increase the risk of high blood pressure. As you age, high blood pressure becomes more common. It is particularly common common in Black people, and it tends to run in families. Other factors that can increase your risk of high blood pressure include being overweight, not getting enough exercise, using tobacco, consuming too much salt (sodium), drinking too much alcohol and experiencing high levels of stress.

 TREATMENT High blood pressure is generally diagnosed after taking blood pressure readings at three or more separate appointments.

This is because your blood pressure varies throughout the day and it can rise during doctor visits.

Primary hypertension is treated with medication. In the case of secondary hypertension, treating the underlying condition may cause your blood pressure to drop.

Types

There are a number of medications to treat high blood pressure. In some cases, a combination of drugs may be used.

Diuretics. Diuretics, sometimes called water pills, act on the kidneys to help your body eliminate sodium and water, reducing blood volume. They are often the first choice in high blood pressure medications.

WHAT'S TOO HIGH?

Blood pressure measurements fall into five basic categories. Systolic pressure refers to the upper (top) number and diastolic pressure to the lower (bottom) number.

Normal blood pressure

Your blood pressure is normal if it's lower than 120/80 millimeters of mercury (mm Hg). Some health care providers recommend 115/75 mm Hg as a better goal.

Elevated

Elevated blood pressure is a systolic pressure ranging from 120 to 129 mm Hg and a diastolic pressure less than 80 mm Hg.

Stage 1 hypertension

In stage 1 hypertension, your systolic pressure ranges from 130 to 139 mm Hg or your diastolic pressure ranges from 80 to 89 mm Hg.

Stage 2 hypertension

Stage 2 hypertension is a systolic pressure of 140 mm Hg or higher, or a diastolic pressure of 90 mm Hg or higher, or both.

Hypertensive crisis

In this condition, your systolic pressure is higher than 180 mm Hg, or your diastolic pressure is higher than 120 mm Hg, or both.

H

Angiotensin-converting enzyme (ACE) inhibitors. They help relax blood vessels by blocking the formation of a natural chemical that narrows them. People with chronic kidney disease may benefit from ACE inhibitors as one of their medications.

Angiotensin II receptor blockers (ARBs). These medications help relax blood vessels by blocking the action, not the formation, of a natural chemical that narrows them. People with chronic kidney disease may benefit from ARBs.

Calcium channel blockers. These medications help relax the muscles of your blood vessels and some slow your heart rate. For older people and people of African heritage, calcium channel blockers may work better than ACE inhibitors alone.

Other medications your health care provider may prescribe include:

- **Alpha blockers.** These drugs reduce nerve impulses to blood vessels, reducing the effects of natural chemicals that narrow blood vessels.
- **Alpha-beta blockers.** In addition to reducing nerve impulses to blood vessels, alpha-beta blockers slow the heartbeat to reduce the amount of blood that must be pumped through the vessels.
- **Beta blockers.** These medications reduce the workload on the heart and dilate blood vessels, causing the heart to beat slower and with less force. Beta blockers tend to be most effective when combined with other blood pressure drugs.
- **Central-acting agents.** These medications prevent the brain from signaling the nervous system to increase heart rate and narrow blood vessels.
- **Vasodilators.** They work on the muscles in artery walls, preventing them from tightening and the arteries from narrowing.
- **Aldosterone antagonists.** They block the effect of a natural chemical that can lead to salt and fluid retention.
- **Renin inhibitors.** Aliskiren (Tekturna) slows the production of renin, an enzyme produced by the kidneys that starts a chain of chemical steps that increases blood pressure. It shouldn't be taken with ACE inhibitors or ARBs.

 LIFESTYLE Your provider may recommend several lifestyle changes, including eating a healthier diet with less salt, exercising regularly, losing weight, quitting smoking, limiting alcohol and managing stress.

High cholesterol

WHAT IS IT? Cholesterol is a waxy substance found in the fats (lipids) in the blood. The body needs cholesterol to build healthy cells, but having too much cholesterol can increase the risk of diseased arteries.

Cholesterol is carried through the blood attached to proteins. This combination of proteins and cholesterol is called a lipoprotein. You may have heard of different types of cholesterol, based on what type of cholesterol the lipoprotein carries. They are:

- **Low-density lipoprotein (LDL).** LDL (the "bad") cholesterol transports cholesterol particles throughout your body. LDL cholesterol builds up in the walls of your arteries, making them hard and narrow.
- **Very-low-density lipoprotein (VLDL).** This type of lipoprotein contains the most triglycerides, a type of blood fat. VLDL cholesterol makes LDL cholesterol larger in size.
- **High-density lipoprotein (HDL).** HDL (the "good") cholesterol picks up excess cholesterol and takes it back to your liver.

When your cholesterol level is high, fatty deposits may develop in your blood vessels. Eventually, these deposits make it difficult for blood to flow through your arteries. A dangerous accumulation of cholesterol and other deposits (plaques) may form on your artery walls, creating a condition called atherosclerosis. Your heart may not get as much oxygen-rich blood as it needs, increasing the risk of a heart attack. Decreased blood flow to your brain can cause a stroke.

WHAT'S THE CAUSE? High cholesterol can be inherited, but it's often the result of unhealthy lifestyle choices. High cholesterol has no symptoms. A blood test is the only way to detect it.

These risk factors increase your risk of high cholesterol:

- **Tobacco use.** Cigarette smoking damages the walls of your blood vessels, making them more likely to accumulate fatty deposits.
- **Obesity.** Having a body mass index (BMI) of 30 or greater puts you at increased risk.
- **Large waist circumference.** Your risk increases if you are a man with a waist circumference of at least 40 inches or a woman with a waist circumference of at least 35 inches.

- **Poor diet.** Foods that are high in cholesterol, such as red meat and full-fat dairy products, can increase your total cholesterol. Foods containing saturated fat and trans fats also can raise your cholesterol level.
- **Lack of exercise.** Exercise helps boost HDL cholesterol while lowering LDL cholesterol.
- **Diabetes.** High blood sugar contributes to higher LDL cholesterol and lower HDL cholesterol. It also damages your arteries.

TREATMENT Lifestyle changes are the first line of treatment for high cholesterol. If they're ineffective, medication is prescribed. The specific drug or combination of drugs you take will depend on a variety of factors, including your age, your current health and possible side effects of the medication.

Statins. They are the commonly prescribed medications to treat high cholesterol. Statins work by blocking a substance your liver needs to make cholesterol. This causes your liver to remove cholesterol from your blood. Statins may also help your body reabsorb cholesterol from built-up deposits on your artery walls. Choices include atorvastatin (Lipitor), fluvastatin (Lescol XL), pravastatin, rosuvastatin (Crestor) and simvastatin (Zocor).

Bile-acid-binding resins. Your liver uses cholesterol to make bile acids, needed for digestion. The medications cholestyramine (Prevalite), colesevelam (Welchol) and colestipol (Colestid) lower cholesterol by affecting the production of bile acids.

Cholesterol absorption inhibitors. Your small intestine absorbs cholesterol from your diet and releases it into your bloodstream. The drug ezetimibe (Zetia) reduces blood cholesterol by limiting the absorption of dietary cholesterol.

Bempedoic acid. This newer drug works in much the same way as statins but is less likely to cause muscle pain. A combination pill containing both bempedoic acid and ezetimibe (Nexlizet) also is available.

PCSK9 inhibitors. These injections can help the liver absorb more LDL cholesterol, which lowers the amount of cholesterol in your blood. They might be used for people who have a genetic condition that causes very high levels of LDL or in people with heart disease who can't take other cholesterol medications. However, they are expensive.

If you also have high triglycerides, your health care provider may prescribe other medications.

Fibrates. The drugs fenofibrate (TriCor, Fenoglide, others) and gemfibrozil (Lopid) reduce your liver's production of VLDL cholesterol and speed the removal of triglycerides from your blood.

Niacin. Niacin (Niacor) limits your liver's ability to produce LDL and VLDL cholesterol. Most providers recommend it only for people who can't take statins.

Omega-3 fatty acid supplements. Omega-3 fatty acids may help lower triglycerides. Supplements are available by prescription or over-the-counter. Talk with your provider before taking them without a prescription.

Tolerance to cholesterol medications varies from person to person. Common side effects are muscle pains, stomach pain, constipation, nausea and diarrhea. You may have periodic liver function tests to monitor the medication's effect on your liver.

LIFESTYLE Lifestyle changes also are essential to improve your cholesterol level. To bring your numbers down, lose excess weight if you're overweight. Eat a healthy diet that's low in cholesterol, saturated fat and trans fat. Exercise most days of the week for at least 30 minutes. And quit smoking if you use tobacco.

KNOW YOUR NUMBERS

Your personal health history and your risk of heart disease are taken into account in determining the best cholesterol levels for you. In general, aim for these numbers to reduce your risk of possible complications from high cholesterol.

- **Total cholesterol:** Below 200 mg/dL* is best.
- **LDL cholesterol:** 100 mg/dL to 129 mg/dL is near ideal. Lower numbers are better if you have heart disease or are at risk.
- **HDL cholesterol:** 60 mg/dL and above is best.
- **Triglycerides:** Below 150 mg/dL is best.

*Cholesterol is measured in milligrams of cholesterol per deciliter (mg/dL) of blood.

HIV/AIDS

WHAT IS IT? Acquired immunodeficiency syndrome (AIDS) is a chronic, potentially life-threatening condition caused by the human immunodeficiency virus (HIV). By damaging your immune system, HIV interferes with your body's ability to fight organisms that cause disease.

HIV infection occurs when infected blood, semen or vaginal secretions enter your body. You can't become infected through hugging, kissing, dancing or shaking hands with someone who has HIV or AIDS. HIV can't be transmitted through the air or water or via insect bites.

Vaginal, anal or oral sex with an infected partner is a common route of HIV transmission. The virus may be spread through needles and syringes contaminated with infected blood. HIV can spread from mother to child during pregnancy, childbirth or breastfeeding. It also can be transmitted through blood transfusions. However, U.S. hospitals and blood banks now screen for HIV antibodies, so this risk is very small.

It can take years before HIV weakens your immune system to the point that you have AIDS.

SYMPTOM CHECKER Signs and symptoms of HIV and AIDS vary depending on the phase of infection. The majority of people develop a flu-like illness within a month or two after the virus enters the body. Known as primary, or acute, HIV infection, this stage may last for a few weeks. Possible signs and symptoms include fever, headache, muscle aches, chills, sore throat, rash and swelling of lymph nodes, mainly in the neck.

The next stage is called clinical latent infection, which can last 8 to 10 years. Some people stay in this stage longer; others progress to more-severe disease sooner. During this stage, there may be no symptoms. Some people experience swelling of the lymph nodes.

As the virus continues to multiply and destroy immune cells, you may develop mild infections and experience chronic fever, fatigue, diarrhea and cough. Without treatment, HIV infection progresses to AIDS in about 10 years.

By this time, your immune system has been severely damaged, making you susceptible to infections and diseases that wouldn't trouble a healthy person. These infections may cause you to experience soaking night sweats, shaking chills, persistent fever, cough, shortness of breath, fatigue, weight loss and skin rashes.

TREATMENT HIV is often diagnosed by testing your blood or saliva for antibodies to the virus, but it can take up to 12 weeks for your body to develop the antibodies. Newer tests can check for a protein produced by the virus (HIV antigen) or the actual viral load in your blood (nucleic acid tests), both of which can be detected soon after infection. Additional blood tests can help determine what stage of the disease you have.

There's no cure for HIV/AIDS, but a variety of drugs used in combination can control the virus and prevent complications. These are called antiretroviral therapy (ART). Each class of drugs blocks the virus in a different way. The goal of therapy is to achieve an undetectable viral load.

Types

There are different classes of anti-HIV drugs.

Non-nucleoside reverse transcriptase inhibitors (NNRTIs). NNRTIs disable a protein needed by HIV to make copies of itself. Examples include efavirenz (Sustiva), etravirine (Intelence) and nevirapine (Viramune).

Nucleoside reverse transcriptase inhibitors (NRTIs). NRTIs are faulty versions of building blocks that HIV needs to make copies of itself. Examples include abacavir (Ziagen), and the combination drugs emtricitabine and tenofovir (Truvada) and lamivudine and zidovudine (Combivir).

Protease inhibitors (PIs). PIs disable protease, another protein HIV needs to make copies of itself. Examples include atazanavir (Reyataz), darunavir (Prezista), fosamprenavir (Lexiva) and ritonavir (Norvir).

Entry or fusion inhibitors. These drugs block HIV's entry into specific cells. Examples include enfuvirtide (Fuzeon) and maraviroc (Selzentry).

Integrase inhibitors. Raltegravir (Isentress) disables integrase, a protein the virus uses to insert its genetic material into specific cells.

Hyperthyroidism

WHAT IS IT? The thyroid is a butterfly-shaped gland in the neck. It makes two main hormones — triiodothyronine (T3) and thyroxine (T4). They influence every cell in the body and certain vital functions, such as body temperature and heart rate. Hyperthyroidism occurs when the thyroid releases too much of these hormones.

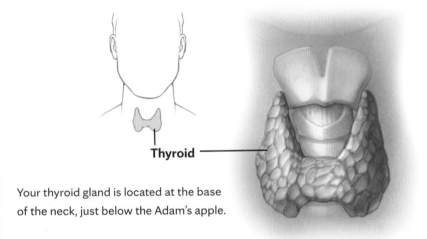

Thyroid

Your thyroid gland is located at the base of the neck, just below the Adam's apple.

WHAT'S THE CAUSE? A number of conditions can cause the thyroid to make or release too much thyroid hormone. They include:

- **Graves' disease.** This is the most common cause of hyperthyroidism. With this disorder, the immune system stimulates your thyroid to make too much T4.
- **Thyroid nodules.** These are often benign lumps that can cause the thyroid to get bigger. It then produces too much T4.
- **Thyroiditis.** Your thyroid can become inflamed after pregnancy, or because of an immune system problem or for an unknown reason. Then too much thyroid hormone can leak into the bloodstream.

SYMPTOM CHECKER Hyperthyroidism can be difficult to diagnose because it can mimic other conditions. It can also cause a wide variety of symptoms, including:

- Eye problems linked to Graves' disease, such as bulging eyeballs; dry, red or swollen eyes; discomfort; light sensitivity; blurry or double vision; inflammation; or reduced eye movement

- Unintentional weight loss, even if you eat the same or more food than usual
- Rapid heartbeat (tachycardia) – commonly more than 100 beats a minute
- Pounding of your heart (palpitations)
- Increased appetite
- Nervousness, anxiety and irritability
- Tremors in the hands and fingers
- Sweating
- Changes in menstrual patterns
- Feeling hot more easily (increased sensitivity to heat)
- Changes in bowel patterns, especially more-frequent bowel movements
- Enlargement of the thyroid gland (goiter)
- Fatigue, muscle weakness
- Trouble sleeping
- Skin thinning
- Fine, brittle hair

Older people are more likely to have no symptoms or only subtle ones, such as a high heart rate, heat intolerance and tiredness during ordinary activities.

Risk factors

Your risk of hyperthyroidism is increased if you're female or if you have a family history of thyroid disease, and particularly of Graves' disease. A personal history of certain chronic illnesses, such as type 1 diabetes, pernicious anemia and primary adrenal insufficiency, also increases your risk.

WHAT TESTS TO EXPECT A medical history, physical exam and blood tests are done to diagnose hyperthyroidism. The provider may check your fingers for a tremor, your eyes and your skin. Your thyroid gland also will be examined as you swallow to see if it's big, bumpy or tender. Your pulse will be checked to see if it's rapid or irregular.

Blood and other tests

If your health care provider thinks you have hyperthyroidism, your blood will be tested to measure levels of T4 and thyroid-stimulating hormone (TSH). If the results show that your hormone levels are too high, you may need another test to see why your thyroid is overactive.

- **Radioiodine uptake test.** For this test, you swallow a small amount of radioactive iodine (radioiodine). You'll be checked after four, six or 24 hours — and sometimes at all three points — to see how much of the radioiodine your thyroid gland collects (the uptake). If your thyroid gland uptake is high, you probably have Graves' disease or thyroid nodules. If uptake is low, you may have thyroiditis.
- **Thyroid scan.** For this test, a radioactive isotope is injected into a vein in your elbow or hand. Then you lie on a table while a special camera takes an image of your thyroid gland. This test shows how iodine collects in your thyroid.
- **Thyroid ultrasound.** This test uses high-frequency sound waves to make images of the thyroid. It may be better at detecting thyroid nodules than other tests, and it doesn't expose you to radiation.

TREATMENT Getting treatment for hyperthyroidism is important. If it's not treated, you can develop heart problems, brittle bones, eye problems and discolored, swollen skin.

The best treatment for you will depend on your age, physical condition, and the cause and severity of your hyperthyroidism. Among possible treatments are:

- **Radioactive iodine.** This is taken by mouth and absorbed by the thyroid gland, causing the thyroid to shrink. Your symptoms may take several months to go away. Radioactive iodine can slow down your thyroid so much that you'll need to take medication to replace T4.
- **Anti-thyroid medications.** Medications such as methimazole and propylthiouracil can be used to prevent the thyroid from producing too much of the thyroid hormones. Symptoms usually improve within weeks to months.
- **Beta blockers.** These drugs can relieve symptoms such as tremor, rapid heart rate and palpitations while your thyroid levels adjust.
- **Surgery (thyroidectomy).** Surgery may be an option if you're pregnant, if you can't take anti-thyroid drugs or don't want to, or if you can't have radioactive iodine. People who have a thyroidectomy need to take levothyroxine (Levoxyl, Synthroid, others) because their bodies can no longer produce thyroid hormone.

If the cause of hyperthyroidism is Graves' disease, your provider may recommend a steroid medication. Some people need eye surgery to improve their vision, correct double vision or help their eyes go back to the usual position.

Hypothyroidism

WHAT IS IT? Hypothyroidism occurs when your thyroid, a butterfly-shaped gland in your neck, doesn't make enough of the hormones thyroxine (T4) and triiodothyronine (T3).

WHAT'S THE CAUSE? Usually, your thyroid releases the right amount of hormones. Several conditions can cause it to make too little. They include:

- **Autoimmune disease.** The most common cause of hypothyroidism is Hashimoto disease. It occurs when your immune system makes antibodies that attack your own tissues. That can include the thyroid gland.
- **Over-response to hyperthyroid treatment.** People whose thyroid gland makes too much T4 (hyperthyroidism) often take radioactive iodine or anti-thyroid drugs. These medications are supposed to restore thyroid function. But sometimes, they end up making hormone levels too low. The result is permanent hypothyroidism.
- **Thyroid surgery.** Removing the thyroid gland, or part of it, can lower or stop hormone production. In that case, you need to take thyroid hormone for the rest of your life.
- **Radiation therapy.** Radiation used to treat cancers of the head and neck can affect your thyroid gland, leading to hypothyroidism.
- **Medications.** Some medications can contribute to hypothyroidism. One example is lithium, which is used to treat certain psychiatric disorders.

Less commonly, some people have hypothyroidism from birth (congenital hypothyroidism). Some babies are born without a thyroid gland, or their thyroid gland doesn't work properly. These babies often have no symptoms, but the problem can be identified during newborn screening that is required in most states.

Other rare causes of hypothyroidism include pituitary disorder, pregnancy and iodine deficiency.

Hypothyroidism can affect anyone, but women, people over 60 and those with a family history of thyroid disease have a greater risk of developing it. Other risk factors include:

- Autoimmune disease, such as type 1 diabetes or celiac disease
- Treatment with radioactive iodine or anti-thyroid medications
- Radiation to the neck or upper chest
- Thyroid surgery
- Pregnancy or delivery of a baby within the past six months

SYMPTOM CHECKER Signs and symptoms of hypothyroidism vary, depending on how low the hormone levels get. Problems tend to develop slowly over years. In adults, they include:

- Fatigue
- Increased sensitivity to cold
- Constipation
- Dry skin
- Weight gain
- Puffy face
- Hoarseness
- Muscle weakness
- High cholesterol
- Pain, stiffness or swelling in joints
- Heavier than usual or irregular menstrual periods
- Thinning hair
- Slowed heart rate
- Depression
- Impaired memory
- Enlarged thyroid gland (goiter)

In addition to the above symptoms, children and teens with hypothyroidism may also have:

- Poor growth, resulting in short stature
- Delayed development of permanent teeth
- Delayed puberty
- Poor mental development

Symptoms of hypothyroidism in a baby include:

- Yellowing of the skin and whites of the eyes
- Large, protruding tongue
- Difficulty breathing
- Hoarse cry
- Umbilical hernia

- Constipation
- Poor muscle tone
- Excessive sleepiness

WHAT TESTS TO EXPECT If a health care provider suspects hypothyroidism based on symptoms, your blood will be tested for thyroid-stimulating hormone (TSH) and sometimes T4.

A low level of T4 and a high level of TSH mean your thyroid gland is sluggish. Your pituitary is producing more TSH to stimulate your thyroid gland to make more thyroid hormone.

TSH tests are also important in managing hypothyroidism. They can help your health care provider determine the right dosage of medication, initially and over time.

TREATMENT Hypothyroidism is usually treated with a synthetic hormone medication that you take by mouth every day.

Levothyroxine (Levo-T, Synthroid, others) is the standard treatment for hypothyroidism. It's taken daily to restore adequate hormone levels and reverse symptoms of hypothyroidism. It gradually lowers cholesterol levels and may reverse weight gain.

Because levothyroxine is a lifelong treatment, it may take time to find the right dosage for you. Once you've been taking it for 6 to 8 weeks, your TSH levels will be rechecked. After that, you'll need to have them checked every year because hormone levels that are too high (hyperthyroidism) also can cause symptoms.

It's important to get treatment for hypothyroidism. Left unchecked, low levels of thyroid hormones can lead to serious problems. They include heart disease, heart failure, damage to nerves in the arms and legs, infertility, birth defects, and a rare condition called myxedema, which can be life-threatening.

LIFESTYLE Certain medications, supplements and even some foods may affect your body's ability to absorb levothyroxine. Talk to your provider if you eat large amounts of soy products, have a high-fiber diet or take other medications.

IBD
(inflammatory bowel disease)

WHAT IS IT? IBD is the umbrella term for diseases that produce chronic inflammation of all or part of the digestive tract. The most common are ulcerative colitis and Crohn's disease.

Ulcerative colitis causes long-lasting inflammation and sores (ulcers) in the innermost lining of the large intestine (colon) and rectum. Crohn's disease causes inflammation of the lining of the digestive tract — the large intestine, small intestine or both — that may spread deep into affected tissues. The most common areas affected by Crohn's disease are the last part of the small intestine and the colon.

The exact cause of IBD remains unknown. Diet and stress were once suspected, but health care providers now know that these factors may aggravate but don't cause IBD. One possible cause is an immune system malfunction. When your immune system tries to fight off an invading virus or bacterium, an abnormal response causes it to attack the cells in the digestive tract too.

SYMPTOM CHECKER Symptoms vary and may range from mild to severe. Signs and symptoms common to both Crohn's disease and ulcerative colitis include:

- **Diarrhea.** Diarrhea is a common problem for people with IBD.
- **Abdominal pain and cramping.** Inflammation and ulceration can affect the movement of contents through the digestive tract, causing pain and cramping and sometimes nausea and vomiting.

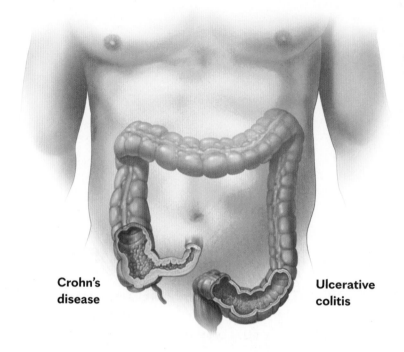

Crohn's disease

Ulcerative colitis

In ulcerative colitis, the lining of the large intestine (colon) becomes inflamed and develops open sores (ulcers). Crohn's disease can affect any part of the gastrointestinal tract, and it may spread deeper to all layers of tissue.

- **Fever and fatigue.** Many people experience a low-grade fever. You may also feel tired or have low energy.
- **Blood in your stool.** You might notice bright red blood in the toilet bowl or darker blood mixed with your stool.
- **Reduced appetite.** Abdominal pain and cramping, as well as inflammation, can affect your appetite.
- **Weight loss.** You may lose weight and even become malnourished because you can't properly digest and absorb food.

TREATMENT A diagnosis of IBD is often made after ruling out other possible causes for your signs and symptoms.

The goal of treatment is to reduce the inflammation that's triggering your signs and symptoms. In the best cases, this may also lead to long-term remission. Drug therapy and surgery are the main treatments for ulcerative colitis and Crohn's disease.

Anti-inflammatory medications

These medications are often the first step in the treatment of IBD.

- **Aminosalicylates.** They include the medications sulfasalazine (Azulfidine) and mesalamine (Delzicol, Rowasa, others), balsalazide (Colazal), and olsalazine (Dipentum), which are available in both oral and enema or suppository forms. The form you take depends on the area of your colon that's affected.
- **Corticosteroids.** They include prednisone and hydrocortisone and are generally reserved for moderate to severe IBD that doesn't respond to other treatments. They're given orally, intravenously, or by enema or suppository. Because corticosteroids have numerous side effects, they generally aren't used long term.

Immune system suppressors

They reduce inflammation by suppressing the immune response that releases inflammation-inducing chemicals in the intestinal lining. For some people, a combination of these drugs works best.

- **Azathioprine (Azasan, Imuran) and mercaptopurine (Purixan, Purinethol).** They're the most widely used immunosuppressants for treatment of IBD. You need to have your blood checked regularly to look for possible side effects.
- **Cyclosporine (Gengraf, Neoral, Sandimmune).** This drug is typically reserved for people with ulcerative colitis who haven't responded well to other medications. It has the potential for serious side effects and isn't for long-term use.
- **Infliximab (Remicade), adalimumab (Humira) and golimumab (Simponi).** Called tumor necrosis factor-alpha (TNF-alpha) inhibitors, or "biologics," these medications neutralize a protein produced by your immune system. They're generally recommended for people with moderate to severe IBD who don't respond to or can't tolerate other treatments.
- **Methotrexate (Trexall).** This drug, used mainly to treat cancer, psoriasis and rheumatoid arthritis, may be used in people with Crohn's disease who don't respond to other medications.
- **Natalizumab (Tysabri) and vedolizumab (Entyvio).** These drugs are prescribed for people with moderate to severe IBD who don't respond well to other medications. Vedolizumab doesn't appear to have the risk of brain infection that natalizumab does.
- **Ustekinumab (Stelara).** It's used to treat psoriasis but may be used to treat Crohn's disease when other medical treatments fail.

Other medications

Other medications may be prescribed to control signs and symptoms such as fever, pain, diarrhea and vitamin deficiencies.

Surgery

If medications aren't effective, surgery may be necessary.

Surgery for ulcerative colitis. Surgery can often eliminate ulcerative colitis, but it usually means removing your entire colon and rectum. A pouch is constructed from the end of your small intestine and attached directly to your anus. This allows you to expel waste relatively normally. If a pouch isn't possible, a permanent opening is created in your abdomen (ileal conduit) through which stool passes for collection in an attached bag.

Surgery for Crohn's disease. Up to half of people with Crohn's disease require at least one surgery. During surgery, the damaged portion of your digestive tract may be removed and the healthy sections reconnected. Surgery may also be performed to treat complications of Crohn's, such as closing abnormal connections (fistulas), draining abscesses or widening narrowed sections in the intestines. Unfortunately, the benefits of surgery are often temporary.

LIFESTYLE Certain foods and beverages can aggravate your symptoms. Here are some suggestions that may help:

- **Limit dairy products.** Many people with IBD find that problems such as diarrhea, abdominal pain and gas improve when they limit or cut out dairy products.
- **Try low-fat foods.** If you have Crohn's disease of the small intestine, you may not be able to digest or absorb fat well. Avoid butter, margarine, cream sauces and fried foods.
- **Pay attention to fiber.** High-fiber foods, such as fresh fruits and vegetables and whole grains, may make your symptoms worse.
- **Avoid other problem foods and beverages.** Stay away from spicy foods. Alcohol and beverages that contain caffeine stimulate your intestines and can make diarrhea worse.
- **Eat small meals.** You may find that you feel better eating five or six small meals a day rather than two or three larger ones.
- **Drink plenty of liquids.** Water is best. Avoid carbonated drinks that produce gas.

IBS (irritable bowel syndrome)

WHAT IS IT? IBS is a common disorder affecting the large intestine (colon) that can cause a variety of symptoms, including abdominal pain and diarrhea or constipation.

For most people, IBS is a chronic condition, although there may be times when the signs and symptoms are worse and times when they improve or even disappear completely. Signs and symptoms may vary widely from person to person and resemble those of other diseases. Among the most common are:

- Abdominal pain or cramping
- A bloated feeling
- Gas
- Diarrhea or constipation, sometimes alternating bouts of each
- Mucus in the stool

Unlike ulcerative colitis and Crohn's disease, IBS doesn't cause bowel tissue changes that increase your risk of serious complications.

WHAT'S THE CAUSE? It's not known exactly what causes IBS. A variety of factors may play a role. For example, muscle contractions in the intestine help food move through the digestive tract. In a person with IBS, the contractions may be stronger and last longer, causing pain, or they may be too weak and slow the passage of food.

Abnormalities in the gastrointestinal nervous system also may play a role. Abdominal stretching from the production of gas or stool may produce discomfort that's not typical. Poorly coordinated signals between the intestines and the brain may cause the body to overreact to regular digestive events. Genes also may play a role. Studies suggest that if one family member has IBS, others may be at increased risk of the condition.

Factors that may trigger symptoms of IBS include:

- **Food.** Many people have more-severe symptoms when they eat certain things. A wide range of food has been implicated — chocolate, spices, fats, fruits, beans, cabbage, cauliflower, broccoli, milk, carbonated beverages and alcohol.

- **Stress.** Most people with IBS find that their signs and symptoms are worse or more frequent during periods of increased stress.
- **Hormones.** Because women are twice as likely as are men to have IBS, hormonal changes likely play a role. Signs and symptoms are often worse during or around menstruation.
- **Other illnesses.** Another illness, such as a bout of gastroenteritis (the "stomach flu"), may trigger symptoms.

WHAT TESTS TO EXPECT There are no specific markers to definitively identify IBS, so making a diagnosis is often a process of ruling out other conditions.

Certain signs and symptoms must be present to receive a diagnosis of IBS. The most important are abdominal pain and discomfort lasting at least three days a month over the last three months. The discomfort must be associated with two or more of the following: pain relief after a bowel movement, changes in the frequency of bowel movements or changes in the consistency of stool. Mucus in the stool may be another indication of possible IBS.

TREATMENT Because there isn't a known cause, the focus of treatment is on relieving symptoms.

Medications
If your symptoms are moderate to severe, your health care provider may recommend:

Fiber supplements. Taking fiber supplements, such as psyllium (Metamucil) or methylcellulose (Citrucel), with fluids may help control constipation.

Anti-diarrheal medications. Over-the-counter medications, such as loperamide (Imodium A-D), may help if diarrhea is a regular symptom. Some people benefit from prescription drugs called bile acid binders, such as cholestyramine (Prevalite), colestipol (Colestid) or colesevelam (Welchol), but they can lead to bloating.

Anticholinergic and antispasmodic medications. These medications, such as hyoscyamine (Levsin) and dicyclomine (Bentyl), can help relieve painful bowel spasms. They're sometimes used to treat bouts of diarrhea, but they can worsen constipation.

I-K

Antidepressant medications. A tricyclic antidepressant or a selective serotonin reuptake inhibitor (SSRI) may help relieve symptoms in people with depression. They also inhibit the activity of neurons that control the intestines.

Several medications are specifically approved for IBS, including:

Alosetron. Alosetron (Lotronex) relaxes the colon and slows the movement of waste through the lower bowel. Because of the potential risk of serious side effects, only health care providers enrolled in a special program can prescribe it. It's intended for severe cases of diarrhea-predominant IBS in women who haven't responded to other treatments. Alosetron isn't approved for men.

Lubiprostone. Lubiprostone (Amitiza) increases fluid secretion in the small intestine to help with the passage of stool. It's approved for women who have constipation and who haven't responded to other treatments. The medication isn't approved for men.

Linaclotide (Linzess). Linaclotide also can increase fluid secretion in your small intestine to help you pass stool.

Eluxadoline (Viberzi). This can ease diarrhea by reducing muscle contractions and fluid secretion in the intestine, and increasing muscle tone in the rectum.

Rifaximin (Xifaxan). This can decrease bacterial overgrowth and diarrhea.

LIFESTYLE In many cases, simple dietary or lifestyle changes may help relieve symptoms.

- **Avoid problem foods.** These may include alcohol, chocolate, coffee and sodas, beans, cabbage, cauliflower and broccoli, and fatty foods.
- **Eat at regular times.** Small, more-frequent meals also may help.
- **Take care with dairy products.** If you're lactose intolerant, use an enzyme product to help break down lactose.
- **Try probiotics.** These "good" bacteria are found in some yogurts, and are available as dietary supplements.
- **Drink plenty of liquids.** Water is best.
- **Exercise regularly.** It helps relieve stress, and it stimulates contractions of the intestines.
- **Find ways to reduce stress.** Try a warm bath or listening to music.

Infertility

WHAT IS IT? Infertility is a common issue among couples trying to have a baby. It's usually diagnosed when a couple hasn't gotten pregnant after a year of frequent, unprotected sex. For women who are 35 or older, the diagnosis may be made much sooner.

Nearly 1 in 7 couples is infertile. The inability to conceive a child can be stressful, but there are treatments available, which vary depending on what's causing the infertility.

WHAT'S THE CAUSE? In about one-third of couples, the cause is related to the woman's health. In another one-third of couples, it's related to the man. And for others, the cause may be related to both people, or the reason for infertility can't be found.

Female and male reproductive organs

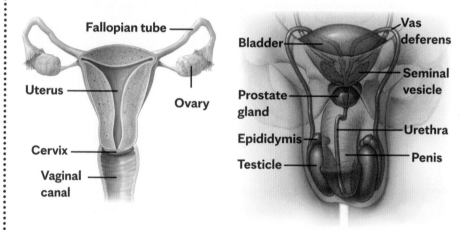

In women, factors that can disrupt fertility include:

- **Lack of ovulation because of a hormone imbalance.** This can happen if you have polycystic ovary syndrome or your pituitary gland doesn't produce reproductive hormones.
- **Damage to or blockage of the fallopian tubes (the tube that carries eggs).** This may make it hard for a fertilized egg to pass through the fallopian tube into the uterus.
- **Endometriosis.** If you've had surgery to remove extra tissue in the uterus, that can make it hard for an egg to implant.

- **Polyps or tumors in the uterus or cervix.** These benign growths can keep the egg from traveling and implanting in the uterus.
- **Congenital issues.** Some women are born with an unusually shaped uterus. That can make it hard to become or stay pregnant.

In men, factors that can lead to infertility include:

- **Producing no or very few sperm.** Fewer than 15 million sperm per milliliter of semen is considered a low count.
- **Abnormal sperm function.** Sperm that are sluggish or move erratically may not be able to reach the egg.
- **Lack of ejaculation.** The tubes that carry the sperm can be blocked by an injury, infection or other reason.
- **Medical issues.** Some health problems, such as having mumps in childhood, can make a man infertile.

Other risk factors for infertility include being older, and having a history of chlamydia or gonorrhea, which can damage the fallopian tubes. In men, testicular or epididymal infections or an undescended testicle can make infertility more likely. An abnormally high or low testosterone level can too.

Smoking, being overweight, excessive use of alcohol and misuse of drugs such as marijuana can reduce the likelihood of conception for anyone.

WHAT TESTS TO EXPECT If you've been unable to get pregnant within a reasonable period of time, seek help from your health care provider for evaluation and treatment of infertility. Your provider will take a detailed medical history and conduct a physical exam.

Fertility tests for women might include:

- **Ovulation testing.** A blood test for progesterone — the hormone produced after ovulation — can show if you're ovulating.
- **Hysterosalpingography.** During this test, X-ray contrast is injected into the uterus and an X-ray is taken to check the inside of the organ. If problems are found, further evaluation may be needed.
- **Ovarian reserve testing.** This helps determine the quality and number of eggs left in the ovaries.
- **Other hormone testing.** Levels of other ovulatory hormones and hormones produced by the thyroid and pituitary glands also may be checked.

- **Imaging tests.** A pelvic ultrasound looks for disease in the uterus or fallopian tubes. Sometimes a sonohysterogram, also called a saline infusion sonogram, or a hysteroscopy is used to see details inside a woman's uterus that aren't visible on a regular ultrasound.

Fertility tests for men might include:

- **Semen analysis.** This test measures the volume and pH of semen, the concentration of sperm, and how well the sperm swim (motility).
- **Hormone testing.** If your semen analysis is repeatedly abnormal, your levels of testosterone and other hormones necessary for fertility may be tested.
- **Ultrasonography.** This type of imaging uses radio waves. It's done if you're not producing sperm or if your physical exam shows an abnormality, such as a testicular mass.

Some people who are infertile have genetic testing to see whether changes in their genes may be causing the problem.

TREATMENT The way infertility is treated depends on the results of a person's physical exam and testing. Age also is a factor.

Because infertility is complex, medications and surgeries for it can be expensive. It also may take a lot of time and energy to overcome. Sometimes, treatment isn't possible or successful. But for some people, fertility treatment can result in pregnancy.

Medications
It can take as long as six months for medication to improve a couple's fertility. Sometimes, the full benefit isn't seen for more than a year.

Medications given to women include:

- **Clomiphene citrate.** This drug is given mostly to women younger than age 39 who don't have polycystic ovary syndrome (PCOS). It's taken by mouth.
- **Gonadotropins (Menopur, Gonal-F, Follistim AQ, Bravelle).** These injectable medications are given to stimulate ovulation.
- **Metformin.** This drug helps the body use insulin better. Taking it may make someone with PCOS more likely to ovulate.

- **Letrozole (Femara).** This drug works like clomiphene. It's usually used for women younger than age 39 who have PCOS.
- **Bromocriptine (Cycloset, Parlodel).** Women whose infertility is caused by a problem with the pituitary gland are given this drug.

Medications given to men to improve the number or motility of sperm include clomiphene citrate and aromatase inhibitors.

Surgery

Sometimes, women need surgery to improve their chances of getting pregnant. Procedures that may help include:

- **Laparoscopy or hysteroscopy.** These surgeries can be used to correct issues with uterine anatomy or remove polyps or fibroids (benign tumors).
- **Tubal surgeries.** Surgery to open up the fallopian tubes may be recommended for women whose tubes are blocked or scarred.

Surgery to restore fertility in men includes:

- **Varicocelectomy.** This surgery corrects a varicocele (repair of enlarged veins in the sac around the testicles).
- **Epididymectomy.** This removes a blockage in the epididymis (coiled tube that stores and carries sperm).
- **Vasectomy reversal.** If you've had a vasectomy, this procedure can reconnect each tube (vas deferens) that carries sperm from a testicle into the semen.

Reproductive assistance

Some couples are referred to specialists in infertility for treatment. Methods to help them conceive include:

- **Intrauterine insemination (IUI).** During IUI, healthy sperm are placed inside the uterus around the time a woman is ovulating.
- **In vitro fertilization (IVF).** Mature eggs are retrieved from a woman, and then fertilized with a man's sperm in a dish in a lab. The resulting embryos then are returned to the woman's uterus.
- **Intracytoplasmic sperm injection (ICSI).** With ICSI, a single healthy sperm is injected into a mature egg. The resulting embryo then is returned to the woman's uterus. ICSI is often used if a man has very few sperm or IVF has not worked.

I-K

Insomnia

WHAT IS IT? Insomnia is a persistent disorder that can make it hard to fall asleep, hard to stay asleep or both.

If you have insomnia, it may take you 30 minutes or more to fall asleep, and you may get less than six hours of sleep most nights of the week. You may awaken feeling unrefreshed, which can lead to daytime sleepiness and take a toll on your ability to function.

WHAT'S THE CAUSE? Common causes include:

- **Stress.** Concerns about work, school, health or family can keep your mind active at night, making it difficult to sleep. Stressful life events — such as the death or illness of a loved one, divorce, or a job loss — may lead to insomnia.
- **Anxiety.** Everyday anxieties as well as anxiety disorders may disrupt your asleep.
- **Depression.** You might either sleep too much or have trouble sleeping.
- **Medical conditions.** Conditions such as chronic pain, breathing difficulties or a need to urinate frequently can lead to insomnia.
- **Change in your environment or work schedule.** Travel or working a late or early shift can disrupt your body's circadian rhythms, making it difficult to sleep.
- **Poor sleep habits.** These include an irregular sleep schedule, stimulating activities before bed and an uncomfortable sleep environment.
- **Medications.** Many prescription and over-the-counter drugs can interfere with sleep.
- **Caffeine, nicotine and alcohol.** Caffeine-containing drinks are well-known stimulants. Nicotine is also a stimulant. Alcohol prevents deeper stages of sleep and may cause you to awaken in the middle of the night.
- **Eating too much late at night.** You may feel physically uncomfortable, making it difficult to get to sleep.

TREATMENT Changing your sleep habits and addressing any underlying causes of insomnia, such as medical conditions or medications, can restore restful sleep for many people.

I-K

Behavior therapies

You learn new sleep behaviors and ways to improve your sleep.

- **Sleep habits education.** Good habits include a regular sleep schedule, relaxing before bed and a comfortable sleep environment.
- **Cognitive behavioral therapy.** It helps you control or eliminate negative thoughts and worries that keep you awake.
- **Relaxation techniques.** Progressive muscle relaxation, biofeedback and breathing exercises can reduce anxiety at bedtime.
- **Stimulus control.** You limit the time you spend awake in bed and associate your bed and bedroom only with sleep and sex.
- **Sleep restriction.** You decrease the time you spend in bed, causing partial sleep deprivation, making you more tired. Once your sleep has improved, your time in bed is gradually increased.
- **Remaining passively awake.** You try to keep yourself awake rather than try to fall asleep.

Medications

Prescription sleeping pills may help you get to sleep. But using them for more than a few weeks is generally not recommended, because of dependence and possible side effects.

Nonprescription sleep medications contain antihistamines that can make you drowsy. But antihistamines may reduce the quality of your sleep, and they can cause side effects, such as daytime sleepiness, dizziness, urinary retention, dry mouth and confusion.

LIFESTYLE Here are some suggestions to manage insomnia and help you sleep better:

- **Exercise.** Exercise daily at least 5 to 6 hours before bedtime.
- **Avoid or limit naps.** Naps can make it harder to fall asleep at night.
- **Pay attention to caffeine, alcohol and nicotine.** Avoid caffeine after lunchtime, limit alcohol and don't smoke.
- **Stick to a schedule.** Keep your bedtime and wake time consistent.
- **Avoid large meals before bed.** A light snack is fine.
- **Don't read, work or eat in bed.** Save your bed for sleep and sex.
- **Make your bedroom comfortable.** Create a calming background noise, and keep the room dark and the temperature cool.
- **Hide bedroom clocks.** Set your alarm, then hide all clocks so that you don't worry about what time it is.

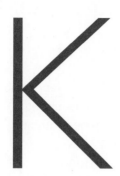

Kidney cysts

WHAT IS IT? Kidney cysts are round pouches of fluid that form in the kidneys. Rarely, they're associated with serious disorders that can impair kidney function. More commonly, kidney cysts are simple cysts that don't cause complications.

It's not clear what causes simple kidney cysts. One theory suggests that kidney cysts develop when the surface layer of the kidney weakens and forms a pouch. The pouch fills with fluid and develops into a cyst. Typically, only one cyst occurs on the surface of a kidney, but multiple cysts can affect one or both kidneys.

Simple kidney cysts are different from the cysts that form with polycystic kidney disease. Polycystic kidney disease is an inherited disorder in which clusters of cysts develop primarily within the kidneys. The disease causes a variety of serious complications, including high blood pressure.

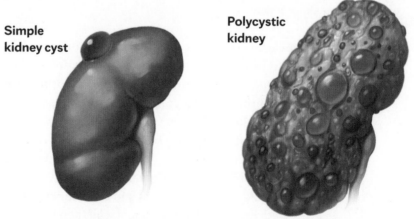

Simple kidney cyst

Polycystic kidney

A kidney cyst is a round or oval fluid-filled pouch that typically grows on the surface.

SYMPTOM CHECKER Simple cysts typically don't cause problems. If a simple cyst grows large enough, signs and symptoms may include dull pain in your back or side, fever, and upper abdominal pain.

Occasionally, complications can occur, including an infected cyst, a cyst that bursts or a cyst that obstructs urine flow. Symptoms of polycystic kidney disease may include high blood pressure, back or side pain, headaches, abdominal swelling, and frequent urination.

TREATMENT Tests and procedures used to diagnose simple kidney cysts include imaging tests, such as an ultrasound or computerized tomography (CT) scan. They can help determine whether a kidney mass is a cyst or a tumor. A blood test may reveal whether a cyst is impairing kidney function.

If a simple kidney cyst causes no signs or symptoms and doesn't interfere with your kidney function, no treatment may be needed.

Types
Treatment for simple kidney cysts that cause symptoms include:

Puncturing and draining the cyst. To shrink a cyst, a long, thin needle is inserted through your skin and the wall of the kidney cyst. Fluid is drained from the cyst. Your health care provider may fill the cyst with an alcohol solution to prevent it from re-forming. Because cysts often re-form after this type of procedure, it's reserved for certain situations.

Surgery to remove the cyst. A large or symptomatic cyst may require surgery to drain and remove it. The surgery can often be performed laparoscopically, with several small incisions rather than one large incision. After the fluid is drained, the walls of the cyst are cut or burned away.

With polycystic kidney disease, the focus of treatment is on controlling symptoms in their early stages and keeping the kidneys as healthy as possible. In addition to managing high blood pressure, your provider may recommend eating a low-sodium diet, maintaining a healthy weight, getting regular exercise and stopping smoking if you smoke.

For severe disease that leads to kidney failure, dialysis or a kidney transplant may be necessary.

Kidney stones

WHAT IS IT? Kidney stones are small, hard deposits that form inside the kidneys. The stones are made of minerals and acid salts. They develop when your urine contains more crystal-forming substances than the fluid in your urine can dilute.

A kidney stone may not cause symptoms until it moves in your kidney or passes into the tube connecting the kidney and bladder (ureter). Signs and symptoms may include:

- Severe pain in the side and back, below the ribs
- Pain that spreads to the lower abdomen and groin
- Pain that comes in waves and fluctuates in intensity
- Pain on urination
- Pink, red or brown urine
- Cloudy or foul-smelling urine
- Nausea and vomiting
- Persistent urge to urinate
- Urinating more often than usual

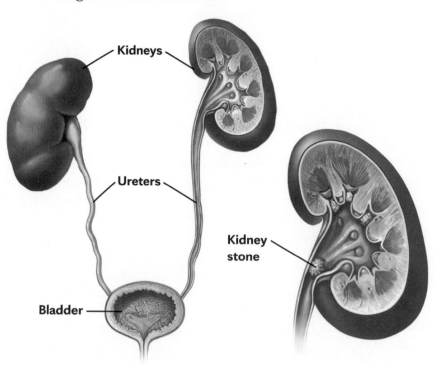

Kidney stones form in the kidneys and can move into the ureters. Symptoms often develop or become more severe once a stone enters a ureter.

I-K

WHAT'S THE CAUSE? Often, stones form when urine becomes concentrated and minerals crystallize and stick together.

Types

Knowing the type of kidney stone helps determine the cause and may give clues on how to reduce your risk of more stones.

Calcium stones. Most kidney stones are calcium stones, usually in the form of calcium oxalate. Oxalate is a naturally occurring substance in food. Some fruits and vegetables, as well as nuts, chocolate and iced tea, have high oxalate levels. Your liver also produces oxalate.

Struvite stones. Struvite stones form in response to an infection, such as a urinary tract infection. They can grow quickly and become quite large, sometimes with little warning.

Uric acid stones. These stones may form in people who don't drink enough fluids, who lose too much fluid, who eat a high-protein diet or who have gout. Genetic factors also may increase the risk of uric acid stones.

Cystine stones. They can form in people with a hereditary disorder that causes the kidneys to excrete too much of certain amino acids.

Other stones. They include more-rare types of kidney stones.

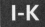

I-K

WHAT TESTS TO EXPECT If your health care provider suspects that you have a kidney stone, you may undergo one or more tests.

- **Blood tests.** Blood tests may reveal too much calcium or uric acid in your blood.
- **Urine tests.** A 24-hour urine collection may show that you're excreting too many stone-forming minerals or too few stone-preventing substances.
- **Imaging tests.** Imaging tests are used to identify kidney stones in your urinary tract.
- **Stone analysis.** You may be asked to urinate through a strainer to catch stones you may pass. Lab analysis reveals their makeup.

TREATMENT Treatment for kidney stones varies, depending on the type of stone and the cause.

Conservative therapies

Most kidney stones don't require invasive treatment. The following may help pass a small stone:

- **Water.** Drink as much as 2 to 3 quarts a day to flush out your urinary system. Also, stones can't form as easily in diluted urine.
- **Pain relievers.** Over-the-counter pain relievers can treat mild pain.
- **Medication.** Your health care provider may prescribe an alpha blocker to relax the muscles in your ureter so that you can pass the stone more quickly and with less pain.

Invasive treatment

When conservative measures aren't helpful, options include:

Sound wave therapy. A procedure called extracorporeal shock wave lithotripsy uses sound waves to create strong vibrations (shock waves) that break the stones into tiny pieces that can be passed in your urine.

Scope procedure. To remove a smaller stone, your provider may pass a thin, flexible tube (ureteroscope) through your urethra and bladder to your ureter. Special tools snare the stone or break it into pieces that will pass in your urine. A small tube (stent) may be placed in the ureter to relieve swelling and promote healing.

Surgery. A kidney stone is removed through a small incision in your back. Your health care provider may recommend this approach if sound wave therapy is unsuccessful or the stone is very large.

Parathyroid gland surgery. Some calcium stones are caused by too much calcium in the blood, due to overactive parathyroid glands (hyperparathyroidism). A small, benign tumor in one of your parathyroid glands may be responsible. Removing the tumor stops the formation of kidney stones.

Medication

Medications can control the amount of minerals and acid in your urine and may help people who form certain kinds of stones. The medication your health care provider prescribes will depend on the kind of kidney stones you have. For calcium stones, a thiazide diuretic or a phosphate-containing preparation is often used.

Knee pain

WHAT'S THE CAUSE? Knee pain is a common complaint. The pain may be the result of an injury, a mechanical problem or arthritis. Signs and symptoms that may accompany your knee pain include:

- Swelling and stiffness
- Redness and warmth to the touch
- Weakness or instability
- Popping or crunching noises
- Inability to fully straighten the knee

Injury

A knee injury can affect any of the ligaments, tendons or fluid-filled sacs (bursae) that surround the knee joint as well as the bones, cartilage and ligaments that form the joint. Common knee injuries include:

- **ACL injury.** An ACL injury is the tearing of the anterior cruciate ligament (ACL) — one of four ligaments that connect your shinbone to your thighbone. An ACL injury is particularly common in people who play a sport that requires sudden changes in direction.
- **Torn meniscus.** The meniscus is the cartilage that acts as a shock absorber between your shinbone and thighbone and is formed of tough, rubbery tissue. It can tear if you suddenly twist your knee while bearing weight on it.
- **Knee bursitis.** Some knee injuries cause inflammation in the small sacs of fluid (bursae) that cushion the outside of the knee joint.
- **Patellar tendinitis.** Runners, skiers and people involved in jumping activities are prone to develop inflammation in the patellar tendon, which connects the quadriceps muscle on the front of the thigh to the shinbone.

Mechanical problems

Mechanical problems that can cause knee pain include:

- **Loose body.** A piece of bone or cartilage breaks off and floats in the joint space. If the piece interferes with knee joint movement, the effect is something like a pencil caught in a door hinge.

I-K

- **Iliotibial band syndrome.** The ligament that extends from the outside of your pelvic bone to the outside of your tibia becomes so tight that it rubs against the outer portion of your femur. Distance runners are especially susceptible to this problem.
- **Dislocated kneecap.** The triangular bone (patella) that covers the front of your knee slips out of place, usually to the outside of your knee.
- **Change in gait.** If you have hip or foot pain, you may change the way you walk. The altered gait can place more stress on your knee joint.

Arthritis

Osteoarthritis and rheumatoid arthritis are the most common causes of arthritis-related knee pain. Gout or pseudogout can also affect the joint.

TREATMENT It's dependent on the cause of the pain.

Medications. Nonprescription pain relievers can often treat mild knee pain. Prescription medications may help relieve pain from conditions such as rheumatoid arthritis or gout. In some cases, medication may be injected directly into the knee joint:

- **Corticosteroids.** An injection may help reduce the symptoms of an arthritis flare and provide pain relief for a few months.
- **Supplemental lubricant.** A thick fluid, similar to the fluid that naturally lubricates joints, may be injected into your knee to improve mobility and ease pain.

Physical therapy. Strengthening the muscles around your knee will make it more stable. Arch supports may help shift pressure away from the side of the knee most affected by osteoarthritis.

Surgery. Surgery may be performed to remove loose bodies, remove or repair damaged cartilage, or reconstruct torn ligaments. All or part of a damaged joint may be replaced with artificial parts.

Self-care. Practice R.I.C.E. (see page 335). If you're overweight, losing weight may reduce the pain and related symptoms. You may also need to change the way you exercise. Consider switching to swimming, water aerobics or other low-impact activities.

L

Lactose intolerance

WHAT IS IT? Lactose intolerance means you aren't able to fully digest the milk sugar (lactose) in dairy products. A deficiency of lactase — an enzyme produced by the lining of your small intestine — is usually responsible for lactose intolerance.

Signs and symptoms usually begin 30 minutes to 2 hours after eating or drinking foods that contain lactose. Symptoms include:

- Diarrhea
- Nausea, and sometimes, vomiting
- Abdominal cramps
- Bloating and gas

TREATMENT Most people find relief by altering their diets and using special products made for people with this condition.

- **Eat smaller servings.** Try not to eat more than 4 ounces of dairy at a time. The smaller the serving, the less likely it is to cause problems.
- **Save milk for mealtimes.** Drinking milk with other foods slows the digestive process and may lessen symptoms.
- **Experiment.** Hard cheeses have small amounts of lactose and generally cause no symptoms. You may be able to eat cultured milk products, such as yogurt, because the bacteria used in the culturing process produce an enzyme that breaks down lactose.
- **Buy lactose-reduced or lactose-free products.** You can find them at most supermarkets in the refrigerated dairy section.
- **Use tablets or drops.** Products containing the lactase enzyme (Dairy Ease, Lactaid, others) may help you digest lactose.

Laryngitis

WHAT IS IT? Laryngitis is an inflammation or irritation of your voice box (larynx) from overuse, irritation or infection, often a viral upper respiratory infection. Swelling of the vocal cords causes your voice to sound hoarse. Other symptoms may include a tickling in your throat, a dry throat and a dry cough.

Most cases of laryngitis are temporary and improve after the underlying cause resolves. Laryngitis that lasts longer than three weeks may be related to irritants, such as allergens, smoke or acid reflux.

TREATMENT Self-care measures such as these can relieve symptoms and reduce the strain on your voice:

- **Breathe moist air.** Use a humidifier to keep the air in your home or office moist. Inhale steam from a hot shower.
- **Rest your voice.** Don't talk or sing too loudly or for too long.
- **Drink plenty of fluids.** Fluids help keep the mucus in your throat thin and easy to clear. Avoid alcohol and caffeine.
- **Moisten your throat.** Suck on lozenges, gargle with salt water or chew gum.
- **Avoid decongestants.** They can dry out the throat.
- **Avoid whispering.** It puts more strain on your voice than normal speech does.
- **Avoid secondhand smoke.** Smoke dries your throat and irritates your vocal cords.
- **Try not to clear your throat.** It causes a harsh vibration of your vocal cords and increases swelling. Clearing your throat also causes your throat to secrete more mucus and feel more irritated, making you want to clear your throat again.

Medications may be prescribed in certain cases.

Antibiotics. An antibiotic won't do any good for a viral infection, but if you have a bacterial infection your care provider may prescribe one.

Corticosteroids. Sometimes they can help reduce vocal cord inflammation. However, corticosteroids carry side effects, so they're used only when there's an urgent need to treat laryngitis — for example, if a toddler has laryngitis associated with croup.

L

Leukemia

WHAT IS IT? Leukemia is cancer of the body's blood-forming tissues, including the bone marrow and the lymphatic system. Scientists don't understand the exact causes of leukemia. It appears to develop from a combination of genetic and environmental factors.

Leukemia usually starts in the white blood cells, which are potent infection fighters. Among people with leukemia, the bone marrow produces white blood cells that don't function properly. Changes in these cells cause them to grow and divide more rapidly and to continue living when other cells would die. Over time, the irregular white blood cells crowd out healthy blood cells in the bone marrow, leading to fewer healthy blood cells and causing the signs and symptoms of leukemia. Other cell changes may also play a part.

Classification

Many types of leukemia exist. Some forms are more common in children. Others occur mostly in adults.

Leukemia is classified based on its speed of progression and the type of cells involved.

- **Acute leukemia.** In acute leukemia, the abnormal white blood cells are immature blood cells. They can't carry out their usual work, and they multiply rapidly, so the disease worsens quickly.
- **Chronic leukemia.** This type of leukemia involves more-mature white blood cells. The blood cells can function as usual for a period of time. Some forms of chronic leukemia may produce no early symptoms and can go unnoticed or undiagnosed for years.
- **Lymphocytic leukemia.** This type of leukemia affects the lymphoid cells (lymphocytes), which form lymphatic tissue that makes up your immune system.
- **Myelogenous leukemia.** This type of leukemia affects the myeloid cells, which eventually give rise to red blood cells, white blood cells and platelet-producing cells. Irregular immature white cells interfere with the bone marrow's ability to produce healthy white cells, red cells and platelets.

There are four major types of leukemia, which are known as:

- **Acute lymphocytic leukemia (ALL).** This is the most common type of leukemia in young children. It rarely occurs in adults.
- **Acute myelogenous leukemia (AML).** AML is the most common type of acute leukemia in adults. It can also occur in children.
- **Chronic lymphocytic leukemia (CLL).** It's the most common chronic adult leukemia. You may feel well for years without needing treatment.
- **Chronic myelogenous leukemia (CML).** This type mainly affects adults. You may have few or no symptoms for months or years before entering a phase in which the leukemia cells begin to grow more quickly.

Other, more-rare types of leukemia exist, including hairy cell leukemia, myelodysplastic syndromes and myeloproliferative disorders.

SYMPTOM CHECKER Leukemia signs and symptoms vary, depending on the type of leukemia. They include:

- Fever or chills
- Persistent fatigue, weakness
- Frequent or severe infections
- Losing weight without trying
- Swollen lymph nodes, enlarged liver or spleen
- Easy bleeding or bruising
- Recurrent nosebleeds
- Tiny red spots in your skin (petechiae)
- Excessive sweating, especially at night
- Bone pain or tenderness

TREATMENT Leukemia is most often diagnosed with a blood test that shows unusual levels of white blood cells or blood platelets. A bone marrow test may reveal certain characteristics of the disease. Your health care provider also may look for physical signs of leukemia, such as pale skin from anemia and swelling of the lymph nodes, liver and spleen.

Types of treatment

Treatment for leukemia depends on many factors. Your health care provider will determine your treatment options based on your age and overall health, the type of leukemia you have, and whether it has spread to other parts of your body. Common treatments used to fight leukemia include:

Chemotherapy. Chemotherapy is the most common form of treatment for leukemia. Depending on the type of leukemia you have, you may receive a single drug or a combination of drugs. Some chemotherapy drugs come in pill form. Others are injected directly into a vein.

Biological therapy. Biological therapy works by helping your immune system recognize and attack leukemia cells.

Targeted therapy. Targeted therapy uses drugs that attack specific vulnerabilities within your cancer cells. For example, the drug imatinib (Gleevec) stops the action of a protein within the leukemia cells of people with chronic myelogenous leukemia. This can help control the disease.

Targeted therapy drugs used in treating other types of leukemia include rituximab (Rituxan), alemtuzumab (Campath), ofatumumab (Arzerra), dasatinib (Sprycel) and nilotinib (Tasigna).

Radiation therapy. Radiation therapy uses X-rays or other high-energy beams to damage leukemia cells and stop their growth. You may receive radiation in one specific area of your body where there's a collection of leukemia cells, or you may receive radiation over your whole body. Radiation therapy may be used to prepare for a stem cell transplant.

Stem cell transplant. A stem cell transplant is a procedure to replace your diseased bone marrow with healthy bone marrow. It is very similar to a bone marrow transplant.

Before having a stem cell transplant, you receive high doses of chemotherapy or radiation therapy to destroy your diseased bone marrow. Then you receive an infusion of blood-forming stem cells that help to rebuild your bone marrow. You may receive stem cells from a donor, or in some cases you may be able to use your own stem cells.

LIFESTYLE People with chronic myelogenous leukemia may live with the disease for years. Many will continue treatment with medication indefinitely. Some days, you may feel sick even if you don't look sick. And some days you may just be sick of having cancer.

If you're having problems coping or you're bothered by medication side effects, talk to your health care provider.

Lice

WHAT IS IT? Lice are tiny, wingless, parasitic insects that feed on your blood. They're easily spread through close personal contact and by sharing belongings. Several types of lice exist:

- **Head lice.** These lice develop on your scalp. They're easiest to see at the nape of your neck and over your ears.
- **Body lice.** These lice live in clothing and on bedding and move onto your skin to feed. Body lice most often affect people who aren't able to bathe or launder clothing regularly.
- **Pubic lice.** Commonly called crabs, they occur on the skin and hair of your pubic area and, less frequently, on body hair, such as chest hair, eyebrows or eyelashes.

SYMPTOM CHECKER Signs and symptoms include:

- Intense itching
- A tickling feeling from movement of hair
- Insects about the size of a sesame seed or slightly larger on your scalp, body, clothing, or pubic or other body hair
- Eggs (nits) that resemble tiny pussy willow buds on hair shafts
- Small, red bumps on the scalp, neck and shoulders

TREATMENT Treatment often involves the use of medicated shampoos or lotions. Steps taken at home also are important.

Head lice

Use medications as directed. Applying too much can cause red, irritated skin.

Over-the-counter products. Shampoos containing pyrethrin or permethrin (Nix) are often the first option to combat lice. You may need to repeat the treatment in 7 to 10 days. These products typically aren't recommended for children younger than age 2.

In some geographical locations, lice have grown resistant to the ingredients in over-the-counter products. If these products don't work, ask your health care provider to prescribe shampoos or lotions that contain different ingredients.

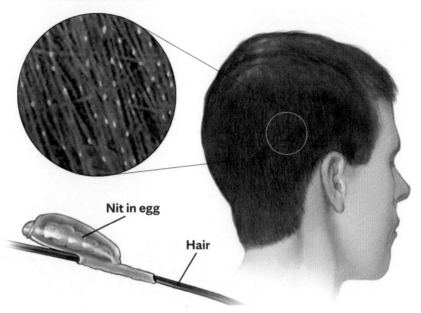

Nits attached to hair

Nit in egg

Hair

Prescription medications. They include malathion, a lotion, and spinosad, a liquid, and are applied to your hair and scalp. You may need to repeat the treatment.

Self-care. Make sure all nits are removed and all clothing, bedding, personal items and furniture are decontaminated.

- **After shampoo treatment, rinse hair with vinegar.** Grasp a lock of hair with a cloth saturated with vinegar and strip the lock downward to remove nits. Treat all the hair in this way. Or soak the hair with vinegar and leave it on a few minutes before combing. Use a fine-toothed or nit comb to physically remove lice and nits from wet hair. Repeat every 3 to 4 days for at least two weeks.
- **Wash contaminated items.** Wash bedding, stuffed animals, clothing and hats with hot, soapy water and dry them at high heat.
- **Seal unwashable items.** Put them in an airtight bag for two weeks.
- **Soak combs and brushes.** Soak them in hot, soapy water or rubbing alcohol for an hour. Another option is to buy new ones.

Body lice and pubic lice

Body lice generally don't need treatment. If self-care measures fail to get rid of the lice, your health care provider might recommend medication. Pubic lice can be treated with the same nonprescription and prescription treatments used for head lice.

Lung cancer

WHAT IS IT? Lung cancer is cancer that begins in the lungs. These organs in your chest take in oxygen when you inhale and release carbon dioxide when you exhale.

There are two general types of lung cancer: small cell lung cancer (SCLC) and non-small cell lung cancer (NSCLC). SCLC is seen mostly in smokers. It's more common than NSCLC.

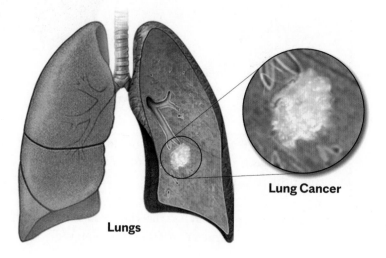

Lung Cancer

Lungs

Lung cancer begins in the cells of your lungs.

WHAT'S THE CAUSE? Smoking is the most common cause of lung cancer. The longer someone smokes and the more cigarettes smoked, the higher the risk of getting lung cancer. If you smoke, the most important thing you can do to prevent the disease is to stop.

Other risk factors for lung cancer include:

- Exposure to secondhand smoke
- Previous radiation therapy
- Exposure to radon gas
- Exposure to asbestos and other carcinogens
- Family history of lung cancer

If you have risk factors for lung cancer, your doctor may recommend annual screening with a CT scan imaging test. It's often done in older adults who have smoked heavily for many years or have quit in the past 15 years.

SYMPTOM CHECKER In the early stages, lung cancer usually doesn't cause symptoms. They're more likely to start when the disease is advanced and may include:

- A new cough that doesn't go away
- Coughing up even a small amount of blood
- Shortness of breath
- Chest pain
- Hoarseness
- Loss of weight without trying
- Bone pain
- Headaches

WHAT TESTS TO EXPECT If there's reason to think you have lung cancer, your health care provider can order tests to look for cancerous cells and rule out other conditions.

Test options include:

- **X-ray.** An X-ray of your lungs may show an abnormal mass or nodule.
- **Computerized tomography (CT).** A CT scan can reveal small lesions in the lung that might not be seen on an X-ray.
- **Sputum cytology.** If you cough up material when you cough hard, looking at the material (sputum) under the microscope can sometimes reveal the presence of cancer cells.
- **Tissue sample (biopsy.)** For a biopsy, some abnormal cells are taken from a person's lung. This can be done in several ways. A lighted tube can be passed down the throat and into the lungs (bronchoscopy). Alternatively, an incision can be made at the base of the neck so that surgical tools can take tissue samples. This may be done if your doctor wants to biopsy a lymph node. Another option is a needle biopsy, in which X-ray or CT images guide a needle through your chest wall and into lung tissue.

Analysis of cells from a biopsy of the lung will reveal whether you have cancer and what type. If lung cancer is diagnosed, the cells are studied carefully. Their characteristics can help determine your prognosis and guide treatment.

Once the cancer has been diagnosed, you may also have additional tests to determine the extent (stage). If an X-ray or CT shows lung cancer, a test called positron emission tomography may be done to see whether the disease has spread throughout your body (metastasized). Magnetic resonance imaging (MRI) may be done to see if there is cancer in the brain.

TREATMENT Treatment of lung cancer depends on its stage and a person's general health. The stage is indicated using numbers 1 to 4. Often, Roman numerals I to IV are used. Stage 1 is noninvasive, meaning it hasn't spread. Each higher numeral is increasingly invasive.

Non-small cell lung cancer
Stage 1 and Stage 2 disease are treated with surgical removal (resection).

With a wedge resection, the cancer and a margin of healthy tissue around it are removed. Some people need to have the lobe of the lung removed (lobectomy) or the entire lung (pneumonectomy).

People who have lung cancer surgery sometimes are given medication (chemotherapy) or radiation before to shrink the tumor or after to keep the disease from recurring.

Stage 3 disease is typically treated with chemotherapy and radiation therapy.

Stage 4 NSCLC is considered incurable. However, people with this diagnosis may receive chemotherapy and radiation therapy to ease their symptoms.

Small cell lung cancer
Most people diagnosed with SCLC have disease that has metastasized. Doctors commonly use a combination of chemotherapy and radiation therapy for SCLC, and it tends to respond well to treatment.

Some people are given a type of treatment that stimulates their own immune system to fight the cancer (immunotherapy).

Lupus

WHAT IS IT? Lupus is a chronic inflammatory disease in which your body's immune system attacks its own tissues and organs. Inflammation caused by lupus can affect many different body systems, including your joints, skin, kidneys, blood cells, brain, heart and lungs.

The most distinctive sign of lupus — a facial rash that resembles the wings of a butterfly unfolding across both cheeks — occurs in many but not all cases.

Lupus is more common in women. Although the disease affects people of all ages, it's most often diagnosed between the ages of 15 and 45. It's likely that lupus results from a combination of genetics and the environment. However, the exact cause of lupus in most cases is unknown. Some potential triggers include:

- **Sunlight.** Exposure to the sun may produce lupus skin lesions or trigger an immune response that can affect internal organs.
- **Infections.** Experiencing an infection can initiate lupus or cause a relapse.
- **Medications.** Certain types of anti-seizure medications, blood pressure medications and antibiotics may trigger the disease. People with drug-induced lupus usually see their symptoms go away when they stop taking the medication.

SYMPTOM CHECKER No two cases of lupus are exactly alike. Signs and symptoms may come on suddenly or develop slowly; they may be mild or severe; and they may be temporary or permanent.

Most people with lupus have mild disease characterized by episodes (flares) when signs and symptoms worsen for a while, then improve or even disappear completely for a time.

The most common signs and symptoms include:

- Joint pain, stiffness and swelling
- Butterfly-shaped rash on the face that covers the cheeks and bridge of the nose
- Skin lesions that appear or worsen with sun exposure (photosensitivity)

- Fatigue and fever
- Fingers and toes that turn white or blue when exposed to cold or during stressful periods (Raynaud's phenomenon)
- Shortness of breath
- Chest pain
- Dry eyes
- Headaches, confusion and memory loss

WHAT TESTS TO EXPECT Diagnosing lupus is difficult because signs and symptoms vary considerably from person to person. In addition, they may vary over time and overlap with those of other disorders.

No one test can diagnose lupus. The combination of signs and symptoms, blood and urine tests, and findings on a physical examination generally leads to the diagnosis.

If your health care provider suspects that lupus is affecting your lungs or heart, he or she may suggest an imaging test, such as an X-ray or echocardiogram. In some cases, it's necessary to remove (biopsy) a small sample of kidney tissue to check for kidney damage and determine the best course of treatment. The sample can be obtained with a needle or through a small incision.

TREATMENT Treatment for lupus depends on your signs and symptoms. As they flare and subside, you and your health care provider may find that you'll need to change medications or dosages.

Medications

Medications most commonly used to control lupus include:

Nonsteroidal anti-inflammatory drugs (NSAIDs). Over-the-counter NSAIDs, such as naproxen sodium (Aleve) and ibuprofen (Advil, Motrin IB, others), may be used to treat pain, swelling and fever associated with lupus. Stronger NSAIDs are available by prescription.

Antimalarial drugs. Medications commonly used to treat malaria, such as hydroxychloroquine (Plaquenil), also can help control lupus.

Corticosteroids. Prednisone and other types of corticosteroids can counter the inflammation of lupus, but they often produce long-term side effects — including weight gain, easy bruising, thinning bones (osteoporosis), high blood pressure, diabetes and an increased risk of infection. The risk of side effects increases the more you take and the longer you take them.

Immunosuppressants. Drugs that suppress the immune system may be helpful in serious cases of lupus, such as in the case of severe kidney disease. Examples include azathioprine (Imuran, Azasan), mycophenolate (CellCept), leflunomide (Arava) and methotrexate (Trexall). These drugs carry a risk of serious side effects including liver damage and an increased risk of cancer.

Biologics. The biologic medication belimumab (Benlysta) may reduce lupus symptoms in some people. For those who have not been helped by other medications, another biologic, rituximab (Rituxan, Truxima), may be beneficial.

LIFESTYLE Take steps to care for your body if you have lupus. Simple measures can help you prevent lupus flares, should they occur, and help you better cope with the symptoms you experience.

- **Get adequate rest.** People with lupus often experience persistent fatigue that's different from typical tiredness and that isn't necessarily relieved by rest. For that reason, it can be hard to judge when you need to slow down. Get plenty of sleep at night and naps or breaks during the day as needed.
- **Be sun smart.** Because ultraviolet light can trigger a flare, wear protective clothing — such as a hat, long-sleeved shirt and long pants — and use sunscreens with a sun protection factor (SPF) of at least 55 when you go outside.
- **Get regular exercise.** Exercise can help you recover from a flare, reduce your risk of a heart attack and other complications, and promote general well-being.
- **Eat a healthy diet.** For good health, eat a diet that emphasizes fruits, vegetables and whole grains. If you have high blood pressure or kidney damage, follow dietary recommendations.
- **Don't smoke.** Smoking increases your risk of cardiovascular disease and can worsen the effects of lupus on your heart and blood vessels.
- **See your health care provider regularly.** Having regular checkups instead of only seeing your provider when your symptoms worsen may help prevent flares as well as reduce your risk of serious complications.

Lyme disease

WHAT IS IT? Lyme disease is the most common tick-borne illness in North America and Europe. It's caused by the bacterium *Borrelia burgdorferi*. Deer ticks, which feed on the blood of animals and humans, can harbor the bacteria and spread it when feeding.

Only a minority of deer tick bites lead to Lyme disease. The longer the tick remains attached to your skin, the greater your risk of getting the disease. In most cases, to transmit Lyme disease, a deer tick must be attached for 36 to 48 hours. If you find an attached tick that looks swollen, it may have fed long enough to transmit bacteria.

Signs and symptoms of Lyme disease vary and usually affect more than one body system. The skin, joints and nervous system are affected most often.

SYMPTOM CHECKER These signs and symptoms may occur within a month after you've been infected:

- **Rash.** A small, red bump may appear at the site of the tick bite. This bump is typical after a tick bite and doesn't indicate Lyme disease. However, over the next few days, the redness may expand, forming a rash in a bull's-eye pattern with a red outer ring surrounding a clear area. This rash is one of the hallmarks of Lyme disease. In some people, the rash may spread to other parts of the body.
- **Flu-like symptoms.** Fever, chills, fatigue, body aches and a headache may accompany the rash.

Several weeks to months after infection, you may experience:

- **Joint pain.** You may develop bouts of severe pain and swelling. Your knees are especially likely to be affected, but the pain can shift from one joint to another.
- **Neurological problems.** Less frequently, symptoms may include inflammation of the membranes surrounding your brain (meningitis), temporary paralysis of one side of your face (Bell's palsy), numbness or weakness in your limbs, and impaired muscle movement.

Other less common signs and symptoms include heart problems, eye inflammation, liver inflammation (hepatitis) and severe fatigue.

TREATMENT Lab tests to identify antibodies to the *Borrelia burgdorferi* bacteria may be used to help confirm the diagnosis. These tests are most reliable a few weeks after an infection, after your body has time to develop antibodies.

If you're treated with appropriate antibiotics in the early stages of the disease, you're likely to recover completely. In later stages, response to treatment may be slower, but the majority of people with Lyme disease recover completely with appropriate treatment.

Antibiotics

Oral antibiotics are the standard treatment for early-stage Lyme disease. They include the drugs doxycycline, amoxicillin, cefuroxime and azithromycin. A 14- to 21-day course is usually recommended. Some studies suggest a shorter course may be equally effective.

If the disease involves the central nervous system, your health care provider may recommend treatment with an intravenous antibiotic for 14 to 28 days. This is usually effective in eliminating infection, but it may take some time to recover from your symptoms.

After treatment, a small number of people still experience some symptoms, such as muscle aches and fatigue. The cause of these continuing symptoms is unknown, and treatment with more antibiotics doesn't help.

BISMACINE

The Food and Drug Administration warns against the use of bismacine, an injectable compound prescribed by some alternative practitioners to treat Lyme disease. Bismacine, also known as chromacine, contains high levels of the metal bismuth. Bismuth is safely used in some oral medications for stomach ulcers, but it's not approved for use in injectable form or as a treatment for Lyme disease. It can lead to bismuth poisoning, which may cause heart and kidney failure.

Lymphedema

WHAT IS IT? Lymphedema refers to swelling that generally occurs in one of your arms or legs. Sometimes both arms or both legs swell.

The condition is most commonly caused by the removal of or damage to your lymph nodes as a part of cancer treatment. The condition results from a blockage in your lymphatic system, which is part of your immune system. The blockage prevents lymph fluid from draining properly. Fluid builds up and causes swelling.

SYMPTOM CHECKER Signs and symptoms of lymphedema in an affected arm or leg may include:

- Swelling
- A feeling of heaviness or tightness
- Restricted range of motion
- Aching or discomfort
- Recurring infections
- Hardening and thickening of the skin (fibrosis)

The swelling may range from mild, barely noticeable changes in the size of your arm or leg to extreme changes that make the limb heavy and hard to use.

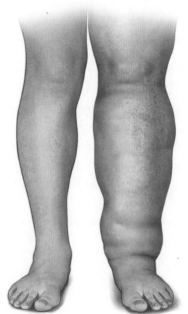

Lymphedema is swelling in an arm or a leg caused by a buildup of lymph fluid.

TREATMENT Treatment focuses on reducing the swelling.

Exercise. Light exercises in which you move the affected limb may encourage lymph fluid drainage. The exercises should focus on gentle contraction of the muscles in your arm or leg.

Wrapping the affected arm or leg. Bandaging your entire limb encourages lymph fluid to flow back toward the trunk of your body. The bandage should be tightest around your fingers or toes and loosen as it moves up your arm or leg.

Massage. A special massage technique called manual lymph drainage may encourage the flow of lymph fluid out of your arm or leg. Have it done by someone specially trained in the technique.

Pneumatic compression. A sleeve is worn over your affected arm or leg. It connects to a pump that intermittently inflates the sleeve, putting pressure on your limb and moving lymph fluid away from your fingers or toes.

Compression garments. Long sleeves or stockings made to compress your arm or leg encourage the flow of the lymph fluid out of your affected limb. Get help from a professional to make sure you obtain a correct fit.

In cases of severe lymphedema, your health care provider may consider surgery to remove excess tissue in your arm or leg to reduce swelling.

L

PREVENTION

To reduce your risk of lymphedema after cancer treatment:

- *Protect your arm or leg.* Avoid injury to your affected limb. Cuts and burns can invite infection. If possible, avoid procedures such as blood draws and vaccinations in the affected limb. Have your blood pressure taken in your other arm.
- *Rest your arm or leg.* After cancer treatment, exercise and stretching are encouraged. Avoid strenuous activity until you've recovered from surgery or radiation.
- *Avoid cold and heat.* Don't apply ice or heat, such as a heating pad, to the limb.
- *Elevate.* When possible, keep the affected limb above the level of your heart.
- *Avoid clothes that constrict the limb.* It's OK to wear compression garments.

Lymphoma

WHAT IS IT? Lymphoma is a cancer of the body's disease-fighting network (lymphatic system). The lymphatic system includes white cells called lymphocytes, lymph nodes (lymph glands), the spleen, thymus gland and bone marrow. Lymphoma can affect these as well as other organs throughout the body.

Many types of lymphoma exist, with the two main types being Hodgkin lymphoma and non-Hodgkin lymphoma. The main difference between Hodgkin and non-Hodgkin lymphoma is in the specific type of white blood cell (lymphocyte) involved.

Doctors and researchers can tell the difference between Hodgkin and non-Hodgkin lymphoma by examining the cancer cells under a microscope. If a large, irregular cell called a Reed-Sternberg cell is found, the lymphoma is classified as Hodgkin. If the Reed-Sternberg cell isn't present, the lymphoma is classified as non-Hodgkin.

Hodgkin lymphoma

Most often, Hodgkin lymphoma (formerly known as Hodgkin's disease) occurs when an infection-fighting cell called a B cell develops a change (mutation) in its DNA. The mutation tells the B cells to divide rapidly and to continue living when a typical, healthy cell would die. In turn, that causes a large number of oversized, irregular B cells to accumulate in the lymphatic system, where they crowd out healthy cells in your lymph nodes. This causes the lymph nodes, spleen and liver to swell and causes the symptoms of Hodgkin lymphoma.

Hodgkin lymphoma is most often diagnosed in people between the ages of 15 and 30 and those older than age 55. It is slightly more common in men, and having a close family member who's had lymphoma increases your risk. People who've had illnesses caused by the Epstein-Barr virus, such as infectious mononucleosis, are more likely to develop Hodgkin lymphoma than are people who haven't had the virus. Having a compromised immune system, such as from HIV/AIDS or from the use of immunosuppressive medications following an organ transplant, also increases your risk.

There are various subtypes of Hodgkin lymphoma.

Non-Hodgkin lymphoma

Non-Hodgkin lymphoma is more common than Hodgkin lymphoma. Similar to Hodgkin lymphoma, non-Hodgkin lymphoma occurs when your body produces too many irregular lymphocytes that continue to grow and divide. The disease may arise in infection-fighting B cells or T cells.

Non-Hodgkin lymphoma can occur at any age, but the risk increases with age. The disease is most common in people in their 60s or older. Similar to Hodgkin disease, use of immunosuppressive medications and certain infections, including the Epstein-Barr virus and HIV, may increase your risk of the disease.

Many different subtypes of non-Hodgkin lymphoma exist.

SYMPTOM CHECKER Signs and symptoms of lymphoma may include:

- Swollen lymph nodes in your neck, armpits or groin
- Fatigue
- Fever and chills
- Night sweats
- Abdominal pain or swelling
- Unexplained weight loss
- Loss of appetite
- Itching
- Chest pain, coughing or trouble breathing

WHAT TESTS TO EXPECT Tests and procedures used to diagnose lymphoma include a physical exam, blood tests, and imaging tests such as a computerized tomography (CT) scan or positron emission tomography (PET).

Minor surgery may be done to remove (biopsy) all or part of an enlarged lymph node for testing. A bone marrow biopsy may be used to look for signs of cancer in the bone marrow.

TREATMENT If your lymphoma appears to be slow growing (indolent), a wait-and-see approach may be an option. Indolent lymphomas that don't produce signs and symptoms may not require treatment for years. Your health care provider will likely schedule regular checkups every few months to monitor your condition and to ensure that your cancer isn't advancing.

If your lymphoma is aggressive or it causes signs and symptoms, your care provider may recommend treatment. Treatment options include the following:

Chemotherapy. Chemotherapy drugs may be taken in pill form or they may be administered through a vein in your arm. The medications may be given alone or they may be combined together. They also may be combined with other treatments, such as radiation therapy, monoclonal antibodies or a stem cell transplant. Several combinations of chemotherapy drugs are used to treat lymphoma.

Radiation therapy. Radiation therapy uses high-powered energy beams to kill cancerous cells and shrink tumors. Radiation therapy may be used alone or in combination with other cancer treatments. In the treatment of lymphoma, radiation therapy often follows chemotherapy.

Stem cell transplant. This treatment is intended to replace your diseased bone marrow with healthy stem cells that help you grow new bone marrow. During a stem cell transplant, your own blood stem cells are removed, frozen and stored for later use. You then receive high-dose chemotherapy and radiation therapy to destroy cancerous cells in your body. When those treatments are complete, the stem cells are thawed and injected into your body to help build healthy bone marrow, which in turn will produce healthy blood cells.

Biologic medications. These drugs help your body's immune system fight the cancer. Rituximab (Rituxan) is a type of monoclonal antibody that attaches to B cells and makes them more visible to your immune system, which can then attack the cancer cells. Rituximab lowers the number of B cells, including your healthy B cells, but your body produces new healthy B cells. The cancerous B cells are less likely to recur.

Radioimmunotherapy drugs. These medications are made of monoclonal antibodies that carry radioactive isotopes. The antibody attaches to cancer cells and delivers radiation directly to the cells. The radioimmunotherapy drug ibritumomab (Zevalin) is used to treat lymphoma.

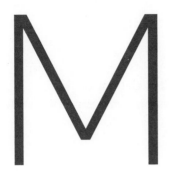

Macular degeneration

WHAT IS IT? Macular degeneration is a leading cause of vision loss in older adults. The disease affects the layer of tissue in the center of the retina (macula), and it destroys your sharp, central vision. There are two types — dry and wet.

Dry macular degeneration. Dry macular degeneration is marked by deterioration of the macula. It's the most common form of the disease and it's generally less severe. Dry macular degeneration typically develops with age — likely because over time, tissue in the macula may thin and break down. Dry macular degeneration can progress to wet macular degeneration, which is typically more severe and can cause rapid vision loss.

Wet macular degeneration. In this form of the disease, blood vessels grow under the retina in the back of the eye, leaking blood and fluid and damaging the macula. It's not clear exactly what causes wet macular degeneration. The condition almost always develops in people who've had dry macular degeneration. The risk may be higher for people who are white, those who are over 55 or obese, or those who smoke or have a family history of the condition.

SYMPTOM CHECKER Macular degeneration may produce the following vision changes:

- The need for brighter light when reading or doing close work
- Increasing difficulty adapting to low light levels
- Increasing blurriness of printed words
- A decrease in the intensity or brightness of colors

- Difficulty recognizing faces
- Decreased central vision
- Crooked central vision
- A blurred or blind spot in the center of the field of vision
- Visual distortions, such as straight lines appearing wavy or street signs looking lopsided

TREATMENT Dry macular degeneration usually progresses slowly, and many people who have it can live relatively typical, productive lives, especially if only one eye is affected. In the case of wet macular degeneration, early diagnosis may slow its progression and reduce the amount of vision loss.

Vitamins. A high-dose formulation of antioxidant vitamins and zinc may reduce the progression of dry macular degeneration. Your health care provider also may recommend eating more fruits, vegetables and other foods that contain nutrients believed to contribute to eye health. Omega-3 fatty acids found in some types of fish may help reduce macular degeneration-related vision loss.

Surgery. For some people with advanced dry macular degeneration in both eyes, surgery to implant a telescopic lens in one eye may be an option. The telescopic lens is equipped with lenses that magnify your field of vision and may improve both distance and close-up vision.

Medication. Medications may be prescribed for wet macular degeneration to help stop the growth of new blood vessels. Medications used to treat wet macular degeneration include bevacizumab (Avastin), ranibizumab (Lucentis), aflibercept (Eylea) and brolucizumab (Beovu). The drugs are injected directly into the eye.

Photodynamic therapy. If other medications aren't an option or aren't effective, this is occasionally used to treat wet macular degeneration. In this procedure, you're given a medication and then focused light from a special laser is directed at the irregular blood vessels in your eye. The light activates the medication causing the irregular blood vessels in your eye to close, which stops the leakage.

Laser therapy. Also a treatment for the wet form of the disease, a high-energy laser beam destroys irregular blood vessels under the macula. This procedure generally isn't an option if you have irregular blood vessels directly under the center of the macula.

M

Menopause

WHAT IS IT? Menopause is a natural biological process in women that marks the end of menstruation. It's diagnosed after 12 months without a period. Most women reach menopause in their 40s or 50s and may notice symptoms of hormone shifts for several years before and after. The phase of months or years leading up to menopause is called perimenopause.

Some women experience only mild symptoms during this time. Others are bothered by significant changes that can affect daily life. Symptoms that can accompany perimenopause and menopause include:

- Irregular periods
- Vaginal dryness
- Hot flashes
- Night sweats
- Sleep problems
- Mood changes
- Weight gain and slowed metabolism
- Thinning hair and dry skin

Surgery that removes both your uterus and your ovaries causes menopause without any transitional phase. You're likely to have hot flashes and other menopausal symptoms, which can be severe because the hormonal changes occur abruptly rather than over several years.

Common conditions

Changes in hormone levels that occur with menopause can result in a variety of conditions. Some of the more common conditions associated with menopause include:

Hot flashes. Hot flashes are sudden feelings of warmth, which are usually most intense over the face, neck and chest. Your skin may change color, as if you're blushing. Hot flashes can also cause profuse sweating and may leave you chilled. Hot flashes are likely related to several factors including changes in reproductive hormones and changes in your body's thermostat, which becomes more sensitive to slight changes in body temperature.

Urinary incontinence. As the tissues of your vagina and urethra lose elasticity, you may experience frequent, sudden, strong urges to urinate,

M

followed by an involuntary loss of urine (urge incontinence), or the loss of urine with coughing, laughing or lifting (stress incontinence). You may experience urinary tract infections more often.

Changes in sexual function. Vaginal dryness from decreased moisture production and loss of elasticity can cause discomfort and slight bleeding during sexual intercourse. Decreased sensation may reduce your desire for sexual activity.

Weight gain. Weight gain is common after menopause because hormone changes can slow metabolism.

TREATMENT Treatment for menopause focuses mainly on relieving symptoms. Options include:

Hormone therapy. Estrogen therapy is the most effective treatment for relieving menopausal hot flashes. Depending on your personal and family medical history, your health care provider may recommend estrogen for a period of time to provide symptom relief. Estrogen also helps prevent bone loss. If you still have your uterus, you'll also need progestin to decrease the risk of endometrial cancer. Long-term use of hormone therapy may have some cardiovascular and breast cancer risks, but starting hormones around the time of menopause has shown benefits for some women.

Vaginal estrogen. Estrogen can be administered directly to the vagina using a vaginal cream, tablet or ring. This treatment releases just a small amount of estrogen, which is absorbed by the vaginal tissues. Estrogen can help relieve vaginal dryness, discomfort with intercourse and some urinary symptoms.

Low-dose antidepressants. A class of drugs called selective serotonin reuptake inhibitors (SSRIs) may decrease menopausal hot flashes. The medication may be helpful for women who can't or don't want to take estrogen or for women who need an antidepressant for a mood disorder.

Gabapentin (Gralise, Horizant, Neurontin). This drug, which is approved to treat seizures, has also been shown to reduce hot flashes.

LIFESTYLE Many of the symptoms associated with menopause are temporary and often can be relieved with simple self-care measures.

For hot flashes

To manage hot flashes, dress in layers so you can easily shed clothes if you need to. Have a cold glass of water when you feel hot flashes coming on. Go somewhere cooler, if possible. Try to pinpoint what triggers your hot flashes. For many women, triggers include hot beverages, caffeine, spicy foods, alcohol, stress, hot weather and even a warm room. Once you know your triggers, try to avoid them or be prepared for how to deal with them.

For vaginal discomfort

To reduce pain and discomfort during intercourse, use nonprescription, water-based vaginal lubricants (Astroglide, K-Y jelly, others) or moisturizers (Replens, others). Choose products that don't contain glycerin, which can cause burning or irritation in women who are sensitive to that chemical. Staying sexually active also helps by increasing blood flow to the vagina.

For urinary incontinence

Pelvic floor muscle exercises, called Kegel exercises, can improve some forms of urinary incontinence by strengthening key muscles. Practice Kegels daily (see page 361).

For sleep troubles

There are several things you can do to improve sleep. Avoid caffeine, which can make it difficult to get to sleep. Don't drink too much alcohol, which can wake you up in the middle of the night. Exercise will help you sleep better, but don't exercise in the evening before bedtime. If hot flashes wake you up during the night, talk to your health care provider about treatment to reduce or relieve them. Practicing relaxation techniques also may help with sleep and other symptoms.

For weight gain

The best approach for losing weight or maintaining your weight is to eat a healthy diet that includes a variety of fruits, vegetables and whole grains. Limit saturated fats, oils and sugars, including alcohol. Exercise for at least 30 minutes most days of the week. In addition to helping you manage your weight, a healthy diet and regular exercise help protect against heart disease, osteoporosis and other conditions that become more common after menopause.

M

Mononucleosis

WHAT IS IT? Infectious mononucleosis, also called mono, is a disease that results from the Epstein-Barr virus. It most commonly affects adolescents and young adults.

The virus is transmitted through saliva, so you can get it through kissing or sharing utensils with someone who has mono. You may also be exposed through a cough or sneeze. However, mononucleosis isn't as contagious as some infections, such as the common cold.

Symptoms of mononucleosis may include:

- Fatigue
- Feeling unwell (malaise)
- Sore throat, but unlike bacterial strep throat, it doesn't get better with antibiotics
- Fever
- Swollen lymph nodes in the neck and armpits
- Swollen tonsils
- Headache
- Skin rash
- Soft, swollen spleen

The virus has an incubation period of approximately 4 to 6 weeks, although in young children this period may be shorter. Symptoms such as fever and sore throat usually lessen within a couple of weeks. Fatigue, enlarged lymph nodes and a swollen spleen may last for a number of weeks longer.

TREATMENT Your health care provider may suspect mononucleosis based on your signs and symptoms, how long they've lasted, and a physical examination.

Blood tests that check for antibodies to the Epstein-Barr virus can confirm the diagnosis. Your provider may use other blood tests to look for an elevated number of white blood cells (lymphocytes) or irregular-looking lymphocytes.

There's no specific therapy to treat infectious mononucleosis. Antibiotics don't work against viral infections such as mono. Treatment mainly

M

involves bed rest and addressing severe symptoms or other problems that may arise.

Self-care

In addition to bed rest, these steps may help relieve symptoms of mononucleosis:

Drink plenty of liquids. Water and fruit juice are best. Fluids help reduce fever, soothe a sore throat and prevent dehydration.

Take pain relievers. Over-the-counter pain relievers, such as acetaminophen (Tylenol, others) or ibuprofen (Advil, Motrin IB, others) may be taken as needed to relieve a fever or pain from a sore throat. Although aspirin is approved for use in children older than age 3, children and teenagers recovering from flu-like symptoms should never take aspirin. That use has been linked to Reye's syndrome, a rare but potentially life-threatening condition.

Gargle with salt water. Do this several times a day to relieve a sore throat. Mix a teaspoon of salt in 8 ounces of warm water.

Medications

Occasionally, a streptococcal (strep) infection accompanies the sore throat of mononucleosis. You may also develop a sinus infection or an infection of your tonsils (tonsillitis). You may need treatment with antibiotics for these bacterial infections.

To ease more-severe symptoms, such as severe swelling of your throat and tonsils, your health care provider may prescribe a corticosteroid medication such as prednisone.

Most symptoms of mononucleosis ease within a few weeks, but it may be 2 to 3 months before you feel completely recovered. The more rest you get, the sooner you should recover. Returning to your usual schedule too soon can increase the risk of a relapse.

Mononucleosis can cause enlargement of the spleen, which needs time to heal. To avoid risk of rupturing your spleen, wait until your health care provider says it's safe to return to contact sports, heavy lifting or vigorous activities. Your provider can recommend a gradual exercise program to help you rebuild strength as you recover.

M

Morton neuroma

WHAT IS IT? Morton neuroma is a painful condition that occurs on the bottom of your foot and affects the ball of your foot. You may feel as if you're standing on a pebble in your shoe or on a fold in your sock.

Morton neuroma involves a thickening of the tissue around one of the nerves leading to your toes. It can cause a sharp, burning pain on the bottom of your foot that may radiate into your toes. Your toes may also sting, burn or feel numb. Typically, there's no outward sign of this condition, such as a lump.

Factors that appear to contribute to Morton neuroma include:

- **High heels.** High-heeled shoes or shoes that are tight or ill fitting can place extra pressure on your toes and the ball of your foot.
- **Certain sports.** High-impact athletic activities such as running may subject your feet to repetitive trauma. Sports that feature tight shoes, such as snow skiing or rock climbing, can put pressure on your toes.
- **Foot deformities.** People with bunions, hammertoes, high arches or flat feet are at higher risk of developing Morton neuroma.

WHAT TESTS TO EXPECT
There is no specific test for the condition.

In making a diagnosis, your health care provider may press on your foot to feel for a mass or tender spot. There may also be what feels like a rubbing or "clicking" between the bones of your foot. Sometimes an imaging test may be helpful.

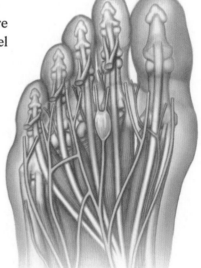

Morton neuroma involves the thickening of the tissue around one of the nerves leading to the toes.

M

TREATMENT Treatment depends on the severity of your symptoms. Your provider will likely recommend trying conservative approaches first.

Self-care

To help relieve the pain associated with Morton neuroma and allow the nerve to heal, consider the following self-care tips:

- **Take anti-inflammatory medications.** Over-the-counter nonsteroidal anti-inflammatory medications, such as ibuprofen (Advil, Motrin IB, others) and naproxen sodium (Aleve), can reduce swelling and relieve pain.
- **Try ice massage.** Freeze a water-filled paper cup or plastic foam cup and roll the ice over the painful site.
- **Change your footwear.** Avoid high heels or tight shoes. Choose shoes with a broad toe box and extra depth.
- **Take a break.** For a few weeks, reduce activities such as running, aerobic exercise or dancing that subject your feet to high impact.

Therapy

Your doctor or a physical therapist may prescribe an arch support or foot pad that fits inside your shoe and helps reduce pressure on the nerve. Arch supports or foot pads can be purchased without a prescription, or you can purchase a custom-made, individually designed shoe insert to fit the exact contours of your foot.

Injections

Some people are helped by the injection of steroids into the painful area. This can relieve the swelling and inflammation of the nerve.

Surgery

If conservative treatments don't help, your health care provider might recommend one of the following:

- **Decompression surgery.** A surgeon may be able to relieve pressure on the nerve by cutting nearby structures, such as the ligament that binds together some of the bones in the front of the foot.
- **Removal of the nerve.** Surgical removal of the neuroma may be necessary if other treatments don't provide pain relief. Surgery is usually successful, but it can result in permanent numbness in the affected toes.

Multiple sclerosis

WHAT IS IT? Multiple sclerosis (MS) is a disease in which the immune system attacks the protective sheath (myelin) that covers nerves. This causes a disruption in communication between the brain and the rest of the body. Ultimately, the nerves themselves may deteriorate.

It isn't clear why MS develops in some people and not others. Factors that may increase your risk include a family history of the disease and being female. Women are about twice as likely as men are to develop MS. A variety of viruses also have been linked to MS, including Epstein-Barr, the virus that causes mononucleosis.

White people, especially those of Northern European descent, are at highest risk of developing MS. The disease is more common in regions further from the equator, including Canada, the northern United States, New Zealand, southeastern Australia and Europe. Having low exposure to sunlight and low levels of vitamin D also increases the risk.

SYMPTOM CHECKER Symptoms vary widely, depending on the amount of damage and which nerves are affected. Some people lose the ability to walk, while others experience long periods of remission. Symptoms may include:

- Numbness or weakness in one or more limbs that often occurs on one side of your body at a time
- Partial or complete loss of vision, usually in one eye at a time
- Double vision or blurring of vision
- Tingling or pain in parts of your body
- Electric-shock sensations that occur with certain neck movements
- Tremor, lack of coordination or unsteady gait
- Slurred speech
- Fatigue
- Dizziness
- Problems with bowel and bladder function

Most people with MS have a relapsing-remitting course, with new symptoms (relapse) that develop over days or weeks and that improve partially or completely, followed by a quiet period (remission) that can last months or years. About 60% to 70% of people with relapsing-remitting MS eventually develop a steady progression of symptoms.

M

NERVE

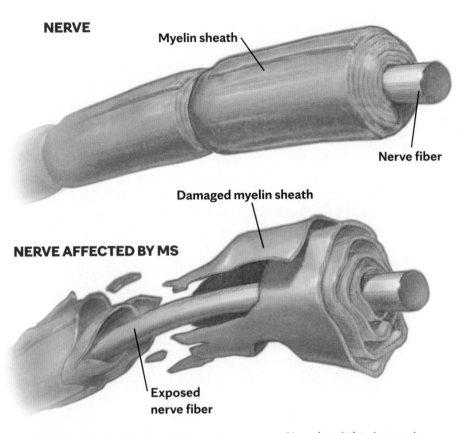

Myelin sheath

Nerve fiber

Damaged myelin sheath

NERVE AFFECTED BY MS

Exposed nerve fiber

In multiple sclerosis, the protective coating on nerve fibers (myelin) is damaged, disrupting brain communication. Ultimately, the nerves may deteriorate.

TREATMENT Treatment of multiple sclerosis typically focuses on speeding recovery from disease flares, slowing the progression of the disease and managing its symptoms. In some instances, people have such mild symptoms that no treatment is necessary.

Manage attacks

To treat disease flares, your health care provider may recommend:

- **Corticosteroids.** Medications such as prednisone or methylprednisolone are prescribed to reduce nerve inflammation.
- **Plasma exchange (plasmapheresis).** The liquid portion of part of your blood (plasma) is removed and separated from your blood cells. The blood cells are then mixed with a protein solution (albumin) and put back into your body. Plasma exchange may be used if your symptoms are new and severe and haven't responded to steroids.

Modify progression

No therapies have shown benefit for slowing disease that follows a steadily progressive course. For disease that includes periods of remission (relapsing-remitting MS), certain medications may lower the relapse rate and reduce the formation of new lesions, particularly early on. Medications that may reduce the relapse rate include:

- **Interferon beta medications.** They're injected under the skin or into muscle. You'll need regular blood tests to monitor for liver disease.
- **Glatiramer acetate (Copaxone, Glatopa).** This is injected beneath the skin and may help block the immune system's attack on myelin.
- **Dimethyl fumarate (Tecfidera).** This is an oral medication you take twice daily.
- **Fingolimod (Gilenya).** This is an oral medication. You'll need to have your heart rate monitored for six hours after the first dose because your heart rate may slow.
- **Teriflunomide (Aubagio).** This medication is taken daily.
- **Natalizumab (Tysabri).** It's generally given to people with more-severe MS or those who can't tolerate other treatments.
- **Mitoxantrone.** This also is used only to treat severe, advanced MS.

Manage symptoms

Treatments used to manage symptoms may include:

- **Physical therapy.** A physical therapist can teach you stretching and strengthening exercises to help maintain muscle flexibility.
- **Muscle relaxants.** They help control muscle stiffness or spasms, particularly in the legs. Muscle relaxants include the drugs baclofen (Lioresal, Gablofen) and tizanidine (Zanaflex).
- **Other medications.** Medications may be prescribed to treat fatigue, depression, pain, and bladder or bowel control problems associated with MS.

LIFESTYLE To help relieve the signs and symptoms:

- **Get plenty of rest.** Rest is important for managing symptoms.
- **Exercise.** For mild to moderate MS, regular exercise can help improve strength, muscle tone, balance and coordination.
- **Eat a balanced diet.** A diet low in saturated fat and high in omega-3 fatty acids may be beneficial.
- **Relieve stress.** Stress may trigger or worsen symptoms.

N

Nasal polyps

WHAT IS IT? Nasal polyps are soft, painless, noncancerous growths on the lining of the nasal passages or sinuses. They result from chronic inflammation due to asthma, recurring infection, allergies, drug sensitivity or certain immune disorders.

Small nasal polyps may not cause any problems. Larger growths or groups of nasal polyps can block the nasal passages or lead to breathing problems, a lost sense of smell and frequent infections.

SYMPTOM CHECKER Signs and symptoms include:

- Persistent stuffiness
- Postnasal drip
- Decreased sense of smell and taste
- Facial pain or pressure, headache, pain in the upper teeth
- Snoring
- Itching around the eyes

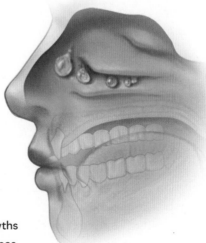

Nasal polyps are noncancerous growths that hang down like teardrops or grapes.

TREATMENT Treatment is aimed at reducing the size of the polyps or eliminating them entirely.

Medications

Drug treatments may include:

Nasal corticosteroids. A corticosteroid nasal spray that reduces inflammation may shrink the polyps or eliminate them completely.

Oral and injectable corticosteroids. Injectable corticosteroids may be used if nasal polyps are severe. An oral corticosteroid, such as prednisone, may be prescribed for a brief period. Oral corticosteroids can cause serious side effects.

Other medications. Antihistamines to treat allergies or antibiotics to treat a chronic or recurring infection may be recommended. Some people benefit from aspirin desensitization therapy and treatment.

Surgery

If drug treatment isn't effective, you may need surgery to remove the polyps and correct problems with your sinuses that make them prone to inflammation and polyp development. Surgery is typically performed by inserting a small tube with a magnifying lens or tiny camera (endoscope) into your nostrils and sinus cavities. Tiny instruments are used to remove the polyps and other obstructions that block the flow of fluids from your sinuses. Your surgeon may also enlarge the openings leading from your sinuses to your nasal passages.

Self-care

To slow the growth of nasal polyps, try the following strategies:

- **Manage allergies and asthma.** They can worsen symptoms.
- **Avoid nasal irritants.** As much as possible, avoid breathing substances that can cause inflammation such as allergens, tobacco smoke, chemical fumes and dust.
- **Humidify your home.** Keeping your breathing passages moistened may improve the flow of mucus from your sinuses.
- **Use a nasal rinse or nasal lavage.** Use a saltwater (saline) spray or nasal lavage to rinse your nasal passages. This may improve mucus flow and remove allergens and other irritants. You can purchase over-the-counter saline sprays or nasal lavage kits.

Neck pain

WHAT'S THE CAUSE? Neck muscles can be strained from poor posture — whether it's leaning into your computer at work or hunching over your workbench at home. Wear-and-tear arthritis also can result in neck pain. Rarely, neck pain is a symptom of a more serious problem.

Common causes of neck pain include:

- **Muscle strain.** Overuse, such as too many hours hunched over a steering wheel, can trigger muscle strain. Even such minor things such as reading in bed or gritting your teeth can strain your neck muscles.
- **Arthritic joints.** Just like all the other joints in your body, your neck joints tend to undergo wear and tear with age, which can cause osteoarthritis in your neck or cervical spondylosis. Cervical spondylosis is a general term for age-related wear and tear affecting the spinal disks in your neck.
- **Nerve compression.** Herniated disks or bone spurs in the vertebrae of your neck can take up too much space and press on the nerves branching out from the spinal cord.
- **Injuries.** Rear-end auto collisions can result in whiplash injuries, which occur when the head is jerked backward and then forward, stretching the soft tissues of the neck beyond their limits.
- **Diseases.** Neck pain can sometimes stem from diseases such as rheumatoid arthritis or meningitis.

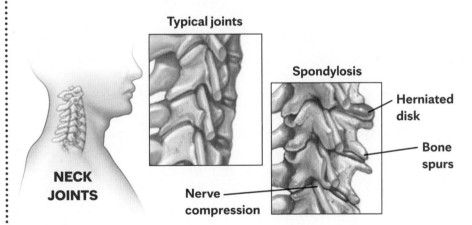

Cervical spondylosis is a general term for age-related wear and tear affecting the joints in the neck. Disks may bulge (herniate) and bone spurs may form, pressing on spinal nerves.

N-O

WHAT TESTS TO EXPECT In addition to doing a physical exam, your health care provider may order imaging tests to get a better picture of what might be causing the pain. These may include:

- **X-rays.** X-rays can reveal areas in your neck where your nerves or spinal cord may be pinched by bone spurs or a bulging disk.
- **Computerized tomography (CT) scan.** A CT scan provides detailed views of the internal structures of your neck.
- **Magnetic resonance imaging (MRI).** An MRI may be used to get detailed views of the spinal cord and the nerves coming from the spinal cord.

If your provider suspects that your neck pain may be related to a pinched nerve, you may have a test called electromyography (EMG). It involves inserting very fine needles through your skin into a muscle to determine whether specific nerves are functioning properly.

Blood tests may be ordered if an infection or inflammation is thought to be at fault. If you have a stiff neck and a fever and meningitis is suspected, your provider may recommend a lumbar puncture (spinal tap) to analyze your spinal fluid.

TREATMENT Most neck pain responds well to self-care. If the pain persists, your provider may recommend other treatments.

Self-care

Steps you can take on your own to relieve neck pain include:

Over-the-counter pain relievers. These include ibuprofen (Advil, Motrin IB, others), naproxen sodium (Aleve) and acetaminophen (Tylenol, others).

Heat and cold. To reduce inflammation, apply cold to your neck for up to 20 minutes several times day. You can use an ice pack or ice wrapped in a towel. You might alternate the cold treatment with heat, such as a heating pad on the low setting. Heat can help relax sore muscles, but it sometimes can make inflammation worse, so use it with caution.

Rest. Lie down from time to time during the day to give your neck a rest from holding up your head. But avoid prolonged rest. Too much inactivity can cause increased stiffness in your neck muscles.

N-O

Gentle stretching. Gently move your neck to one side and hold it for about 30 seconds. Then move it to another position. Stretch your neck in as many directions as your pain allows.

Medications

If nonprescription medications aren't helpful, your health care provider may prescribe stronger pain medicine. Muscle relaxants or tricyclic antidepressant medications also may be used to treat pain.

Therapy

Possible treatments include:

Neck exercises and stretching. A physical therapist can teach you about neck exercises and stretches. Exercises may improve pain by restoring muscle function, optimizing posture to prevent overload of muscle, and increasing the strength and endurance of your neck muscles.

Transcutaneous electrical nerve stimulation (TENS). Electrodes placed on your skin near the painful areas deliver tiny electrical impulses that may relieve pain.

Traction. Traction uses weights and pulleys to gently stretch your neck and keep it immobilized. This therapy, under supervision of a medical professional and physical therapist, may provide relatively fast relief of some neck pain, especially pain related to nerve root irritation.

Short-term immobilization. A soft collar that supports your neck can take pressure off the structures in your neck. If used for more than 1 to 2 weeks, however, a collar may do more harm than good.

Surgery and other procedures

Possible treatments include:

Steroid injections. Corticosteroid medications may be injected near the nerve roots, into the small facet joints in the bones of the cervical spine or into the muscles in the neck to help with pain. Numbing medications, such as lidocaine, also can be injected to relieve neck pain.

Surgery. Surgery is rarely needed for neck pain, but it may be an option for relieving nerve root or spinal cord compression.

Nonallergic rhinitis

WHAT IS IT? Nonallergic rhinitis, also called vasomotor rhinitis, is a condition characterized by chronic sneezing or having a congested, drippy nose with no apparent cause. The symptoms of nonallergic rhinitis are similar to those of hay fever (allergic rhinitis), but there's no identifiable allergic reaction involved.

Although nonallergic rhinitis is more annoying than harmful, it can make you miserable. Triggers of nonallergic rhinitis include certain odors or irritants in the air, changes in the weather, some medications, certain foods, and chronic health conditions.

SYMPTOM CHECKER Signs and symptoms of nonallergic rhinitis may include:

- Stuffy nose
- Runny nose
- Sneezing
- Mucus (phlegm) in the throat (postnasal drip)

Nonallergic rhinitis doesn't usually cause itchy nose, eyes or throat — symptoms associated with allergies such as hay fever.

A diagnosis of nonallergic rhinitis is generally made based on your symptoms and by ruling out other causes, especially allergies. You may need to undergo allergy testing, which may involve skin or blood tests. Your health care provider may also look inside your nasal passages and sinus cavities to make sure your symptoms aren't caused by a problem such as a deviated septum or nasal polyps. This is done with a thin, fiber-optic viewing instrument called an endoscope.

TREATMENT Treatment of nonallergic rhinitis depends on how much it bothers you. For mild cases, home treatment and avoiding triggers may be enough. For symptoms that are hard to tolerate, certain medications may provide relief.

Saline nasal sprays. Use a nonprescription saline nasal spray or homemade saltwater solution to flush the nose of irritants and help thin the mucus and soothe the membranes in your nose.

Corticosteroid nasal sprays. A nonprescription corticosteroid nasal spray, such as fluticasone (Flonase Allergy Relief) or triamcinolone (Nasacort Allergy 24 Hour), helps prevent and treat inflammation associated with some types of nonallergic rhinitis. Prescription nasal sprays also are available.

Antihistamine nasal sprays. Oral antihistamines don't seem to help nonallergic rhinitis. But an antihistamine in the form of a nasal spray — azelastine (Astepro) or olopatadine hydrochloride (Patanase) — may reduce symptoms in some people.

Anti-drip anticholinergic nasal sprays. The prescription drug ipratropium in nasal spray form can be helpful if a runny, drippy nose is your main complaint.

Oral decongestants. The over-the-counter drugs pseudoephedrine (Sudafed 12 Hour) and phenylephrine help narrow blood vessels, reducing congestion in the nose.

Decongestant nasal sprays. These include oxymetazoline (Afrin, others). Don't use these over-the-counter products for more than three or four days, as that can actually cause symptoms to worsen.

Self-care

These tips can help reduce discomfort and relieve the symptoms of nonallergic rhinitis. For people with mild symptoms, self-care may be all the treatment that's needed.

- **Rinse your nasal passages.** Nasal irrigation involves rinsing out your sinuses with a salt-and-water solution. You can use a neti pot or a specially designed squeeze bottle to flush out thickened mucus and irritants from your nose. When performed daily, this is one of the most effective treatments for nonallergic rhinitis. Rinse the device after each use with distilled or sterile water and leave open to air-dry.
- **Humidify.** Set up a humidifier at home or work. Breathe in the steam from a warm shower to help loosen the mucus.
- **Stay hydrated.** Drink plenty of liquids, especially water. Avoid caffeinated beverages, which can cause dehydration and aggravate your symptoms.
- **Avoid your triggers.** If you are able to identify things that cause or worsen your symptoms, try to avoid them.

Nosebleeds

TREATMENT Many people experience a nosebleed on occasion. A nosebleed may be scary, but generally it's a minor annoyance. Most nosebleeds stop on their own or stop after a few self-care steps.

Sit upright and lean forward. By remaining upright, you reduce blood pressure in the veins of your nose. This discourages further bleeding. Sitting forward will help you avoid swallowing blood, which can irritate your stomach.

Pinch your nose. Use your thumb and index finger to pinch both nostrils shut, even if only one side is bleeding. Breathe through your mouth. Continue to pinch for 5 to 10 minutes. This maneuver puts pressure on the bleeding point on the nasal septum and often stops the flow of blood.

Repeat. If the bleeding doesn't stop, repeat these steps for up to a total of 15 minutes.

After the bleeding has stopped, to keep it from starting again, don't pick or blow your nose and don't bend down for several hours. Keep your head higher than the level of your heart.

Talk to your health care provider if you're having frequent nosebleeds, even if you can stop them fairly easily. Frequent nosebleeds are those that occur more than once a week. It's important to determine what's causing them.

EMERGENCY CARE

Some nosebleeds require immediate care. See a health care provider if the bleeding:

- Is severe
- Lasts longer than 30 minutes
- Interferes with your breathing
- Follows an injury, such as a fall or a car accident

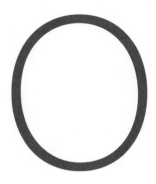

Obesity

WHAT IS IT? Obesity is a complex disorder involving an excessive amount of body fat. Obesity increases the risk of many health problems, including heart disease, diabetes and high blood pressure.

You're considered obese when your body mass index (BMI) is 30 or higher. Your body mass index is calculated by dividing your weight in kilograms (kg) by your height in meters (m) squared. For most people, BMI is a reasonable estimate of body fat. But some people, such as muscular athletes, may have a BMI in the obese category even though they don't have excess body fat.

WHAT'S THE CAUSE? Although there are genetic, hormonal, behavioral and metabolic influences on body weight, obesity typically occurs when you take in more calories than you burn through exercise and usual daily activities. Your body stores these excess calories as fat. Obesity usually results from a combination of factors. Some of the more common factors include:

- **Family inheritance and influence.** Your genes may affect the amount of body fat you store and where that fat is distributed. Genetics may also play a role in how efficiently your body converts food into energy and how your body burns calories during exercise. In addition, family members may share similar eating and activity habits.
- **Lifestyle choices.** If you're not very active, you can easily take in more calories every day than you burn. You're also more likely to be obese if your diet is high in calories, lacks fruits and vegetables, includes a lot of fast food, and is laden with high-calorie beverages and oversized portions. All contribute to weight gain.

- **Lack of sleep.** Too little sleep can cause changes in hormones that increase your appetite. You may also crave foods high in calories and carbohydrates, which can contribute to weight gain.
- **Social and economic issues.** Avoiding obesity is difficult if you don't have safe areas to walk or exercise, you were never taught healthy ways of cooking, or you don't have access to healthy foods.
- **Certain medications.** Some medications are associated with weight gain. They include some antidepressants, anti-seizure medications, diabetes medications, antipsychotic medications, corticosteroids and beta blockers.
- **Medical problems.** Obesity can sometimes be traced to a medical cause, such as Prader-Willi syndrome or Cushing syndrome. Some medical problems, such as arthritis, can lead to decreased activity, which may result in weight gain.
- **Microbiome.** Your gut bacteria are affected by what you eat and may contribute to weight gain or difficulty losing weight.

TREATMENT The goal of treatment is to reach and stay at a healthy weight. Weight-loss therapies include:

Dietary changes

Reducing calories and eating healthy foods are vital to overcoming obesity. Slow and steady weight loss over a longer period of time is considered the safest way to lose weight and the best way to keep it off. You and your health care provider can determine how many calories you should consume each day to lose weight, but a typical amount is 1,200 to 1,500 calories for women and 1,500 to 1,800 for men. Aim to adopt healthy-eating habits you can stick with for the long term.

Exercise and activity

People who are able to lose weight and maintain their weight loss for more than a year generally get regular exercise. Aim for at least 150 minutes a week of moderate-intensity physical activity. To achieve more-significant weight loss, you may need to exercise more. Extra movement throughout the day also helps burn calories.

Behavior changes

A behavior modification program examines your habits to find out what factors or situations may have contributed to your obesity and helps you make changes. Therapy can be one-on-one or in a support group.

Prescription medications

If other methods haven't worked, several medications approved for weight loss may be an option.

- **Bupropion-naltrexone (Contrave).** This medication combines two drugs that work together in the brain to reduce hunger signals and control cravings. Common side effects include nausea, headache and constipation.
- **Orlistat (Xenical).** It blocks the digestion and absorption of fat in the stomach and intestines. Unabsorbed fat is eliminated in the stool, which can cause unpleasant side effects. A reduced-strength version of orlistat (Alli) is sold without a prescription.
- **Liraglutide (Saxenda).** Liraglutide is also used to manage diabetes. Unlike other weight-loss drugs, liraglutide is given by injection. Nausea is a common complaint.
- **Phentermine-topiramate (Qsymia).** It combines a short-term weight-loss drug with a medication used to control seizures.
- **Semaglutide (Ozempic, Wegovy).** This newer drug is given by weekly injections. In people with obesity caused by certain conditions, this medication may be used together with diet and exercise to help lose weight and keep the weight off.

Surgery

Weight-loss surgery can help you lose much of your excess body weight. Some weight-loss procedures can now be done endoscopically, in which flexible tubes are inserted through the mouth and throat instead of needing surgical incisions. But to keep the weight off, you still need to make lifestyle changes. Weight-loss surgeries include:

- **Gastric bypass surgery.** A surgeon creates a small pouch at the top of your stomach. The small intestine is cut a short distance below the main stomach and connected to the new pouch. Food and liquid flow directly from the pouch into the small intestine, bypassing most of your stomach.
- **Gastric sleeve.** Part of the stomach is removed, creating a smaller reservoir for food. It's a less complicated surgery than gastric bypass.
- **Adjustable gastric banding.** Your stomach is separated into two pouches with an inflatable band. Pulling the band tight, like a belt, the surgeon creates a tiny channel between the two pouches. The band keeps the opening from expanding. This procedure has become less common than other procedures because the results typically aren't as good.

Obsessive-compulsive disorder

 WHAT IS IT? Obsessive-compulsive disorder (OCD) is a pattern of unwanted thoughts and fears (obsessions) that lead to repetitive behaviors (compulsions). These obsessions and compulsions interfere with daily activities and cause significant distress.

 WHAT'S THE CAUSE? The cause of OCD isn't fully understood. Biology and genetics may each play a role. Obsessive fears and compulsive behaviors can be learned from watching family members or gradually learned over time.

Factors that may increase your risk of developing OCD or can trigger it include:

- Family history of OCD
- Stressful life events
- Other mental health disorders, such as anxiety disorder, depression, substance misuse or tic disorders

 SYMPTOM CHECKER People with OCD usually have both obsessions and compulsions that last at least six months. Some people have only obsessions or only compulsions. These behaviors can take up a lot of time and make it difficult to function in social situations, at school or at work.

Common examples of obsessive behaviors linked with OCD are being afraid to touch objects that others have touched or doubting that you've locked a door or turned off the stove.

Obsessions often have themes to them, such as:

- Fear of contamination or dirt
- Doubting and having difficulty tolerating uncertainty
- Needing things orderly and symmetrical
- Thoughts about being aggressive, losing control and harming yourself or others
- Unwanted thoughts about sexual or religious objects

Compulsions are repetitive behaviors you feel driven to perform. They're meant to reduce your anxiety about your obsessions or prevent something bad from happening. However, engaging in compulsions doesn't make you happy and may not relieve your anxiety for long.

Common examples of compulsive behaviors linked with OCD are washing your hands until the skin becomes raw, checking doors repeatedly to make sure they're locked, and counting in certain patterns. Themes common to compulsions include:

- Washing and cleaning
- Checking
- Counting
- Orderliness
- Following a strict routine
- Demanding reassurance

TREATMENT See your health care provider if your obsessions or compulsions are affecting your quality of life. There's a difference between being a perfectionist and having OCD. OCD thoughts aren't simply excessive worries about real problems in your life or liking to have things clean or arranged in a certain way.

The two main treatments for OCD are psychotherapy and medications. Often, a combination of these is most effective. Treatment for OCD may not cure the disorder, but it can help bring your symptoms under control so that they don't rule your daily life. If your OCD is severe, you may need long-term, ongoing or more-intensive treatment.

Psychotherapy

Cognitive behavioral therapy (CBT) is effective for many people with OCD. This type of talk therapy helps you become aware of harmful thought patterns so that you can respond to them differently. One form of CBT is exposure and response prevention (ERP). With ERP, you're gradually exposed to a feared object or obsession and you learn ways to resist doing your compulsive rituals. This practice may help improve your quality of life as you learn to manage your symptoms.

Medications

Some psychiatric medications can help control OCD obsessions and compulsions. Usually, the first medication a doctor will use to treat OCD is an antidepressant. Talk to your health care provider about the risks and benefits of using certain medications. Antidepressants approved to treat OCD include:

- Clomipramine (Anafranil)
- Fluoxetine (Prozac)
- Fluvoxamine (Luvox)
- Paroxetine (Paxil, Pexeva)
- Sertraline (Zoloft)

If your OCD doesn't respond to an antidepressant, your doctor may recommend:

- **An intensive outpatient or residential treatment program.** These programs typically last several weeks and emphasize ERP therapy principles. They may be helpful for people with severe OCD symptoms that make it hard for them to function.
- **Deep brain stimulation** (**DBS**). With DBS, electrodes are implanted in your brain. They produce electrical impulses that may help regulate your impulses. DBS is approved by the FDA to treat OCD in adults age 18 years and older who don't respond to traditional treatment approaches.
- **Transcranial magnetic stimulation** (**TMS**). This noninvasive procedure uses magnetic fields to stimulate nerve cells to improve your OCD symptoms. During a TMS session, a device with an electromagnetic coil is placed against your scalp near your forehead. The electromagnet delivers a magnetic pulse that stimulates nerve cells in your brain.

LIFESTYLE Because OCD is a chronic condition, it may always be part of your life. However, there are some things you can do yourself to build on your treatment plan:

- Practice the techniques you learn from your mental health
- provider.
- Take your medications as directed, and don't stop taking them without talking to your doctor.
- Pay attention to warning signs, such as triggers for your OCD symptoms.
- Check with your doctor before taking other medications to avoid interactions with your OCD treatment.
- Explore hobbies and other healthy ways to channel your energy.
- Join a support group to help you cope with the challenges of OCD.

Osteoporosis

WHAT IS IT? Osteoporosis causes bones to become weak and brittle so that even mild stresses such as bending over or coughing can cause a fracture. Osteoporosis-related fractures most commonly occur in the hip, wrist or spine.

Factors that can increase your risk of osteoporosis include:

- **Family history.** Having a parent or sibling with osteoporosis puts you at greater risk.
- **Body frame size.** People with small body frames tend to have a higher risk because they may have less bone mass to draw from as they age.
- **Sex hormones.** Lowered sex hormone levels tend to weaken bone. Reduced estrogen at menopause is a risk factor for women. Men experience a gradual reduction in testosterone with age.
- **Thyroid problems.** Too much thyroid hormone can cause bone loss. This can occur if you have an overactive thyroid or you take too much thyroid medication to treat an underactive thyroid.
- **Other hormone disorders.** Osteoporosis has also been associated with overactive parathyroid and adrenal glands.
- **Low calcium intake.** Too little calcium in your diet increases your risk.
- **Sedentary lifestyle.** People who are inactive are at increased risk.
- **Steroid medications.** Long-term use of oral or injected corticosteroid medications, such as prednisone and cortisone, interferes with the bone-rebuilding process.
- **Gastrointestinal surgery.** Surgery to reduce the size of your stomach or to bypass or remove part of the intestine limits the surface area available to absorb nutrients, including calcium.
- **Malabsorption disorders.** Diseases that interfere with typical absorption of nutrients increase the risk of osteoporosis.

SYMPTOM CHECKER Typically there are no symptoms early on. Once bones are weakened, symptoms may include:

- Back pain, caused by a fractured or collapsed vertebra
- Loss of height over time
- A stooped posture
- A bone fracture that occurs much more easily than expected

Healthy bone

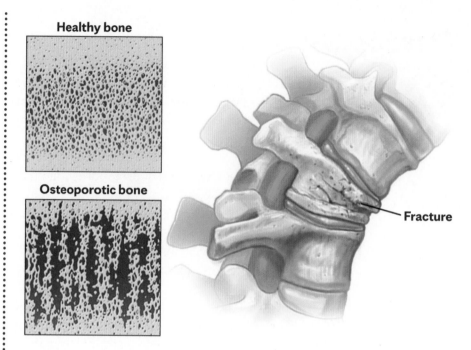

Osteoporotic bone

Fracture

Healthy bone has the appearance of a honeycomb matrix. Osteoporotic bone looks more porous when examined under a microscope.

Osteoporosis is generally diagnosed with a test that measures your bone density. For the test, you lie on a padded table and a scanner passes over part of your body. The scanner uses low levels of X-rays to determine the proportion of mineral in your bones.

TREATMENT The most effective way to combat osteoporosis is with a combination of medication and lifestyle changes. Drugs known as bisphosphonates are often the first line of treatment.

Bisphosphonates

Bisphosphonates are generally preferred because of their effectiveness, cost and long-term safety data. The medications inhibit bone breakdown, preserve bones mass and may even increase bone density. They're taken by mouth or given intravenously. Examples include:

- Alendronate (Binosto, Fosamax)
- Risedronate (Actonel, Atelvia)
- Ibandronate
- Zoledronic acid (Reclast)

Other medications

If you can't tolerate bisphosphonates or if they aren't effective, your health care provider might recommend:

- **Denosumab (Prolia).** This drug slows the bone breakdown process and produces results similar to those of bisphosphonates. Denosumab is delivered via a shot under the skin every six months.
- **Teriparatide (Bonsity, Forteo) and abaloparatide (Tymlos).** Rather than slowing bone loss, these powerful drugs stimulate new bone growth. They are given by injection under the skin and are used only for people with severe osteoporosis.
- **Romosozumab (Evenity).** This newer drug, also given by injection, is the first to work by both slowing bone loss and boosting bone formation. Your doctor may recommend it if you're postmenopausal and you have a high risk of fracture or other treatments haven't worked.

Hormone-related therapy

Estrogen, especially when started soon after menopause, can help maintain bone density. However, estrogen therapy can increase the risk of breast cancer or blood clots, particularly if it's used later or long term. Therefore, its use is limited. The medication raloxifene (Evista) mimics estrogen's beneficial effects on bone density in postmenopausal women, without some of the risks associated with estrogen.

LIFESTYLE To reduce your risk of osteoporosis or a fracture:

- **Get adequate calcium.** People ages 18 to 50 need 1,000 milligrams (mg) of calcium a day. The amount increases to 1,200 mg daily in women older than 50 and in men older than 70. Good sources of calcium include low-fat dairy products, dark green leafy vegetables and calcium-fortified orange juice. If you find it difficult to get enough calcium, consider taking a supplement.
- **Get adequate vitamin D.** Vitamin D improves your body's ability to absorb calcium. Adults should aim for 600 to 800 international units (IU) daily. Sources of vitamin D are sunlight and fortified milk. It's also available as a supplement.
- **Exercise.** Exercise helps build strong bones and slow bone loss. Strength training and weight-bearing exercises, such as walking and running, are especially beneficial.
- **Don't smoke.** It increases bone loss and the chance of a fracture.
- **Avoid excessive alcohol.** Alcohol may decrease bone formation.

Ovarian cysts

WHAT IS IT? Ovarian cysts are fluid-filled sacs or pockets within or on the surface of an ovary. Many women have ovarian cysts at some time during their lives. Most present little or no discomfort, are harmless, and disappear without treatment within a few months.

Ovarian cysts typically develop as a result of the typical function of your menstrual cycle. Your ovaries typically grow cystlike structures called follicles each month. Follicles produce the hormones estrogen and progesterone and release an egg when you ovulate. Sometimes a monthly follicle keeps growing. When that happens, it is known as a functional cyst.

Cysts not related to the typical function of your menstrual cycle — nonfunctional cysts — may contain tissue, such as hair, skin or teeth, because they form from cells that produce human eggs. Or they may be filled with a watery liquid or a mucous material. These are rare.

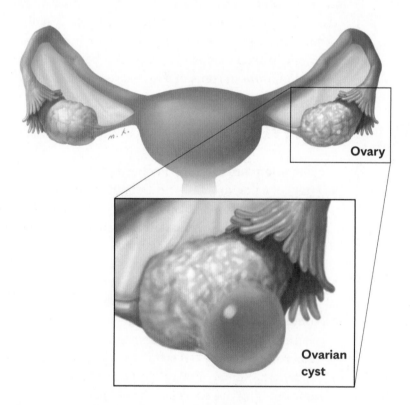

Ovary

Ovarian cyst

An ovarian cyst is a tiny sac filled with fluid located on an ovary. Cysts may form within an ovary, but most often they develop on its surface.

SYMPTOM CHECKER Some ovarian cysts — especially those that have ruptured — can produce symptoms. A large ovarian cyst can cause abdominal discomfort. If a large cyst presses on your bladder, you may feel the need to urinate more frequently because bladder capacity is reduced.

Symptoms of ovarian cysts may include:

- Pelvic or abdominal pain — a dull ache that may radiate to your lower back and thighs
- Pelvic pain shortly before your period begins or just before it ends
- Pelvic pain during intercourse
- Pain during bowel movements or pressure on your bowels
- Nausea, vomiting or breast tenderness similar to that experienced during pregnancy
- Fullness or heaviness in your abdomen
- Pressure on your bladder that causes you to urinate more frequently or makes it difficult to empty your bladder completely

TREATMENT Your health care provider may recommend tests, including an ultrasound exam, to help determine the size and type of cysts. In addition, treatment will depend on your age and your signs and symptoms. Your provider may suggest:

Watchful waiting. In many cases, you can wait to see if the cyst goes away on its own within a few months. This is typically an option if you have no symptoms and the cyst is small and filled with fluid. Your provider will likely recommend follow-up exams to see if the cyst has changed in size.

Birth control pills. Birth control pills can reduce the chance of new cysts developing in future menstrual cycles. They don't treat existing cysts, though.

Surgery. If the cyst is large, it doesn't look like a functional cyst, it's growing, or it persists through two or three menstrual cycles, your provider may recommend surgery. Some cysts can be removed without removing the ovary. In some circumstances, your provider may suggest removing the affected ovary and leaving the other ovary intact. Your provider may also recommend surgery if a cystic mass develops on the ovaries after menopause.

P

Pancreatitis

WHAT IS IT? Pancreatitis is an inflammation of the pancreas. The condition can come on suddenly and last for days (acute pancreatitis), or it can develop gradually and last for months to years (chronic pancreatitis).

Typically, during digestion inactivated pancreatic enzymes move through ducts in the pancreas and travel to the small intestine, where they become activated and aid digestion. In pancreatitis, the enzymes become activated while still in the pancreas. The cells of the pancreas become irritated, causing inflammation and the signs and symptoms associated with pancreatitis. Many conditions can lead to pancreatitis, including alcohol overuse, gallstones and viral illnesses.

SYMPTOM CHECKER Signs and symptoms of pancreatitis vary and depend on which type you experience. Acute pancreatitis generally causes:

- Upper abdominal pain
- Abdominal pain that radiates to your back
- Abdominal pain that feels worse after eating
- Nausea and vomiting
- Tenderness when touching the abdomen

Signs and symptoms of chronic pancreatitis generally include:

- Upper abdominal pain
- Losing weight without trying
- Oily, smelly stools

TREATMENT Treatment for pancreatitis usually requires hospitalization. Initial treatment typically focuses on controlling the inflammation and making you comfortable. This may include:

- **Early eating.** Newer data have suggested that eating as soon as you tolerate food helps heal the pancreas.
- **Pain medications.** Pancreatitis can cause severe pain. You'll receive medications to help control the pain.
- **Intravenous (IV) fluids.** To prevent dehydration, fluids are administered through a vein in your arm.

Once your pancreatitis is under control, the next step is to treat the underlying cause of your pancreatitis. Examples include:

- **Removal of bile duct obstructions.** Pancreatitis caused by a narrowed or blocked bile duct may require procedures to open or widen the duct.
- **Gallbladder surgery.** If gallstones caused your condition, you may need surgery to remove your gallbladder.
- **Pancreas surgery.** Surgery may be necessary to drain fluid from your pancreas or to remove diseased tissue.
- **Alcohol treatment.** If excessive alcohol use is the cause, your health care provider may recommend treatment for alcohol addiction.

Chronic pancreatitis may require additional treatments, including:

- **Pain management.** You may need medications to control chronic pain. Severe pain may be relieved with surgery to block the nerves that send pain signals from the pancreas to the brain.
- **Digestive enzymes.** Pancreatic enzyme supplements help your body break down and process the nutrients in the foods you eat.
- **Dietary changes.** A dietitian can teach you what foods are the easiest to digest.

P

LIFESTYLE Steps you can take at home include:

- **Stop drinking alcohol.** If you can't stop on your own, ask for help.
- **Stop smoking.** If you smoke, quit.
- **Eat a low-fat diet.** A diet that limits fat and emphasizes fresh fruits and vegetables, whole grains, and lean protein is best.
- **Drink more fluids.** Pancreatitis can cause dehydration, so drink plenty of fluids throughout the day.

Parkinson's disease

WHAT IS IT? Parkinson's disease is a disorder of the central nervous system that affects your movement. It develops gradually, sometimes starting with a small tremor in one hand. The disease also commonly causes stiffness or slowing of movement. Symptoms typically worsen as the condition progresses.

With Parkinson's disease, certain nerve cells (neurons) in the brain gradually break down or die. Most symptoms are due to loss of neurons that produce a chemical messenger in your brain called dopamine. When dopamine levels decrease, it causes abnormal brain activity, leading to signs of Parkinson's disease.

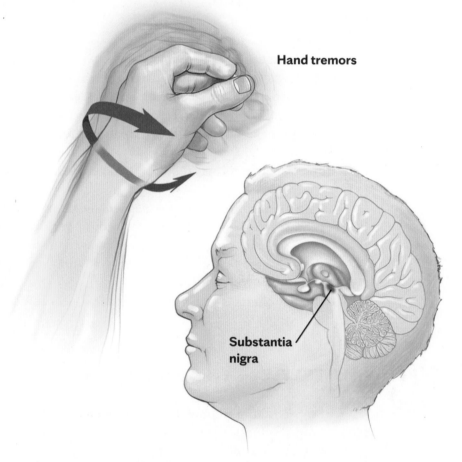

Hand tremors

Substantia nigra

Movement problems associated with Parkinson's, such as tremor, are primarily caused by inadequate levels of dopamine, which transmits messages from the substantia nigra to other parts of the brain.

WHAT'S THE CAUSE? Several factors appear to play a role, but more research is needed. Risk factors include:

- **Genes.** Researchers have identified specific genetic mutations that can cause Parkinson's disease. They're uncommon except in rare cases with many family members affected by the disease.
- **Environmental triggers.** Exposure to certain toxins or environmental factors may increase the risk of later Parkinson's disease, but the risk is relatively small.
- **Age.** Parkinson's disease ordinarily begins in middle or late life.
- **Being male.** Men are more likely to develop Parkinson's disease.

SYMPTOM CHECKER Signs and symptoms may vary from person to person. They may include:

- **Tremor.** You may first notice mild shaking (tremor) of your hand when it's relaxed and at rest.
- **Slowed movement.** Your steps may become shorter when you walk, and you may drag your feet as you try to walk.
- **Rigid muscles.** Muscle stiffness may occur in any part of your body, limiting range of motion.
- **Impaired posture and balance.** Your posture may become stooped, or you may have balance problems.
- **Loss of automatic movements.** Your ability to perform unconscious movements, including blinking, smiling or swinging your arms when you walk, is decreased.
- **Speech changes.** You may speak more softly, slur your words or hesitate before talking. Your speech may be more monotone.

TREATMENT Parkinson's disease can't be cured, but medications and other therapies can help control signs and symptoms.

Medications
Medications to treat Parkinson's disease include:

Carbidopa-levodopa. Levodopa, the most effective Parkinson's disease medication, is a natural chemical that passes into your brain and is converted to dopamine. Levodopa is combined with carbidopa (Sinemet), which protects it from premature conversion to dopamine outside your brain. After years, the benefit from levodopa may become less predictable, with a tendency to "wear off."

P

Dopamine agonists. These drugs mimic dopamine effects in your brain. They aren't as effective as levodopa; however, they last longer and may be used with levodopa to smooth the off-and-on effect of levodopa. Dopamine agonists include pramipexole (Mirapex ER), ropinirole and rotigotine (given as a patch, Neupro).

MAO B inhibitors. These medications include selegiline (Zelapar) and rasagiline (Azilect). They help prevent the breakdown of dopamine by inhibiting the brain enzyme monoamine oxidase B (MAO B), which metabolizes dopamine.

Catechol O-methyltransferase (COMT) inhibitors. Entacapone (Comtan) is the primary medication from this class. It mildly prolongs the effect of levodopa therapy by blocking an enzyme that breaks down dopamine.

Anticholinergics. These medications are used less often because their modest benefits are often offset by serious side effects.

Amantadine. This medication can be given with carbidopa-levodopa therapy during the later stages of Parkinson's disease to control involuntary movements induced by carbidopa-levodopa. It may also be prescribed for mild, early-stage Parkinson's disease.

Deep brain stimulation

In this procedure, surgeons implant electrodes into a specific part of your brain. The electrodes, connected to a generator that's implanted near your collarbone, send electrical pulses to your brain. The pulses help reduce Parkinson's disease symptoms by interfering with abnormal brain activity. Deep brain stimulation is most often offered to people with advanced Parkinson's disease who have unstable medication responses. The surgery can control erratic and fluctuating responses to levodopa or help control involuntary movements that don't improve with medication adjustments. It can also reduce tremor, reduce rigidity and improve slowing of movement. However, this treatment doesn't keep the disease from progressing.

LIFESTYLE Certain lifestyle changes may also help make living with Parkinson's disease easier. Exercise is extremely important. It can increase your muscle strength, flexibility and balance. Your doctor may suggest that you work with a physical therapist to develop an exercise program that works for you.

Peripheral artery disease

WHAT IS IT? Peripheral artery disease (PAD) is a common circulatory problem in which narrowed arteries reduce blood flow to your limbs. When you develop PAD, your extremities — usually your legs — don't receive enough blood flow to keep up with demand. This causes symptoms, most notably leg pain when walking.

PAD is often associated with widespread accumulation of fatty deposits in your arteries (atherosclerosis), which may reduce blood flow to your heart and brain, as well as your legs.

Less commonly, blood vessel inflammation, injury to your limbs, or unusual anatomy of your ligaments or muscles may cause PAD.

SYMPTOM CHECKER Signs and symptoms of PAD include:

- Painful cramping in your hip, thigh or calf muscles during activity that goes away with rest (intermittent claudication)
- Pain when using your arms, such as aching and cramping when knitting, writing or doing other manual tasks
- Leg numbness or weakness
- Coldness in your lower leg or foot, especially when compared with the other side
- Sores on your toes, feet or legs that won't heal
- A change in the color of your legs
- Slower hair growth on your legs
- Shiny skin on your legs
- Slower toenail growth
- No pulse or a weak pulse in your legs or feet
- Erectile dysfunction

Leg pain may vary widely from mild discomfort to debilitating pain. Severe pain can make it difficult for you to walk without stopping to rest or do other types of physical activity. The location of the pain depends on the location of the clogged or narrowed artery. Calf pain is the most common.

Factors that increase your risk of developing PAD include smoking, diabetes, obesity, high blood pressure, high cholesterol and a family history of PAD.

P

TREATMENT Treatment has two major goals. The first is to manage symptoms, such as leg pain, so that you can resume physical activities. The second is to stop the progression of atherosclerosis. Lifestyle changes, including exercise and a healthy diet, may help significantly. Your provider may also recommend medication or a procedure.

Medications

Medications used to treat PAD include:

- **Symptom-relief medications.** The drug cilostazol increases blood flow to the limbs both by preventing blood clots and by widening the blood vessels. It helps relieve symptoms such as leg pain. An alternative to cilostazol is pentoxifylline.
- **Medications to prevent blood clots.** Because PAD reduces blood flow to your limbs, you're at increased risk of blood clots. A blood clot can block an already narrowed blood vessel and cause tissue death. Your provider may prescribe daily aspirin therapy or another medication to prevent blood clots, such as clopidogrel (Plavix).
- **Medications to treat other conditions.** Your provider may prescribe medication to lower your cholesterol level, reduce high blood pressure or treat diabetes that may accompany PAD.

Angioplasty and surgery

In some cases, procedures may be necessary to treat narrowed arteries that cause pain or symptoms such as leg numbness or weakness.

- **Angioplasty.** A small tube (catheter) is threaded through a blood vessel to the affected artery. There, a small balloon on the tip of the catheter is inflated to reopen the artery and flatten the blockage, while stretching the artery to increase blood flow. Your doctor may insert a mesh framework (stent) in the artery to help keep it open.
- **Bypass surgery.** A surgeon creates a graft using a vessel from another part of your body or a blood vessel made of synthetic fabric. This technique allows blood to flow around (bypass) the blocked or narrowed artery.
- **Thrombolytic therapy.** If a blood clot is blocking an artery, a clot-dissolving drug is injected into your artery to break up the clot.

Supervised exercise program

A supervised training program can increase the distance you can walk pain-free. Regular exercise improves symptoms in a number of ways.

Peripheral neuropathy

WHAT IS IT? This condition results from damage to your peripheral nerves — usually those in your hands and feet — that causes weakness, numbness and pain. The pain typically occurs with a tingling feeling.

Your peripheral nervous system sends information from your brain and spinal cord (central nervous system) to the rest of your body. It also transmits information from your body back to your brain.

Peripheral neuropathy causes these messages to become less clear. The condition can result from traumatic injuries, infections, metabolic problems, certain medications, exposure to toxins and alcoholism. One of the most common causes is diabetes. More than half of people with diabetes develop some type of neuropathy.

SYMPTOM CHECKER Signs and symptoms may include:

- Gradual onset of numbness and tingling in your feet or hands, which may spread upward into your legs and arms
- Sharp, jabbing or burning pain
- Extreme sensitivity to touch
- Lack of coordination and falling
- Muscle weakness or paralysis if motor nerves are affected
- Heat intolerance and altered sweating
- Bowel, bladder or digestive problems
- Blood pressure changes, causing dizziness or lightheadedness

A physical exam, your medical history and various tests can help your health care provider make a diagnosis.

TREATMENT The goals of treatment are to manage the condition causing the neuropathy and to relieve symptoms.

Medications
Medications used to relieve peripheral neuropathy pain include:

Pain relievers. Over-the-counter pain medications, such as nonsteroidal anti-inflammatory drugs, can relieve mild symptoms. For more-severe symptoms, your provider may recommend prescription medications.

Anti-seizure medications. Epilepsy drugs such as gabapentin (Gralise, Neurontin) and pregabalin (Lyrica) may relieve nerve pain.

Capsaicin. A cream containing capsaicin, a substance found naturally in hot peppers, may modestly improve symptoms.

Antidepressants. Certain tricyclic antidepressants, such as amitriptyline, doxepin and nortriptyline (Pamelor), may relieve nerve pain by interfering with chemical processes that cause you to feel pain. The medication duloxetine (Cymbalta) and the antidepressant venlafaxine (Effexor XR) also may help ease pain.

Your provider also may prescribe medication to treat the underlying condition that's causing the neuropathy.

Therapies

Other options for treatment include:

Transcutaneous electrical nerve stimulation (TENS). Adhesive electrodes placed on the skin deliver a gentle electric current at varying frequencies to relieve pain. TENS is applied for 30 minutes daily.

Plasma exchange and intravenous immune globulin. People with peripheral neuropathy caused by certain inflammatory conditions may benefit from these procedures.

Physical therapy. If you have muscle weakness, physical therapy can help improve your muscle strength and movements.

Surgery. Rarely, symptoms are caused by pressure on a peripheral nerve, such as from a tumor. In this case, surgery may be necessary.

LIFESTYLE To help you manage symptoms:

- **Eat a balanced diet.** To keep nerves healthy eat plenty of fruits, vegetables, whole grains and lean protein.
- **Exercise regularly.** Try to get 30 minutes to an hour most days of the week.
- **Avoid situations that may worsen nerve damage.** This includes repetitive motions, cramped positions, exposure to toxic chemicals, smoking and excessive alcohol.

Pink eye

WHAT IS IT? Pink eye (conjunctivitis) is an inflammation or infection of the transparent membrane that lines your eyelid and covers the white part of your eyeball. When small blood vessels become inflamed, your eyes appear reddish or pink.

Pink eye is caused by a bacterial or viral infection or an allergic reaction. Viral and bacterial conjunctivitis are often associated with colds or a respiratory infection and are very contagious.

Common pink eye signs and symptoms include:

- Redness in one or both eyes
- A gritty feeling or itchiness in one or both eyes
- Discharge in one or both eyes that forms a crust during the night
- Tearing

TREATMENT Treatment will depend on the cause.

Bacterial conjunctivitis. Your care provider may prescribe antibiotic eye drops or ointment. The infection should go away within several days.

Viral conjunctivitis. There is no treatment. Signs and symptoms should gradually clear on their own in 1 to 2 weeks.

Allergic conjunctivitis. It's treated with eye drops that help control allergic reactions. Try to avoid whatever causes your allergies.

Self-care. To help you cope until your symptoms disappear:

- **Apply a compress to your eyes.** A cool-water compress may be the most soothing, but you can use a warm one if it feels better.
- **Try eye drops.** Over-the-counter eye drops called artificial tears may relieve symptoms. Some products contain medications helpful for people with allergic conjunctivitis.
- **Don't wear contact lenses.** Avoid them until your eyes feel better, and then use a new pair.
- **Practice good hygiene.** Don't touch your eyes with your hands and wash your hands often. Use a clean towel and washcloth daily; don't share them with others. Replace any eye cosmetics.

P

PMS (premenstrual syndrome)

WHAT IS IT? PMS includes mood swings, tender breasts, food cravings, sleep difficulties, fatigue, irritability, anxiety and depression that recur in a predictable pattern in some women around the time of menstruation.

Hormone fluctuations and chemical changes in the brain that occur on a monthly basis are thought to contribute to PMS. Insufficient amounts of the brain chemical serotonin may play a role in mood changes and depression, as well as symptoms such as fatigue, food cravings and sleep problems.

Among women who experience PMS, for some, the symptoms are mild. For others, they can be severe enough to affect their daily lives. A small number of women have disabling symptoms every month. This form of PMS is called premenstrual dysphoric disorder (PMDD). Symptoms of PMDD include depression, mood swings, anger, anxiety, feeling over-whelmed, difficulty concentrating, irritability and tension.

Regardless of their severity, signs and symptoms of PMS generally disappear within about four days of the start of your menstrual period.

TREATMENT For many women, lifestyle changes can help relieve PMS symptoms. A health care provider may prescribe medications for more-severe or troublesome symptoms. The success of medications varies from woman to woman.

Medications
Commonly prescribed medications include:

Nonsteroidal anti-inflammatory drugs (NSAIDs). Taken before or at the onset of your period, NSAIDs such as ibuprofen (Advil, Motrin IB, others) or naproxen sodium (Aleve) can ease cramping and breast discomfort.

Antidepressants. Selective serotonin reuptake inhibitors (SSRIs) — which include fluoxetine (Prozac), paroxetine (Paxil, Pexeva), sertraline (Zoloft) and others — can help reduce mood symptoms. SSRIs are the first line treatment for severe PMS or PMDD. They are generally taken daily. But some people may take them only for the two weeks before menstruation begins.

Diuretics. These prescription medications include the drug spironolactone (Aldactone). Diuretics help your body shed excess fluid. They may be taken to treat swelling and bloating that can accompany PMS.

Hormonal contraceptives. Contraceptives stop ovulation. This may bring relief from PMS symptoms.

LIFESTYLE Oftentimes, you can manage or reduce PMS symptoms with changes in the way you eat, exercise and approach daily life.

Modify your diet
Make these changes to your diet to see if your symptoms improve:

- Eat smaller, more-frequent meals to reduce bloating and the sensation of fullness that can accompany PMS.
- Limit salt and salty foods to help reduce bloating and fluid retention.
- Eat foods high in complex carbohydrates, such as fruits, vegetables and whole grains. Carbohydrates affect serotonin levels. Complex carbs are generally healthier than simple carbs.
- Eat foods rich in calcium. If you can't tolerate dairy products or aren't getting adequate calcium in your diet, a daily calcium supplement may help. Calcium may help reduce some of the physical and psychological symptoms of PMS.
- Avoid caffeine and alcohol.
- Take your vitamins. Magnesium, vitamin E and vitamin B-6 have all been reported to soothe symptoms, though evidence is limited or lacking.

Exercise regularly
Daily exercise can improve your overall health and alleviate symptoms such as fatigue, anxiety and a depressed mood. Try to exercise for 30 minutes to an hour most days of the week.

Reduce stress and learn to relax
This starts with making sure that you get adequate sleep each night. Progressive muscle relaxation or deep-breathing exercises can help reduce headaches, anxiety and stress, and they may improve insomnia. Other techniques for relieving stress and promoting relaxation include yoga, tai chi and massage.

P

Pneumonia

WHAT IS IT? Pneumonia is an infection that inflames the air sacs in one or both lungs. The air sacs may fill with fluid or pus, producing a cough, which may bring up thick phlegm.

A variety of organisms, including bacteria, viruses and fungi, can cause pneumonia. The condition is most serious for infants and young children, people older than age 65, and people with underlying health problems or weakened immune systems. Factors that increase your risk of developing pneumonia include:

- **Certain chronic diseases.** This includes diseases such as asthma, chronic obstructive pulmonary disease, diabetes and heart disease.
- **Weakened or suppressed immune system.** HIV/AIDS, an organ transplant, chemotherapy to treat cancer or long-term steroid use can weaken your immune system.
- **Smoking.** It damages your body's natural defenses against the bacteria and viruses that cause pneumonia.
- **A ventilator.** Being on a ventilator while hospitalized to help you breathe increases the risk of pneumonia.

SYMPTOM CHECKER Signs and symptoms may vary from mild to severe. Mild symptoms often are similar to those of a cold or flu, but they last longer.

- Fever, sweating and shaking chills
- Lower than normal body temperature
- Cough, which may produce thick, sticky fluid
- Chest pain when you breathe deeply or cough
- Shortness of breath
- Fatigue and muscle aches
- Nausea, vomiting or diarrhea
- Headache

Newborns and infants may not show any sign of the infection. Or they may vomit, have a fever and cough, appear restless or tired and without energy, or have difficulty breathing and eating.

Older people with pneumonia sometimes have sudden changes in mental awareness.

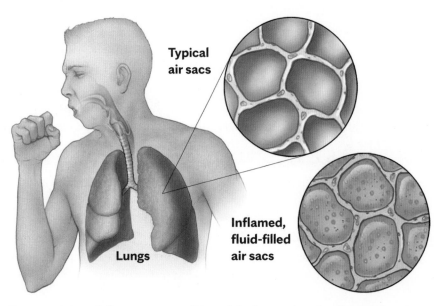

Typical air sacs

Inflamed, fluid-filled air sacs

Lungs

Pneumonia is an inflammatory condition of the lungs primarily affecting the microscopic air sacs. The sacs become inflamed and may fill with fluid or pus.

WHAT TESTS TO EXPECT Your health care provider will likely listen to your lungs with a stethoscope to check for bubbling or crackling sounds that indicate the presence of thick liquid.

If pneumonia is suspected, tests may be performed to make a diagnosis and determine the type of infection. They include a chest X-ray, blood and lung fluid (sputum) tests, and oxygen level measurements.

If you have serious symptoms or an underlying health condition, other tests may include:

- **Pleural fluid culture.** A fluid sample is taken from the thin tissue lining that surrounds the lungs (pleural area) and analyzed to help determine the type of infection.
- **CT scan.** If your pneumonia isn't clearing as quickly as expected, your provider may recommend a chest CT scan to check for complications. This imaging test shows a more detailed image of your lungs than a chest X-ray does.

TREATMENT The goals of treatment are to cure the infection and prevent any complications. Specific treatments depend on the type and severity of your pneumonia, and your age and overall health. The options include:

P

Antibiotics. They're used to treat bacterial pneumonia. Symptoms often improve within three days, although improvement usually takes twice as long in smokers.

Antiviral medications. Antiviral drugs may be used to treat certain types of viral pneumonia. Symptoms generally improve in 1 to 3 weeks.

Fever reducers. These include the over-the-counter medications aspirin, ibuprofen (Advil, Motrin IB, others) or acetaminophen (Tylenol, others).

Cough medicine. Because coughing helps loosen and move fluid from your lungs, it's a good idea not to eliminate your cough completely. Cough medicine may help you rest at night.

Hospitalization may be necessary for severe symptoms or for pneumonia in people older than 65 and very young children.

LIFESTYLE To help you recover more quickly and decrease your risk of complications:

- **Get plenty of rest.** Even when you start to feel better, be careful not to overdo it.
- **Stay home from school or work.** Don't return to your usual schedule until your temperature returns to normal and you stop coughing up mucus. Because pneumonia can recur, don't resume a full workload until you're sure you're well.
- **Drink plenty of fluids.** Fluids, especially water, help loosen mucus in your lungs.
- **Take all your medications.** If you stop medication too soon, your lungs may continue to harbor bacteria that can multiply and cause your pneumonia to recur.

PREVENTION

A vaccine can help prevent some types of pneumonia. Several vaccines are available in the United States. A pneumococcal vaccine is recommended for everyone older than age 65, as well as people living in nursing homes or long-term care facilities, or those who smoke. For adults with certain chronic health conditions or other risk factors, the vaccine may be given earlier. Ask your health care provider about getting these shots.

Poison ivy rash

WHAT IS IT? Poison ivy rash is caused by sensitivity to an oily resin called urushiol, found in the leaves, stems and roots of poison ivy, poison oak and poison sumac. At least 50% of the people who come into contact with these plants develop an itchy rash.

Often, the rash develops in a straight line because of the way the plant brushes against the skin. But if you come into contact with a piece of clothing or pet fur that has urushiol on it, the rash may be more widespread. A reaction usually develops 12 to 48 hours after exposure and typically lasts 2 to 3 weeks.

The severity of the rash depends on the amount of urushiol that gets on your skin. A section of skin with more of the oily resin on it may develop a rash sooner. You can also transfer the oil to other parts of your body with your fingers.

SYMPTOM CHECKER Signs and symptoms of a poison ivy rash include:

- Redness
- Itching
- Swelling
- Blisters

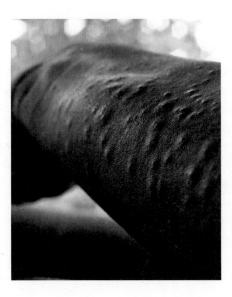 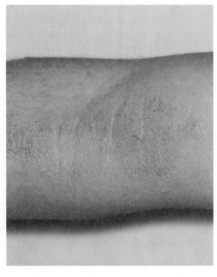

Some people are extra-sensitive to the oil that causes poison ivy rash, and this tendency runs in families. See your care provider if:

- The reaction is severe or widespread
- The rash affects your face or genitals
- Blisters are oozing pus
- You develop a fever greater than 100 F (37.8 C)
- The rash doesn't get better within a few weeks

 TREATMENT Mild cases generally require no medical treatment. For more-severe or widespread rashes — especially if it's on your face or genitals — your health care provider may suggest taking corticosteroid medication, such as prednisone. If the rash has become infected, antibiotics may be prescribed.

Until the rash disappears, to help control the itching:

- Apply an over-the-counter corticosteroid cream the first few days.
- Use calamine lotion.
- Take an oral antihistamine, such as diphenhydramine, which may also help you sleep better.
- Soak in a cool-water bath containing an oatmeal-based product.
- Place cool, wet compresses on the affected area for 15 to 30 minutes several times a day.

PREVENTION

To prevent a poison ivy rash:

- ***Know your plants.*** Learn how to identify poison ivy, poison oak and poison sumac.
- ***Wash your skin.*** Washing your skin with soap within 5 to 10 minutes after exposure may help avert a reaction. After an hour or so the urushiol usually has penetrated the skin. Washing may not prevent a reaction, but it may reduce its severity.
- ***Clean contaminated objects.*** Wearing long pants, socks, shoes and gloves will help protect your skin. Wash your clothing promptly with detergent if you think you've come into contact with poison ivy. Wash any other contaminated items. Urushiol can remain potent for years.
- ***Apply a barrier cream.*** An over-the-counter skin cream containing bentoquatam (Ivy Block) absorbs urushiol and may lessen your skin's reaction to the oil.

Prostate cancer

WHAT IS IT? Prostate cancer is cancer that occurs in the prostate — a small, walnut-shaped gland in males. It produces a fluid called seminal fluid, which nourishes and transports sperm.

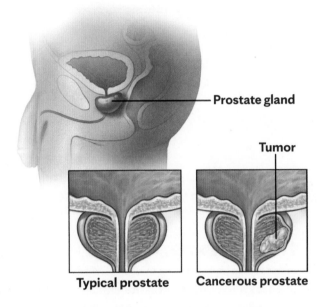

Prostate gland

Tumor

Typical prostate **Cancerous prostate**

The prostate gland is located just below the bladder in males. It surrounds the top portion of the tube that drains urine from the bladder (urethra). As a prostate tumor grows, it can interfere with the urethra and bladder function.

WHAT'S THE CAUSE? Prostate cancer begins when cells in the prostate develop changes (mutations) in their DNA. The changes allow the cells to grow too fast. Experts don't know exactly why these changes occur.

- **Older age.** Prostate cancer is much more common in men after age 50.
- **Race.** Black people have a higher risk of prostate cancer than people of other races do. Prostate cancer is also likely to be more aggressive or advanced in Black people. It's not yet clear why.
- **Family history.** If you have a parent, sibling or child with prostate cancer, your risk of it may be higher. The same may be true if you have a family history of genes that increase the risk of breast cancer (BRCA1 or BRCA2) or a very strong family history of breast cancer.

P

- **Obesity.** In people who are significantly overweight, prostate cancer is more likely to be aggressive and to return after initial treatment.

SYMPTOM CHECKER At first, prostate cancer may cause no signs or symptoms. As it grows and becomes more advanced, you may develop signs and symptoms such as:

- Trouble urinating
- Reduced force in your urine stream
- Blood in your urine
- Bone pain
- Loss of weight without trying
- Erectile dysfunction

If you have any persistent signs or symptoms that worry you, make an appointment with your health care provider.

TESTS TO EXPECT Testing healthy men with no symptoms for prostate cancer is controversial. Men in their 50s may want to discuss the pros and cons of prostate cancer screening with a doctor. If you have risk factors, you might have the discussion at an earlier age.

Prostate screening may include:

- Digital rectal exam (DRE), in which your doctor inserts a gloved, lubricated finger into your rectum to check your prostate
- Prostate-specific antigen (PSA) testing, in which your blood is tested to see how much PSA your prostate gland is producing

If screening finds an abnormal result, your health care provider may recommend more tests, such as:

- Ultrasound, in which sound waves are used to create a picture of your prostate gland
- Magnetic resonance imaging, which can give more-detailed pictures
- Prostate biopsy, in which a thin needle is inserted into the prostate to collect tissue

If a prostate biopsy shows cancerous cells, a lab test will also determine how aggressive the cancer is. Most often, a Gleason score is given. This score ranges from 2 (nonaggressive) to 10 (very aggressive). The cells from the biopsy may also be tested for gene mutations.

TREATMENT Options for treating prostate cancer depend on how fast it's growing, whether it has spread and your overall health. You and your health care provider will also want to consider the potential benefits or side effects of specific treatments.

Low-grade prostate cancer may not need treatment right away, or at all. Instead, your provider may recommend regular follow-up blood tests, rectal exams and prostate biopsies to monitor the cancer. This is called active surveillance.

For cancer that hasn't spread

Treatment options for early-stage prostate cancer include:

Surgery. Cancer that hasn't spread from the prostate may be removed surgically (radical prostatectomy), along with some surrounding tissue and a few lymph nodes. Most prostatectomies are done laparoscopically. With this type of surgery, several small incisions are made in your abdomen and instruments are inserted into them. Then, the surgeon guides a robot in moving the instruments. Prostatectomy also can be done by making one long incision in your abdomen (retropubic surgery).

Radiation therapy. With radiation therapy, high-powered energy is used to kill cancer cells. The radiation therapy may come from outside your body (external beam radiation) or be placed inside your body (brachytherapy). Treatments with external beam radiation usually are done five days a week for several weeks. Brachytherapy involves placing rice-sized radioactive seeds in your prostate tissue. The seeds deliver a low dose of radiation over a long period of time.In some situations, both types of radiation therapy may be recommended.

Ablative therapies. Cold or heat can be used to destroy prostate tissue when a tumor is very small or when surgery isn't possible. Cryoablation or cryotherapy involves using very cold gas to freeze prostate tissue. High-intensity focused ultrasound (HIFU) treatment uses concentrated ultrasound energy to heat the prostate tissue and cause it to die. Researchers are studying whether these techniques might be used to treat cancer in part of the prostate while sparing healthy tissue.

P

For advanced prostate cancer

Treatment options for later-stage prostate cancer include:

Hormone therapy. This treatment stops your body from producing the hormone testosterone. Prostate cancer cells rely on testosterone to grow. There are two types of medication you may be given to stop your testicles from producing testosterone: luteinizing hormone-releasing hormone (LHRH) and gonadotropin-releasing hormone (GnRH) agonists and antagonists. You also may be treated with anti-androgens, which block testosterone from reaching cancer cells. Surgery to remove your testicles (orchiectomy) may be an option.

Chemotherapy. Chemotherapy drugs kill rapidly growing cells, including cancer cells. They can be given through a vein in your arm, in pill form or both. Chemotherapy may be an option if your prostate cancer has spread to other areas in your body or it doesn't respond to hormone therapy.

Immunotherapy. This treatment uses your immune system to fight advanced cancer that doesn't respond to hormone therapy. With one type, your own immune cells are treated in a lab so that they'll fight the cancer. Then they're infused back into your body through a vein. There are also immunotherapy drugs you can take to help your immune system find and attack the cancer cells.

Targeted drug therapy. These medications target specific proteins or other mutations in your cancer cells. Targeted drugs can cause the cancer cells to die without harming healthy cells. Your doctor may recommend targeted drug therapy if you have advanced or recurrent prostate cancer that isn't responding to hormone therapy or your cancer cells have a specific genetic mutation.

LIFESTYLE You can reduce your risk of prostate cancer if you:

- Choose a healthy diet full of fruits and vegetables
- Choose healthy foods over supplements
- Exercise most days of the week
- Maintain a healthy weight

Talk to your health care provider if you have a very high risk of prostate cancer. Medications or other treatments may be an option, but they can present other serious risks.

Prostate gland enlargement

WHAT IS IT? Prostate gland enlargement, also known as benign prostatic hyperplasia (BPH), can produce bothersome urinary symptoms in men. Left untreated, the condition may block the flow of urine, causing bladder, urinary tract or kidney problems.

The prostate gland is located just beneath the bladder. The tube that transports urine from the bladder out of your penis (urethra) passes through the center of the prostate gland. As the gland enlarges, it can press on the urethra and interrupt urine flow.

Most men have continued prostate growth throughout life. It isn't entirely clear what causes the gland to enlarge. Changes in the balance of sex hormones as men age may be one cause. Genetics may play a role. Having a blood relative, such as a father or brother, with prostate problems means you're more likely to have problems, too.

SYMPTOM CHECKER Symptoms tend to gradually worsen over time. Common signs and symptoms include:

- Frequent or urgent need to urinate
- Increased frequency of urination at night
- Difficulty starting urination
- Weak urine stream or a stream that stops and starts
- Dribbling at the end of urination
- Inability to completely empty the bladder

TREATMENT To determine the best option, your health care provider will consider your symptoms, the size of your prostate gland, other health conditions you might have and your preferences.

If your symptoms are tolerable, you might monitor your symptoms to see if they worsen or improve. For some men, symptoms can ease without treatment. Other options include:

Medication
Medication is the most common treatment for mild to moderate symptoms of prostate enlargement.

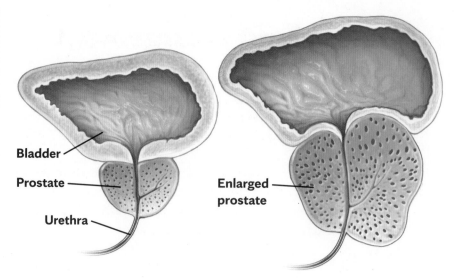

Bladder

Prostate

Urethra

Enlarged
prostate

The prostate gland is about the size and shape of a walnut or golf ball. When enlarged, it may obstruct urine flow from the bladder and out the urethra.

Alpha blockers. Alpha blockers relax the bladder neck muscles and
muscle fibers in the prostate gland, making urination easier. The medications — which include alfuzosin (Uroxatral), doxazosin (Cardura),
tamsulosin (Flomax) and silodosin (Rapaflo) — usually work quickly in
men with relatively small prostates.

5-alpha reductase inhibitors. These drugs shrink your prostate by preventing hormonal changes that cause prostate growth. These medications — which include finasteride (Proscar) and dutasteride (Avodart)
— might take up to six months to become effective.

Combination drug therapy. Your health care provider might recommend taking more than one drug at the same time, such as an alpha
blocker and a 5-alpha reductase inhibitor.

Tadalafil (Cialis). This medication, used to treat erectile dysfunction,
may be prescribed to treat symptoms of prostate enlargement in some
situations. It's not routinely used for this purpose.

Minimally invasive therapy

Minimally invasive therapy might be recommended if your symptoms
are moderate to severe, medication hasn't helped, you have a urinary
tract obstruction or you don't want to take medication daily. A variety
of minimally invasive therapies are used to treat BPH.

Transurethral resection of the prostate (TURP). A thin, lighted instrument is inserted into your urethra, and a surgeon removes all but the outer part of the prostate gland. TURP generally relieves symptoms quickly, and most men have a stronger urine flow afterward.

Transurethral incision of the prostate (TUIP). Instead of removing almost all of the gland, a surgeon makes one or two small cuts in the gland — making it easier for urine to pass through the urethra. It may be an option if you have a small or moderately enlarged prostate.

Transurethral microwave thermotherapy (TUMT). A special electrode is inserted into your prostate gland. Microwave energy from the electrode destroys the inner portion of the gland, shrinking it and easing urine flow. Re-treatment might be necessary over time.

Transurethral needle ablation (TUNA). Using a thin, lighted instrument inserted into your urethra, needles are placed into your prostate gland. Radio waves pass through the needles, heating and destroying prostate tissue that's blocking urine flow. Like TUMT, this procedure might only partially relieve symptoms and is rarely used.

Laser therapy. A high-energy laser reduces overgrown prostate tissue. Laser therapy often relieves symptoms immediately with limited side effects. It's most often used in men who can't undergo other prostate procedures.

Surgery

A surgeon makes an incision in your lower abdomen to reach the prostate gland and remove excess tissue. Surgery may be performed if you have a very large prostate, bladder damage or other complicating factors. The procedure may be performed using traditional surgery or robot-assisted surgery.

LIFESTYLE To help control symptoms:

- **Limit beverages in the evening.** Don't drink anything two hours before bedtime to avoid having to get up at night to urinate.
- **Limit caffeine and alcohol.** They can increase urine production, irritate the bladder and worsen symptoms.
- **Limit decongestants or antihistamines.** They can tighten the band of muscles around the urethra, making it harder to urinate.

Prostatitis

WHAT IS IT? Prostatitis is the name for swelling and inflammation of the prostate gland. It affects men of all ages and often causes painful or difficult urination and pain in the groin.

The condition may result for a number of reasons, including a bacterial infection, immune system disorder, nervous system disorder or injury to the prostate. In many cases, the cause is never identified.

Bacterial prostatitis is often caused by common strains of bacteria. The infection may start when bacteria carried in urine leaks into your prostate. If bacteria aren't eliminated, prostatitis may recur or become difficult to treat. This is called chronic bacterial prostatitis.

Depending on the cause, prostatitis may come on gradually or suddenly. It may get better quickly, either on its own or with treatment. Some types of prostatitis last for months or keep recurring (chronic prostatitis).

SYMPTOM CHECKER Prostatitis symptoms vary depending on the cause. They may include:

- Pain or a burning sensation when urinating
- Difficulty urinating, such as dribbling or hesitant urination
- Frequent urination, particularly at night
- An urgent need to urinate
- Pain in the abdomen, groin or lower back
- Pain in the area between the scrotum and rectum
- Pain or discomfort of the penis or testicles
- Painful orgasms (ejaculations)
- Flu-like symptoms (with bacterial prostatitis)

TREATMENT A diagnosis of prostatitis involves ruling out other conditions that may be causing your symptoms. A digital rectal examination is generally performed to feel the gland. You also may need to undergo blood, urine or bladder tests.

Treatment for prostatitis generally depends on the cause, if the cause is known. Options include medication, massage and self-care.

Antibiotics. This is the most common treatment for prostatitis. The choice of medication is based on the type of bacteria that may be causing your infection. If you have severe symptoms, you may need intravenous (IV) antibiotics.

Alpha blockers. These medications help relax the bladder neck and the muscle fibers where your prostate joins your bladder. This treatment may lessen symptoms, such as painful urination.

Anti-inflammatory agents. Nonsteroidal anti-inflammatory drugs (NSAIDs), such as ibuprofen (Advil, Motrin IB, others) or naproxen sodium (Aleve), may relieve painful symptoms.

Prostate massage. A doctor uses a procedure similar to a digital rectal exam to massage the prostate gland and release prostate fluid into your urethra. A urine sample after the massage expels the prostate fluid for bacterial testing. This may also provide some symptom relief.

Self-care. The following steps may lessen symptoms:

- Soak in a warm bath (sitz bath).
- Limit or avoid alcohol, caffeine, and spicy or acidic foods.
- Avoid prolonged sitting, or sit on a pillow or inflatable cushion to ease pressure on the prostate gland.
- Avoid bicycling, or wear padded shorts and adjust your bicycle to relieve pressure on your prostate.

P

PROSTATITIS, CANCER AND PSA LEVELS

Prostatitis can cause elevated levels of prostate-specific antigen (PSA), a protein produced by the prostate gland. It's the same protein used to screen for prostate cancer. Cancerous cells produce more PSA than do noncancerous cells, so higher levels of PSA in the blood may indicate prostate cancer. However, conditions other than prostate cancer, including prostatitis or a very enlarged prostate gland, also can increase PSA levels. There's no direct evidence that prostatitis can lead to prostate cancer.

Psoriasis

WHAT IS IT? Psoriasis is a common skin condition that causes cells to build up on the surface of the skin, forming thick, silvery scales and itchy, dry patches that are sometimes painful.

The condition is believed to result from an immune system disorder. A type of white blood cell called a T lymphocyte (T cell) is likely involved. Usually, T cells travel throughout the body to detect and fight off foreign substances, such as viruses or bacteria. With psoriasis, the T cells attack healthy skin cells by mistake. Overactive T cells may trigger other immune responses associated with symptoms of the disease.

What causes T cells to malfunction in people with psoriasis isn't clear. Certain genes may play a role. Environmental factors, including stress, cold weather and smoking, may be involved as well.

SYMPTOM CHECKER Signs and symptoms can vary from person to person and may include one or more of the following:

- Red patches of skin covered with silvery scales
- Small scaling spots (commonly seen in children)
- Dry, cracked skin that may bleed
- Itching, burning or soreness
- Thickened, pitted or ridged nails
- Swollen and stiff joints

There may be times when your psoriasis symptoms improve, alternating with times when they get worse.

TREATMENT There are three main treatments for psoriasis: topical treatments, light therapy, and oral or injected drugs.

Topical treatments

Creams and ointments that you apply to your skin can often treat mild to moderate psoriasis. When the disease is more severe, they may be combined with other therapies. Topical treatments include:

- **Topical corticosteroids.** These powerful anti-inflammatory drugs are the most frequently prescribed medications for treating mild to moderate psoriasis. They slow cell turnover by suppressing the immune system, which reduces inflammation and itching.

- **Vitamin D analogues.** These synthetic forms of vitamin D slow down the growth of skin cells. Examples include calcipotriene (Dovonex) and calcitriol (Rocaltrol).
- **Topical retinoids.** Tazarotene (Tazorac, Avage) was developed to treat psoriasis. Like other vitamin A derivatives, it normalizes DNA activity in skin cells and may decrease inflammation.
- **Calcineurin inhibitors.** The drugs tacrolimus (Prograf) and pimecrolimus (Elidel) approved for the treatment of atopic dermatitis, may treat some forms of psoriasis. The medications are thought to disrupt the activation of T cells.
- **Salicylic acid.** Available over-the-counter and by prescription, salicylic acid promotes sloughing of dead skin cells and reduces scaling. Sometimes it's combined with other medications, such as topical corticosteroids or coal tar, to increase its effectiveness.
- **Coal tar.** It's probably the oldest treatment for psoriasis. It reduces scaling, itching and inflammation, but is messy, stains clothing and bedding, and has a strong odor.
- **Anthralin.** This medication is a tar cream that slows skin cell growth. It's thought to normalize DNA activity in skin cells. Anthralin can also remove scales, making the skin smoother, but it stains most anything it touches.

Light therapy (phototherapy)

Natural or artificial ultraviolet light may be used to treat the disease.

- **Sunlight.** When exposed to ultraviolet (UV) rays in sunlight or artificial light, the activated T cells in the skin die. This slows skin cell turnover and reduces scaling and inflammation. Brief, daily exposures to small amounts of sunlight may improve psoriasis.
- **UVB phototherapy.** Controlled doses of UVB light from an artificial light source may improve mild to moderate psoriasis.
- **Narrow band UVB therapy.** It's a newer form of phototherapy administered two or three times a week until the skin improves. Maintenance may require only weekly sessions.
- **Goeckerman therapy.** Some doctors combine UVB treatment and coal tar treatment, which is known as Goeckerman treatment.
- **Photochemotherapy, or psoralen plus ultraviolet A (PUVA).** It involves taking a light-sensitizing medication before exposure to UVA light. UVA light penetrates deeper into the skin than does UVB light, and psoralen makes the skin more responsive to UVA

exposure. This more aggressive treatment is generally used for more-severe cases.

- **Excimer laser.** Used in mild to moderate psoriasis, it treats only the involved skin. A controlled beam of UVB light is directed to the psoriasis plaques to control scaling and inflammation.

Oral or injected medications

These treatments are generally reserved for severe psoriasis or disease that's resistant to other types of treatment.

- **Retinoids.** They reduce the production of skin cells, but signs and symptoms usually return once therapy is discontinued. The medication can produce serious side effects.
- **Biologics.** Medications approved for the treatment of moderate to severe psoriasis include apremilast (Otezla), etanercept (Enbrel), infliximab (Remicade), adalimumab (Humira), ustekinumab (Stelara) and secukinumab (Cosentyx). The drugs block interactions between certain immune system cells and particular inflammatory pathways. They must be used with caution because they may have serious side effects.
- **Methotrexate.** It decreases skin cell production and suppresses inflammation. The drug is generally well tolerated in low doses but when used for long periods can cause serious side effects.
- **Cyclosporine.** It's similar to methotrexate in effectiveness. Like other immunosuppressant drugs, it increases your risk of infection and other health problems.

LIFESTYLE Although self-help measures won't cure psoriasis, they may improve the appearance and feel of damaged skin.

- **Take daily baths.** Bathing helps remove scales and calm inflamed skin. Add bath oil, colloidal oatmeal, Epsom salts or Dead Sea salts to the water and soak. Avoid hot water and harsh soaps.
- **Moisturize.** Blot your skin after bathing and apply a heavy moisturizer while your skin is still moist. During cold, dry weather, you may need to apply moisturizer several times daily.
- **Get some sunlight.** A controlled amount of sunlight can improve lesions, but too much sun can trigger or worsen outbreaks and increase the risk of skin cancer.
- **Avoid triggers, if possible.** Find out what triggers, if any, worsen your psoriasis and take steps to avoid them.

PTSD (post-traumatic stress disorder)

 WHAT IS IT? Post-traumatic stress disorder (PTSD) is a mental health condition that may affect someone after experiencing or witnessing a terrifying event. It's a reaction so severe and prolonged that people with it have difficulty functioning.

With PTSD you may have disturbing memories or flashbacks and changes to your mood. You may also startle more easily or notice other changes in your behavior. Avoiding people or places that may remind you of the event is another common symptom.

 WHAT'S THE CAUSE? Doctors aren't sure why some people get PTSD. It's probably caused by a mix of stressful experiences, inherited mental health risks, your temperament and the way you respond to stress.

Risk factors for PTSD include:

- Experiencing intense or long-term trauma
- Having been abused as a child
- Having a job that puts you at risk of being exposed to traumatic events, such as being in the military or a first responder
- Having other mental health problems
- Having blood relatives with mental health problems
- Not having a good support system of family and friends
- Being an American Indian/Alaska Native

Experiences that more commonly lead to PTSD include an accident, combat exposure, childhood physical abuse, sexual violence or physical assault. Being threatened with a weapon also more often leads to PTSD.

 SYMPTOM CHECKER Many people who go through traumatic events have temporary difficulty adjusting and coping. With time and good self-care, they usually get better. If you have fear, anxiety, anger, depression and guilt months or years after a terrifying event that interferes with your day-to-day functioning, you may have PTSD.

In people who develop long-term PTSD, four general types of symptoms may occur: intrusive memories, avoidance, negative changes in thinking and mood, and changes in physical and emotional reactions.

P

Intrusive memories. If you have PTSD, you may find yourself reliving a traumatic event as if it were happening again (flashbacks). You may have upsetting dreams or nightmares about the event. If something reminds you of it, you may have a strong emotional or physical reaction.

Avoidance. People with PTSD often try not to think or talk about the traumatic event. They may avoid places, activities or people that remind them of it.

Negative changes in thinking and mood. Hopelessness about the future is common in people who have PTSD. You may feel detached from your family and friends, have difficulty maintaining close relationships, and be emotionally numb.

Changes in physical and emotional reactions. People who have PTSD may be easily startled or frightened and always on guard for danger. They may be self-destructive, and they may have angry outbursts or be aggressive. They also may have trouble sleeping.

Symptoms of PTSD can start within one month after a traumatic event, or they may not appear until years later. They can lead you to have problems in social or work situations and in relationships.

PTSD symptoms may vary over time and yours may be different from someone else's. You may find that you have symptom triggers, such as stress or a reminder of the trauma you went through. For example, hearing a car backfire could cause someone who is a military veteran to relive combat experiences.

TREATMENT Talk to your health care provider if you experienced a traumatic event and you've had disturbing thoughts and feelings about it for more than a month or you're having trouble getting your life back under control. Getting treatment for PTSD right away can help prevent your symptoms from worsening.

Untreated PTSD can lead to complications such as:

- Depression
- Anxiety
- Panic disorder
- Drug and alcohol use
- Suicidal thoughts or actions

To diagnose PTSD, your doctor will perform a physical exam and do a psychological evaluation. A diagnosis of PTSD requires exposure to an event that involved the actual or possible threat of death, violence or serious injury. For example, a traumatic event may have happened to you. You also may have seen it happen to someone else or heard that it happened to them. People also can get PTSD if they're exposed to graphic details of traumatic events over and over (such as if they're first responders).

The main treatment for PTSD is psychotherapy, but it can also be combined with medication. Treatment can give you new tools to cope with your symptoms. It can help you think better about yourself, others and the world. Treatment can also help you deal with related problems, such as depression, anxiety, or misuse of alcohol or drugs.

Psychotherapy

Three types of talk therapy are used for PTSD.

- Cognitive therapy can help you recognize ways of thinking that are keeping you stuck.
- Exposure therapy can help with flashbacks and nightmares. It's a way to safely face the situations and memories so you can learn to cope with them.
- Eye movement desensitization and reprocessing (EMDR) therapy combines exposure therapy with guided eye movements to help you process traumatic memories and change how you react.

Medications

Several types of drugs may help treat symptoms of PTSD.

- Selective serotonin reuptake inhibitors such as sertraline (Zoloft) and paroxetine (Paxil) can help depression and anxiety. They're also good for improving sleep problems and concentration.
- Anti-anxiety medications can relieve your anxiety and related problems.
- Some studies suggest that prazosin (Minipress) may reduce or suppress nightmares in some people with PTSD.

It may take some time to find the best medication, with the fewest side effects, for your PTSD symptoms and situation. You may see an improvement in your mood and other symptoms within a few weeks.

R

Raynaud's disease

WHAT IS IT? In Raynaud's disease, smaller arteries that supply blood to your skin narrow, limiting blood circulation to the affected areas — mainly your fingers and toes — causing them to be unpleasantly cold and uncomfortable.

Doctors don't fully understand the cause of Raynaud's disease, but blood vessels in the hands and feet appear to overreact to cold or stress. During an attack, affected areas of your skin usually first turn white and then turn blue and feel cold and numb. As you warm yourself or relieve stress and circulation improves, the affected areas may turn red, throb, tingle or swell.

TREATMENT Dressing for the cold in layers and wearing gloves or heavy socks are often effective for mild symptoms. Medications may be used for more-severe forms of the disease. The goal is to widen (dilate) blood vessels to improve circulation.

For very severe Raynaud's, treatment may include cutting the sympathetic nerves surrounding blood vessels in affected hands or feet or injecting the nerves with chemicals to block their exaggerated responses.

These steps can help decrease attacks.

- **Don't smoke.** Smoking constricts blood vessels.
- **Avoid rapid temperature changes.** Try not to go from a hot environment to an air-conditioned room.
- **Avoid cold.** Wear gloves or mittens when taking food out of the freezer. Use insulated drinking glasses. Wear socks to bed.

Restless legs syndrome

WHAT IS IT? Restless legs syndrome is a condition in which you have creeping or crawling sensations in your legs and an uncontrollable urge to move your legs due to the discomfort. The sensations typically happen in the evenings or while you're sitting still or lying down for extended periods. Moving temporarily eases the discomfort.

Sometimes, restless legs syndrome may be associated with another condition called periodic limb movement of sleep, which causes your legs to twitch and kick, possibly throughout the night, while you sleep.

There's no known cause for restless legs syndrome. Researchers suspect it may result from an imbalance of the brain chemical dopamine, which sends messages to control muscle movement. Sometimes restless legs syndrome runs in families, especially if it starts before age 50. Pregnancy or hormonal changes may temporarily worsen signs and symptoms. Some women get restless legs syndrome for the first time during pregnancy. Signs and symptoms usually disappear after delivery.

SYMPTOM CHECKER People typically describe restless legs syndrome as a condition that involves compelling, unpleasant sensations in their legs or feet. Less commonly, the sensations affect the arms.

The sensations generally occur within the limb rather than on the skin, and are described as:

- Crawling
- Creeping
- Pulling
- Throbbing
- Aching
- Itching

Signs and symptoms can range from barely bothersome to incapacitating. Many people find it difficult to fall asleep at night or to stay asleep during the night. Symptoms also may fluctuate in severity. In some cases, they disappear for periods of time, then recur.

TREATMENT Treatment typically focuses on lifestyle changes, and if those aren't effective, medications may be prescribed.

A variety of medications may help reduce the restlessness in your legs. They include:

Medications that increase dopamine. These drugs reduce movement in your legs by affecting the level of the chemical messenger dopamine in your brain. Ropinirole, rotigotine (Neupro) and pramipexole (Mirapex ER) are approved to treat moderate to severe restless legs syndrome.

Medications that treat neuropathy symptoms. These drugs are thought to interfere with communication between nerves. They include gabapentin (Neurontin) and pregabalin (Lyrica).

Opioids. Narcotic medications may relieve severe symptoms, but they aren't recommended because they can be addicting.

Muscle relaxants and sleep medications. Medications known as benzodiazepines may help you sleep better at night, but they don't eliminate the leg sensations, and they may cause daytime drowsiness.

Some medications may worsen symptoms — certain antidepressants, some antipsychotic medications, some anti-nausea drugs, and some cold and allergy medications.

LIFESTYLE Many times, simple lifestyle changes can help alleviate symptoms.

- **Take warm baths.** Soaking in a warm bath and massaging your legs can relax your muscles.
- **Use warm or cool packs.** Use of heat or cold, or alternating the two, may lessen limb sensations.
- **Try relaxation techniques.** Stress can aggravate restless legs syndrome. Meditation or yoga before bed may be helpful.
- **Stretch and massage.** Begin and end your day with stretching exercises or gentle massage.
- **Exercise.** Moderate, daily exercise may relieve symptoms, but overdoing it or exercising too late in the day may intensify them.
- **Limit or avoid caffeine.** For some people, cutting back on caffeine reduces signs and symptoms.

R

Ringing in the ear (tinnitus)

WHAT IS IT? Tinnitus is a common problem, affecting about 1 in 5 people. Tinnitus isn't a condition itself — rather, it's a symptom of an underlying condition, often age-related hearing loss.

Tinnitus is most commonly caused by problems in your outer, middle or inner ear. It may also be related to the hearing (auditory) nerves or the part of your brain that interprets nerve signals as sound (auditory pathways). Rarely, tinnitus is associated with a blood vessel problem or muscle contractions.

Often, tinnitus results from inner ear cell damage in which the tiny, delicate hairs in your inner ear break or bend. This causes them to "leak" random electrical impulses to your brain, creating ringing sounds and other noises associated with tinnitus.

Tinnitus may stem from age-related hearing loss, exposure to loud noise and earwax blockage. Some medications, including certain antibiotics, some cancer medications, diuretics, quinine medications, certain antidepressants and high doses of aspirin, also may cause or worsen tinnitus.

SYMPTOM CHECKER Tinnitus symptoms include hearing these types of phantom noises, even though no external sound is present:

- Ringing
- Buzzing
- Roaring
- Clicking
- Hissing

The phantom noises may vary in pitch from a low roar to a high squeal, and you may hear the noise in one or both ears. In some cases, the sound can be so bothersome that it interferes with your ability to concentrate or hear.

TREATMENT Treatment for tinnitus typically begins with treating any underlying conditions that may be contributing to the condition. This may include such things as removing impacted earwax, changing medications, treating a blood vessel condition or using hearing aids.

Medications

Drugs can't cure tinnitus, but they may help reduce the severity of the problem and help you cope with your symptoms. For example, tricyclic antidepressants have been used with some success. Because of possible side effects, they're generally reserved for more severe tinnitus. Your health care provider might prescribe other medications for anxiety that often accompanies tinnitus.

Noise suppression

White noise, a constant, low-level noise, may help suppress the ringing sound so it's less bothersome. Noise suppression may include:

- **White noise machines.** These devices produce environmental sounds such as falling rain or ocean waves and may help you sleep. Fans, humidifiers, dehumidifiers and air conditioners in the bedroom also may provide the same benefit.
- **Masking devices.** Worn in the ear and similar to hearing aids, these devices produce a continuous, low-level white noise that suppresses tinnitus symptoms.

Counseling

These options help you change the way you think and feel about your symptoms. Over time, your tinnitus may bother you less.

- **Tinnitus retraining.** A wearable device delivers individually programmed tonal music to mask the tinnitus you experience. Over time, this technique may help you not to focus on it.
- **Cognitive behavioral therapy** (CBT). A licensed mental health professional or psychologist can help you learn coping techniques to make tinnitus symptoms less bothersome.

Self-care

Steps you can take to help reduce symptoms include:

- **Avoiding irritants.** Reduce your exposure to things that may make your tinnitus worse, such as loud noises, caffeine and nicotine.
- **Managing stress.** Stress can make tinnitus worse.
- **Reducing alcohol consumption.** Alcohol increases the force of your blood by dilating your blood vessels, causing greater blood flow, especially in the inner ear area.

Ringworm

WHAT IS IT? Ringworm is a common type of fungal infection. You can get it on your head (tinea capitis) or your body (tinea corporis). Ringworm appears as scaly or inflamed patches that may slowly get bigger. These areas have a clear or scaly area inside the ring.

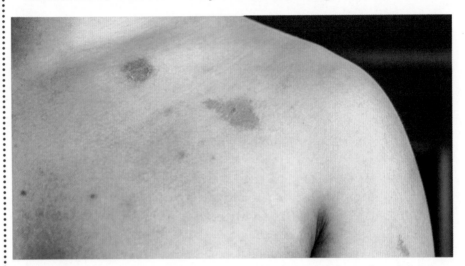

Ringworm of the body is a roughly ring-shaped rash that is itchy, scaly and slightly raised. The rings usually start small and then expand outward.

WHAT'S THE CAUSE? Ringworm is caused by a fungus. No worm is involved. The name comes from the rash's circular appearance.

Many different types of fungus cause ringworm. They come from common mold-like parasites that live on the cells in the outer layer of your skin. Ringworm can be spread in several ways:

- Direct, skin-to-skin contact with someone who has ringworm
- Touching, petting or grooming a dog or cat that has it
- Touching objects or surfaces (clothing, towels, bedding, linens, combs, brushes) that a person or animal with ringworm used

Outbreaks of ringworm are common in schools and child care centers where the infection easily spreads with close contact.

You can also get ringworm by touching soil that's infected with it, but that's rare.

Risk factors for ringworm include:

- Living in a warm climate
- Having close contact with a person or animal with ringworm
- Sharing clothing, bedding or towels with someone who has the infection
- Participating in skin-to-skin sports, such as wrestling
- Wearing tight or restrictive clothing
- Having a weak immune system

SYMPTOM CHECKER Ringworm on the scalp makes hairs break, creating bald spots. It's most common in toddlers and school-age children. On the body, the infection usually appears as an itchy, round rash with clearer skin in the middle.

Signs and symptoms of ringworm on the scalp include:

- One or more round, scaly or red patches where hair has broken off at or near the scalp
- Patches that slowly get bigger and have small, black dots where the hair has broken off
- Brittle or fragile hair you can easily break or pull out
- Tender or painful areas on your scalp

Signs and symptoms of ringworm on the body include:

- A scaly, ring-shaped area on your buttocks, trunk, arms or legs
- Itchiness
- A clear or scaly area inside the ring that may have colored bumps around it (on white skin, the bumps may be red; on Black or brown skin, they may be purple, brown or gray)
- A round, flat patch of itchy skin
- Overlapping rings

TREATMENT For a mild case of body ringworm, you can try applying an over-the-counter antifungal lotion, cream or ointment such as clotrimazole (Lotrimin AF) or terbinafine (Lamisil AT) as directed on the packaging.

Ringworm on the scalp
If your child has hair loss, scaling or itchiness of the scalp, see a health care provider. Nonprescription creams, lotions and powders won't get rid of scalp ringworm.

A provider may prescribe one of the following medications to treat scalp ringworm:

- Griseofulvin (Gris-Peg) (usually the first choice)
- Terbinafine
- Itraconazole (Sporanox, Tolsura)
- Fluconazole (Diflucan)

Your child may need to take one of these medications in pill form for six weeks or more — until hair regrows. With treatment, the bald spots usually fill in and the skin heals with no scarring.

Your health care provider also may recommend washing your child's hair with a prescription-strength antifungal shampoo. The medicated shampoo removes fungus spores and can help prevent the ringworm infection from spreading to other parts of your child's body or other people.

Ringworm on the body

Medications used to treat ringworm on the body include:

- Terbinafine (Lamisil)
- Ketoconazole
- Clotrimazole (Lotrimin AF)

Your child may need to apply one of these creams to the ringworm for 2 to 4 weeks. If the rash doesn't get better, your provider may also prescribe an antifungal drug in a pill. Using a prescription-strength medicated shampoo on your child as a body wash also may be recommended. Doing that can help prevent the ringworm from spreading to other parts of your child's body or other people.

LIFESTYLE It's hard to prevent ringworm because the fungus that causes it is common and can spread before symptoms appear. To lower your child's risk of ringworm, take these steps:

- Educate yourself and your family about ringworm
- Shampoo regularly, especially after haircuts
- Keep skin clean and dry
- Avoid infected animals (look for a patch of skin where fur is missing)

Rosacea

WHAT IS IT? Rosacea, often mistaken for adult acne, is a common skin condition that causes redness in your face and may produce small, red, pus-filled bumps.

Although rosacea can occur in anyone, it most commonly affects middle-aged women who have fair skin. The condition may be mistaken for acne, an allergic reaction or other skin problems.

The cause of rosacea is unknown. It may be due to a combination of genetic and environmental influences. The condition is often aggravated by factors that increase blood flow to the surface of your skin, such as hot foods or beverages; spicy foods; alcohol; temperature extremes; stress, anger or embarrassment; strenuous exercise; and hot baths or saunas.

SYMPTOM CHECKER Rosacea signs and symptoms may flare up for a period of weeks to months and then diminish before flaring again. They include:

- **Facial redness.** Rosacea usually causes a persistent redness in the central portion of your face. Small blood vessels on your nose and cheeks often swell and become visible.
- **Swollen red bumps.** Many people also develop bumps on their face that resemble acne. These bumps sometimes contain pus. Your skin may feel hot and tender.
- **Eye problems.** Some people also experience eye dryness, irritation and swollen, reddened eyelids.
- **Enlarged nose.** Rarely, rosacea can thicken the skin on the nose, causing the nose to appear bulbous. This condition, called rhinophyma, occurs more often in men than in women.

TREATMENT There's no cure for rosacea. A combination of approaches is often most effective in treating the disorder.

Medications
Medications used for rosacea include antibiotics, which also have anti-inflammatory effects. Antibiotics come in the form of creams, gels or lotions that you spread on the affected skin. Oral antibiotics are generally prescribed for short-term use.

Another option is the acne medication isotretinoin (Amnesteem, Claravis, others). This powerful drug is most commonly used to treat severe cystic acne, but it can help clear up acne-like lesions of rosacea. This drug can cause side effects and it shouldn't be used during pregnancy because it can cause serious birth defects.

Minimally invasive procedures

Enlarged blood vessels and other changes due to rhinophyma may become permanent. Procedures such as laser surgery and electrosurgery may reduce the visibility of the blood vessels, remove tissue buildup around your nose and generally improve your appearance.

Self-care

It's important to minimize your exposure to anything that causes a flare-up, such as certain foods or alcohol. In addition:

- Wear sunscreen with an SPF of 30 or higher.
- Protect your face in the winter with a scarf or ski mask.
- Don't irritate your face by rubbing or touching it too much.
- Use a gentle cleanser.
- Avoid facial products that contain alcohol or skin irritants.

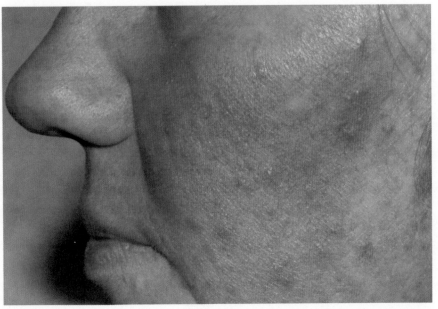

Changes typical of rosacea are redness of the cheeks, nose and central face, with small red bumps or pustules.

Rotator cuff injury

WHAT IS IT? The rotator cuff is a group of muscles and tendons that surround the shoulder joint, keeping the head of your upper arm bone firmly within the socket of the shoulder.

The pain associated with a rotator cuff injury may begin as a dull ache deep in your shoulder and become more severe. It may disturb your sleep, particularly if you lie on or move the affected shoulder. You may find it difficult to reach above your head or behind your back.

Rotator cuff injuries commonly result from:

- **Falling.** Using your arm to break a fall or falling on your arm can bruise or tear a rotator cuff tendon or muscle.
- **Lifting or pulling.** Lifting an object that's too heavy or doing so improperly can strain or tear your tendons or muscles.
- **Repetitive stress.** Repetitive overhead movement of your arms can stress your rotator cuff muscles and tendons, causing irritation, inflammation and tearing.
- **Bone spurs.** An overgrowth of bone can occur on a part of the collarbone that protrudes over the rotator cuff, irritating and damaging the tendon.

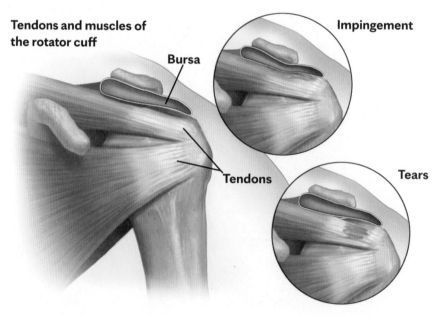

Tendons and muscles of the rotator cuff

Bursa

Impingement

Tendons

Tears

Pinching and irritation of tendons (impingement) and rotator cuff tears are among shoulder problems that become more frequent with age.

TREATMENT Conservative care is often all that's needed to treat an irritated tendon. Other options exist for tears and more severe damage.

Conservative care

Try these steps:

- **Rest your shoulder.** Avoid painful movements and limit heavy lifting or overhead activity until your shoulder pain subsides.
- **Apply ice and heat.** Use a cold pack 15 to 20 minutes every three or four hours. When the inflammation and pain have improved, hot packs or a heating pad may relax tight muscles.
- **Take pain relievers.** Ibuprofen (Advil, Motrin IB, others), naproxen sodium (Aleve) or acetaminophen (Tylenol, others) may help.

Medication

If conservative treatments don't help, your health care provider might recommend a corticosteroid injection into your shoulder joint. While such shots are often helpful, if administered too frequently they can contribute to weakening of the tendon.

Therapy

Physical therapy can help restore flexibility and strength to your shoulder after a rotator cuff injury. Most people exercise the front muscles of the chest, shoulder and upper arm, but it's equally important to strengthen the muscles in the back of the shoulder and around the shoulder blade.

Surgery

Options may include:

- **Bone spur removal.** The excess bone may be removed and the damaged portion of the tendon smoothed.
- **Tendon repair or replacement.** A torn rotator cuff tendon may be repaired and reattached to the upper arm bone. If the torn tendon is too damaged for reattachment, a nearby tendon may be used as a replacement.
- **Shoulder replacement.** Severe injuries associated with arthritis of the shoulder may require shoulder replacement surgery.

R

S

Sexually transmitted infections

WHAT IS IT? Sexually transmitted infections (STIs) include diseases such as chlamydia, gonorrhea, genital herpes, hepatitis B, human papillomavirus (HPV), human immunodeficiency virus (HIV), syphilis and trichomoniasis.

Sexually transmitted infections are generally acquired by sexual contact. The organisms that cause STIs may pass from person to person in blood, semen, or vaginal and other bodily fluids. Some may also be transmitted in other ways, such as from mother to infant during pregnancy or childbirth, or through blood transfusions or shared needles. STIs don't always cause symptoms, and it's possible to get an infection from someone who seems perfectly healthy.

Factors that increase your risk of a sexually transmitted infection include:

- **Unprotected sex.** Vaginal or anal penetration by an infected partner who isn't wearing a latex condom significantly increases the risk of getting an STI. Improper or inconsistent use of condoms also can increase the risk. Oral sex also may transmit infection without some type of protection.
- **Sexual contact with multiple partners.** The more people you have sexual contact with, the greater your overall risk of exposure.
- **A history of STIs.** Being infected with one STI makes it much easier for another STI to take hold. It's also possible to be reinfected by the same infected partner if the partner isn't treated.
- **Alcohol misuse or recreational drug use.** Substance misuse can inhibit your judgment, making you more willing to take part in risky behaviors. Some STIs also can spread by way of contaminated needles.

SYMPTOM CHECKER Sexually transmitted infections have a range of signs and symptoms. These might include:

- Sores or bumps on the genitals or in the oral or rectal area
- Painful or burning urination
- Discharge from the penis
- Unusual or odd-smelling vaginal discharge
- Unusual vaginal bleeding
- Pain during sex
- Sore, swollen lymph nodes, particularly in the groin but sometimes more widespread
- Lower abdominal pain
- Rash over the trunk, hands or feet

Signs and symptoms may appear a few days after exposure. But depending on the organism, symptoms of some STIs may not be noticeable for years after infection.

WHAT TESTS TO EXPECT If your sexual history and signs and symptoms suggest that you have a sexually transmitted infection, lab tests will likely be performed to identify the cause. They may include:

- **Blood tests.** Blood tests can confirm the diagnosis of HIV or later stages of syphilis.
- **Urine samples.** Some infections can be confirmed with a urine sample.
- **Fluid samples.** If you have active genital sores, testing fluid and samples from the sores may be done to diagnose the type of infection. Laboratory tests of material from a genital sore or discharge are used to diagnose the most common bacterial and some viral STIs at an early stage.

S

TREATMENT Treatment usually consists of medication. Sexually transmitted infections caused by bacteria are generally easier to treat. Viral infections can be managed but not always cured.

Antibiotics
Antibiotics, often in a single dose, can cure many sexually transmitted bacterial and parasitic infections, including gonorrhea, syphilis, chlamydia and trichomoniasis. Typically, you'll be treated for gonorrhea and chlamydia at the same time because the two infections often

appear together. Once you start antibiotic treatment, it's crucial to follow through and take all of the medication. It's also important to abstain from sex until you've completed treatment and any sores have healed.

Antiviral drugs

If you have genital herpes, you'll have fewer herpes recurrences if you take daily suppressive therapy with a prescription antiviral drug. Antiviral drugs lessen the risk of infection, but it's still possible to give your partner herpes. For people who have HIV, antiviral drugs can keep the infection in check for many years, although the virus can still be transmitted. The sooner you start treatment, the more effective it is. If you take your medications exactly as directed, it's possible to reduce the viral load in the blood so that it can hardly be detected. Antiviral drugs also are used to treat hepatitis.

If you've had an STI, ask your health care provider how long after treatment you need to be retested. Doing so ensures that the treatment worked and that you haven't been reinfected.

If you are pregnant and have an STI, getting treatment right away can prevent or reduce the risk of your baby becoming infected.

GET VACCINATED

Getting vaccinated early, before sexual exposure, is effective in preventing certain types of sexually transmitted infections. Vaccines are available to prevent HPV, hepatitis A and hepatitis B. The HPV vaccine can prevent more than 90% of cancers caused by HPV infection.

The Centers for Disease Control and Prevention recommends the HPV vaccine for girls and boys ages 11 and 12. If not fully vaccinated at ages 11 and 12, the CDC recommends that teens and young adults through age 26 receive the vaccine. In addition, people ages 27 to 45 who aren't vaccinated against HPV may want to talk with their providers about the risk of HPV and the possible benefit of getting the vaccine.

The hepatitis B vaccine is usually given to newborns, and the hepatitis A vaccine is recommended for 1-year-olds. Both vaccines are recommended for people who aren't already immune to these diseases. They are also recommended for those who are at increased risk of infection, such as men who have sex with men and IV drug users.

S

Shingles

WHAT IS IT? Shingles is a viral infection that causes a painful rash. It is also known as herpes zoster.

Although the rash can occur anywhere on the body, it most often appears as a single stripe of blisters that wraps around either the left or the right side of the torso. Sometimes the shingles rash occurs around one eye or on one side of the neck or face. The infection generally lasts between two and six weeks.

Shingles is caused by the varicella-zoster virus, the same virus that causes chickenpox. After you've had chickenpox, the virus lies inactive in nerve tissue near your spinal cord and brain. Years later, it can reactivate, producing shingles. Among people who get shingles, most get it only once. But it's possible to get shingles more often.

Varicella-zoster is part of a group of viruses called herpes viruses, which includes the viruses that cause cold sores and genital herpes. But the chickenpox and shingles virus isn't the same one responsible for cold sores or genital herpes.

SYMPTOM CHECKER Shingles usually affects only a part of one side of the body. Signs and symptoms may include:

- Pain, burning, numbness or tingling
- Sensitivity to touch
- A red rash that begins a few days after the pain
- Fluid-filled blisters that break open and crust over
- Itching

Some people may experience:

- Fever
- Headache
- Sensitivity to light
- Fatigue

The pain with shingles can be intense. It's even possible to have shingles pain without ever developing the rash. If you have a shingles rash that's widespread and painful, contact your health care provider right away.

S

For some people, shingles pain continues long after the blisters have cleared. This condition is known as postherpetic neuralgia. It occurs when damaged nerve fibers send confused and exaggerated messages of pain from your skin to your brain.

 TREATMENT There's no cure for shingles, but prompt treatment with prescription antiviral drugs can speed healing and reduce the risk of complications. Antiviral medications include acyclovir (Zovirax), vala-cyclovir (Valtrex) and famciclovir.

Your health care provider may also prescribe medication to help relieve the pain associated with shingles.

Taking a cool bath or using cool, wet compresses on your blisters may help relieve itching and pain.

It's especially important to seek treatment right away if you have pain and a rash near an eye. If left untreated, shingles infection can lead to permanent eye damage.

PREVENTION

Two vaccines may help prevent shingles — the chickenpox vaccine and the shingles vaccine.

Chickenpox vaccine. The varicella vaccine is routinely given to children to prevent chickenpox. It's also recommended for adults who've never had chickenpox. Though it doesn't guarantee you won't get chickenpox or shingles, the vaccine reduces your chances of complications and severe disease.

Shingles vaccine. The varicella-zoster vaccine (Shingrix) is approved for use in adults age 50 and older. It's recommended even if you had shingles or you got the Zostavax vaccine, an earlier vaccine for shingles. Like the chickenpox vaccine, the shingles vac-cine doesn't guarantee you won't get an infection. Should you develop shingles, the vaccine will likely reduce its severity, as well as your risk of postherpetic neuralgia.

S

Shin splints

WHAT IS IT? Shin splints refers to pain along the shinbone — the large bone in the front of your lower leg (tibia).

Shin splints are common in runners and dancers. They often occur in athletes who've recently intensified or changed their training routines, causing the muscles, tendons and bone tissue to become overworked and inflamed.

If you have shin splints, you'll likely notice tenderness, soreness or pain along the inner part of your lower leg and mild swelling in your lower leg.

TREATMENT Most cases of shin splints can be treated with rest, ice and other self-care measures.

Rest. Avoid activities that cause pain, swelling or discomfort, but don't give up all physical activity. While you're healing, try low-impact exercises, such as swimming, bicycling or water running.

Ice the affected area. Apply ice packs to the affected shin for 15 to 20 minutes at a time, 4 to 8 times a day for several days. To protect your skin, wrap the ice packs in a thin towel.

Take an over-the-counter pain reliever. Try ibuprofen (Advil, Motrin IB, others), naproxen sodium (Aleve) or acetaminophen (Tylenol, others) to reduce pain.

To help prevent a recurrence of shin splints:

- **Choose the right shoes.** Wear footwear that suits your sport. If you're a runner, replace your shoes about every 350 to 500 miles.
- **Consider arch supports.** Arch supports can help prevent the pain of shin splints, especially if you have flat arches.
- **Lessen the impact.** Cross-train with a sport that places less impact on your shins, such as swimming, walking or biking.
- **Add strength training to your workout.** To strengthen your calf muscles, try toe raises. When they become easy, do the exercises holding progressively heavier weights. Leg presses and other exercises for your lower legs can be helpful, too.

Sinusitis

WHAT IS IT? Sinusitis causes the cavities around your nasal passages (sinuses) to inflame and swell. This interferes with drainage and causes mucus to build up in nasal cavities.

Sinusitis may last for a short period (acute) or persist (chronic). Acute sinusitis is most often caused by the common cold. Chronic sinusitis may stem from an infection. But it is more likely to be associated with allergies, growths in the sinuses (nasal polyps), a deviated nasal septum or airborne pollutants.

SYMPTOM CHECKER Signs and symptoms may include:

- Drainage of thick, yellow or greenish discharge
- Nasal obstruction or congestion, causing difficulty breathing
- Pain, swelling and pressure around your eyes, cheeks or forehead
- Reduced sense of smell and taste
- Headache, ear pain or both
- Aching in your upper jaw and teeth
- Bad breath (halitosis)
- Cough, which may be worse at night

HEALTHY SINUSES   **SINUSITIS**

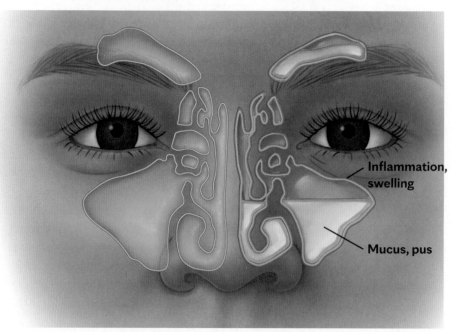

Inflammation, swelling

Mucus, pus

S

TREATMENT Acute sinusitis related to the common cold can often be treated with self-care measures. Antibiotics are generally prescribed only if the infection is severe or persistent and thought to be caused by bacteria.

In addition to getting plenty of rest and fluids, try these measures:

- **Moisten your sinus cavities.** Take a hot shower, breathing in the warm, moist air. This can help ease pain and help mucus drain.
- **Apply warm compresses to your face.** Place warm, damp towels around your nose, cheeks and eyes to ease facial pain.
- **Rinse out your nasal passages.** Use a specially designed squeeze bottle or neti pot to rinse your nasal passages. This home remedy can help clear your sinuses. Rinse the device after each use.
- **Use a saline nasal spray.** Spray it into your nose several times a day to rinse your nasal passages.
- **Try a decongestant.** Nonprescription oral decongestants include Sudafed and Actifed. Decongestant nasal sprays include oxymetazoline (Afrin, others). Nasal decongestants should be used for only a few days at most. Otherwise, they can cause the return of more-severe congestion (rebound congestion).
- **Take a pain reliever.** Acetaminophen (Tylenol, others) or ibuprofen (Advil, Motrin IB, others) may be helpful.

For chronic sinusitis, in addition to self-care measures, your health care provider may recommend one or more of the following:

- **Nasal corticosteroid.** These nasal sprays help prevent and treat inflammation. Examples include fluticasone (Flonase), budesonide (Rhinocort Allergy), triamcinolone (Nasacort Allergy 24 Hour), mometasone (Nasonex Allergy) and beclomethasone (Beconase AQ).
- **Oral or injected corticosteroid.** They're used to relieve inflammation from severe sinusitis, especially if you also have nasal polyps. Examples include prednisone and methylprednisolone.
- **Aspirin desensitization treatment.** This may be recommended if your sinusitis is associated with an allergy to aspirin. The treatment is available only in specialized medical centers.
- **Immunotherapy.** If allergies are contributing to your sinusitis, allergy shots (immunotherapy) that reduce the body's reaction to specific allergens may help treat sinusitis.
- **Surgery.** In some cases, a surgeon may remove scar tissue or a polyp that's causing nasal blockage. Enlarging a narrow sinus opening also may be an option to promote drainage.

S

Skin cancer

WHAT IS IT? Skin cancer — the abnormal growth of skin cells — most often develops on skin exposed to the sun, such as the scalp, face, lips, ears, neck, chest, arms and hands. But this common form of cancer can also occur on areas of your skin not ordinarily exposed to sunlight.

Skin cancer begins in the skin's top layer called the epidermis. The epidermis contains three main types of cells: basal cells, squamous cells and melanocytes. When skin cancer cells begin to form, the type of cancer cells determines the type of skin cancer a person has. The three major types of skin cancer are basal cell carcinoma, squamous cell carcinoma and melanoma.

Basal cell carcinoma

Basal cell carcinoma usually occurs in sun-exposed areas of the body, such as the neck or face. It may appear as:

- A pearly or waxy bump
- A flat, flesh-colored or brown scar-like lesion

Squamous cell carcinoma

Most often, squamous cell carcinoma occurs on sun-exposed areas of the body, such as the face, ears and hands. People with brown or Black skin are more likely to develop squamous cell carcinoma on areas that aren't often exposed to the sun. Squamous cell carcinoma may appear as:

- A firm, red nodule
- A flat lesion with a scaly, crusted surface

Melanoma

Melanoma, the most deadly form of skin cancer, can develop anywhere on your body, in an existing mole that becomes cancerous or separate from any moles. Melanoma most often appears on the face, arms, legs, back and shoulders. It can also occur on skin that hasn't been exposed to the sun. In nonwhite people, it occurs more often on the soles of the feet, on the palms of the hands or under the nails.

S

The most important warning sign for melanoma is a new spot that changes in size, shape or color. Another warning sign is a spot that looks different from all of the other spots on your skin. Another guide to identifying melanoma is the ABCDE rule:

- **Asymmetry.** One side, or half, of a mole or birthmark doesn't match the other.
- **Border.** The edges are irregular, ragged, notched or blurred.
- **Color.** The color isn't the same all over.
- **Diameter.** The spot is larger than the size of a pencil eraser.
- **Evolving.** The mole or spot is changing in size, shape or color.

WHAT'S THE CAUSE? Skin cancer occurs when changes (mutations) occur in the DNA of skin cells. These changes cause the cells to grow out of control and form a mass of cancer cells. Much of the damage to DNA in skin cells results from ultraviolet (UV) radiation found in sunlight and in the lights used in tanning beds.

But sun exposure doesn't explain skin cancers that develop on skin not ordinarily exposed to sunlight. This indicates that other factors may contribute to the risk of skin cancer, such as exposure to toxic substances or having a condition that weakens the immune system.

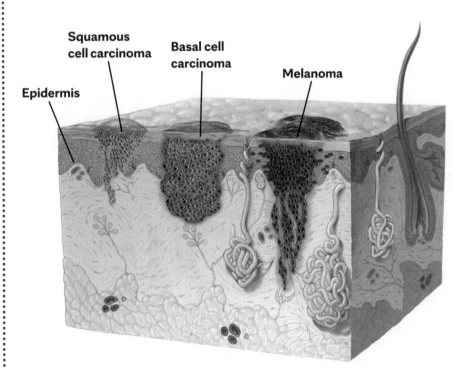

Epidermis

Squamous cell carcinoma

Basal cell carcinoma

Melanoma

S

Factors that may increase your risk of skin cancer include:

- **White skin.** Having less pigment (melanin) in your skin provides less protection from UV radiation. If you have blond or red hair, light-colored eyes, and you freckle or sunburn easily, you're more likely to develop skin cancer than is a person with brown or Black skin.
- **History of sunburns.** Having had one or more blistering sunburns as a child or teenager increases your risk of developing skin cancer as an adult.
- **Excessive sun exposure.** Anyone who spends considerable time in the sun may develop skin cancer, especially if the skin isn't protected by sunscreen or clothing. Tanning, including exposure to tanning lamps and beds, also puts you at increased risk.
- **Sunny or high-altitude climates.** People who live in sunny, warm climates are exposed to more sunlight than are people who live in colder climates. Living at higher elevations, where the sunlight is strongest, also exposes people to more radiation.
- **Moles.** People who have many moles or irregular moles called dysplastic nevi are at increased risk of skin cancer. These moles are typically larger than other moles and are more likely to become cancerous in the future.
- **Precancerous skin lesions.** Skin lesions known as actinic keratosis can increase your risk of developing skin cancer. They typically appear as rough, scaly patches and range in color from brown to dark pink.
- **Family history.** If one of your parents or a sibling has had skin cancer, you may have an increased risk of the disease.

TREATMENT After learning you have skin cancer, additional tests may be needed to determine its stage.

Because superficial skin cancers such as basal cell carcinoma rarely spread, a biopsy that removes the entire growth often is the only test needed to determine the cancer stage. If you have a large squamous cell carcinoma or melanoma, your health care provider may recommend further tests to determine the extent of the cancer.

Stage 1 cancers are small and limited to the area where they began. Stage 4 indicates advanced cancer that has spread to other areas of the body. Sometimes the Roman numerals I through IV are used to indicate a cancer's stage.

Options

Treatment options vary, depending on the size, type, depth and location of the lesion. Small cancers that are limited to the surface of the skin may not require treatment beyond an initial biopsy that removes the growth. If additional treatment is needed, options may include:

Freezing. Your health care provider may destroy actinic keratoses and some small, early skin cancers by freezing them with liquid nitrogen (cryosurgery). The dead tissue comes off when it thaws.

Excisional surgery. This type of treatment may be appropriate for any type of skin cancer. A doctor cuts out (excises) the cancerous tissue and a surrounding margin of healthy skin.

Mohs surgery. This procedure is for larger, recurring or difficult-to-treat skin cancers. It's often used when a person wants to conserve as much skin as possible, such as on the nose. During Mohs surgery, a doctor removes the skin growth layer by layer, examining each layer under the microscope, until no cancerous cells remain. The procedure allows cancerous cells to be removed without taking an excessive amount of surrounding healthy skin.

Curettage and electrodesiccation or cryotherapy. After removing most of a growth, a doctor scrapes away layers of cancer cells using a device with a circular blade (curet). An electric needle destroys any remaining cancer cells. In a variation of this procedure, liquid nitrogen can be used to freeze the base and edges of the treated area.

Radiation therapy. Radiation therapy may be an option when surgery may not completely remove all cancer cells.

Chemotherapy. For cancers limited to the top layer of skin, creams or lotions containing anti-cancer agents may be applied directly to the skin. Oral or intravenous (IV) chemotherapy drugs may be used to treat skin cancers that have spread to other parts of the body.

Photodynamic therapy. This treatment destroys skin cancer cells with a combination of laser light and drugs that makes cancer cells sensitive to light.

Biological therapy. Biological treatments stimulate your immune system to kill cancer cells.

S

Sleep apnea

WHAT IS IT? Sleep apnea is a potentially serious sleep disorder in which breathing repeatedly stops and starts. There are two main types of sleep apnea:

Obstructive sleep apnea

Obstructive sleep apnea occurs when the muscles in the back of your throat relax. Your airway narrows or closes and you aren't able to breathe properly. Your brain senses this inability to breathe and briefly rouses you from sleep so that you can reopen your airway. You may make a snorting, choking or gasping sound. This pattern can repeat itself several times an hour, all night long. The disruptions impair your ability to reach the restful phases of sleep.

People at greater risk of obstructive sleep apnea are those who are overweight, who have a thicker neck or who are bothered by nasal congestion. Men are more likely to develop it than women.

Central sleep apnea

Central sleep apnea, which is much less common, occurs when your brain fails to transmit signals to your breathing muscles while you're sleeping. You may awaken with shortness of breath or have difficulty getting to sleep or staying asleep. Heart disorders, older age, opioid medications and stroke increase the risk of this type of sleep apnea. People with central sleep apnea may be more likely to remember awakening than people with obstructive sleep apnea.

SYMPTOM CHECKER Common signs and symptoms of obstructive and central sleep apnea include:

- Excessive daytime sleepiness
- Loud snoring, usually more prominent in obstructive sleep apnea
- Episodes of breathing cessation during sleep
- Abrupt awakenings with shortness of breath, usually more common with central sleep apnea
- Awakening with a dry mouth or sore throat
- Morning headache
- Difficulty staying asleep
- Attention difficulty

TREATMENT Treatment for obstructive sleep apnea includes:

Continuous positive airway pressure (CPAP). A machine delivers air pressure through a mask placed over your nose while you sleep. The air pressure is somewhat greater than that of the surrounding air — just enough to keep your upper airway passages open. CPAP is the most common and reliable method of treating sleep apnea.

Adjustable airway pressure devices. They automatically adjust the pressure while you're sleeping. Bilevel positive airway pressure (BPAP) units provide more pressure when you inhale and less when you exhale.

Oral appliances. They're designed to keep your throat open. Some open your throat by bringing your jaw forward, which can sometimes relieve snoring and mild obstructive sleep apnea.

Adaptive servo-ventilation (ASV). This newer airflow device learns your regular breathing pattern and stores the information in a built-in computer. After you fall asleep, the machine uses pressure to normalize your breathing pattern and prevent pauses in your breathing.

Surgery. Surgery is usually only an option after other treatments have failed. Surgical options include:

- **Tissue removal.** A surgeon removes tissue from the rear of the mouth and top of the throat. The tonsils and adenoids usually are removed as well. This type of surgery may be more successful in stopping snoring than in treating sleep apnea.
- **Nerve stimulation.** An implanted device stimulates the nerve that controls tongue movement (hypoglossal nerve) to open the airway.
- **Jaw repositioning.** The jaw is moved forward, enlarging the space behind the tongue and soft palate. This makes obstruction less likely.
- **Implants.** Plastic rods are surgically implanted into the soft palate to help keep the airway open.
- **Creating a new air passageway.** In case of life-threatening sleep apnea, a surgeon makes an opening in the neck and inserts a metal or plastic tube to ease breathing. This is called a tracheostomy. The opening stays covered during the day. At night it's uncovered to bypass the blocked airway in the throat.

Treatments for central sleep apnea generally involve treating the underlying medical condition. Using supplemental oxygen while you sleep may help. In some situations, CPAP or BPAP may be helpful.

S

Sprained ankle

WHAT IS IT? A sprained ankle occurs when you roll, twist or turn your ankle in an awkward way, stretching or tearing the tough bands of tissue (ligaments) that help hold your ankle bones together. Most sprained ankles involve injuries to the ligaments on the outer side of the ankle.

Signs and symptoms of a sprained ankle include:

- Pain, especially when bearing weight on the affected foot
- Swelling and, sometimes, bruising
- Restricted range of motion
- A "pop" that's heard or felt at the time of injury, on occasion

After having one ankle sprain or ankle injury, you're more likely to sprain the ankle again.

TREATMENT Treatment for a sprained ankle depends on the severity of your injury. For many sprains, you can treat the injury at home using the R.I.C.E. approach (see page 335). Other treatments include:

Medications. An over-the-counter pain reliever, such as ibuprofen (Advil, Motrin IB, others), naproxen sodium (Aleve) or acetaminophen (Tylenol, others) can help manage the pain.

Devices. Because walking with a sprained ankle might be painful, you may need to use crutches or a removable splint until the pain subsides. If your ankle joint is unstable, you may need a cast or walking boot to immobilize the joint so that it can heal properly.

Therapy. Once the swelling goes down, a physical therapist may help with exercises to restore range of motion, strength, flexibility and balance. If you sprained your ankle while exercising or participating in a sport, talk to your health care provider about when you can resume your activity. You may need to wear an ankle brace or wrap your ankle to protect it from re-injury.

Surgery. In rare cases of severe ligament tears, particularly in elite athletes, surgery may be needed to repair the damage.

TREATING SPRAINS AND STRAINS

For immediate self-care of a muscle or ligament sprain, try the R.I.C.E. approach:

- **Rest.** Avoid activities that cause pain, swelling or discomfort.
- **Ice.** Immediately after injury use an ice pack or slush bath for 15 to 20 minutes and repeat every 2 to 3 hours while you're awake. Cold reduces pain, swelling and inflammation in injured muscles, joints and connective tissues. It may also slow bleeding if a tear has occurred. If you have vascular disease, diabetes or decreased sensation, talk with your health care provider before applying ice.
- **Compression.** Compress the sprained area with an elastic bandage until the swelling stops. Don't interfere with circulation by wrapping too tightly. Begin wrapping at the end farthest from your heart. Loosen the wrap if the pain increases, the area becomes numb or swelling is occurring below the wrapped area.
- **Elevation.** Elevate the injured limb above the level of your heart, especially at night. Gravity helps reduce swelling by draining excess fluid.

Sprain vs. strain

Sprains and strains are common injuries that share similar signs and symptoms, but involve different parts of the body.

A sprain is a stretching or tearing of ligaments — the tough bands of fibrous tissue that connect two bones together in your joints. The most common location for a sprain is in your ankle.

A strain is a stretching or tearing of a muscle or tendon. A tendon is a fibrous cord of tissue that connects muscles to bones. Strains often occur in the lower back and in the hamstring muscle in the back of your thigh.

Initial treatment for both sprains and strains includes rest, ice, compression and elevation (R.I.C.E.). Mild sprains and strains can often be successfully treated at home. Severe sprains and strains sometimes require surgery to repair torn ligaments, muscles or tendons.

After the first two days, gently begin to use the injured area. You should see a gradual, progressive improvement in the joint's ability to support your weight or your ability to move without pain. Mild and moderate injuries usually heal in 3 to 6 weeks.

S

Stomach flu

WHAT IS IT? Stomach flu (viral gastroenteritis) is an infection in your intestines that leads to watery diarrhea, stomach cramps, nausea, vomiting and sometimes fever. Despite its name, the stomach flu is not the same as influenza.

WHAT'S THE CAUSE? Stomach flu is caused by a virus. You can get it by sharing utensils, towels or food with someone who has the virus. Eating food or drinking water contaminated with the virus also can make you sick.

In many cases, the virus is passed when someone with it handles food you eat after using the toilet. Some shellfish, especially raw or under-cooked oysters, also can make you sick.

Norovirus and rotavirus are the viruses that most often cause stomach flu. Norovirus can sweep through families and communities. Rotavirus most often affects young children. In some countries, including the United States, a rotavirus vaccine is available for infants.

Children, older adults, dormitory residents and anyone with a weakened immune system may be at high risk of stomach flu.

SYMPTOM CHECKER Stomach flu attacks your intestines, causing signs and symptoms such as:

- Watery, usually nonbloody diarrhea
- Nausea, vomiting or both
- Stomach cramps and pain
- Occasional muscle aches or headache
- Low-grade fever

Depending on the cause, symptoms may appear within 1 to 3 days after you're infected. They can range from mild to severe. Symptoms usually last just a day or two, but occasionally, they may last up to two weeks.

Because the symptoms are similar, it's easy to confuse diarrhea caused by a virus with diarrhea caused by bacteria such as salmonella or E. coli.

See your health care provider if you experience any of the following:

- You can't keep liquids down for 24 hours
- You've been vomiting or have had diarrhea for more than two days
- You have signs of dehydration, such as excessive thirst, dry mouth, deep yellow urine or little or no urine, and severe weakness, dizziness or lightheadedness
- You see blood in your vomit or bowel movements
- You have severe stomach pain
- Your fever is above 104 F (40 C)

If your child has any of the following signs and symptoms, call your child's health care provider right away:

- Has a fever of 102 F (38.9 C) or higher
- Seems tired or very irritable
- Is in a lot of discomfort or pain
- Has bloody diarrhea
- Has signs of dehydration, such as a dry mouth, thirst and crying without tears

If you have an infant, remember that spitting up, which may be common, is different from vomiting. Call your baby's health care provider right away if your baby has any of these symptoms:

- Frequent vomiting
- No wet diapers in six hours
- Bloody stools or severe diarrhea
- A sunken soft spot (fontanel) on the top of the head
- A dry mouth or crying without tears
- Unusual sleepiness or being unresponsive

TREATMENT There's often no specific medical treatment for stomach flu. Antibiotics don't work for viruses. The best way to recover quickly is through self-care and staying hydrated.

To care for yourself at home with stomach flu, you can try:

- Not eating solid food for a few hours so that your stomach can settle
- Sucking on ice chips or taking frequent small sips of water
- Easing back into eating, as you're able, with bland foods
- Getting plenty of rest

- Taking anti-diarrheal medications, such as loperamide (Imodium A-D) or bismuth subsalicylate (Pepto-Bismol), unless you have bloody diarrhea

If your child has stomach flu, it's important to replace lost fluids and salts. Give your child an oral rehydration solution (Pedialyte, others). Don't give over-the-counter anti-diarrheal medications. They can make it hard for your child's body to get rid of the virus.

Make sure your child gets plenty of rest. Once your child is rehydrated, start offering foods like toast, yogurt, fruits and vegetables. Avoid sugary foods, which can make diarrhea worse.

If your infant is sick, let the baby's stomach settle for 15 to 20 minutes after vomiting or a bout of diarrhea, then offer small amounts of liquid. If you're breastfeeding, let your baby nurse. If your baby is bottle-fed, offer a small amount of an oral rehydration solution or regular formula. Don't dilute your baby's already-prepared formula.

The main complication of stomach flu is a severe loss of water and essential salts and minerals (dehydration). Dehydration shouldn't be a problem if you or your child is healthy and drink enough to replace fluids you lose from vomiting and diarrhea.

LIFESTYLE To help prevent stomach flu, get your children vaccinated against rotavirus and follow these steps to limit the spread of viruses:

- Wash your hands thoroughly for 20 seconds.
- Avoid sharing eating utensils, drinking glasses and plates and use separate towels in the bathroom.
- Prepare food safely, and don't cook if you're sick.
- If someone in your home has stomach flu, disinfect hard surfaces with a mixture of 5 to 25 tablespoons (73 to 369 milliliters) of bleach to 1 gallon (3.8 liters) of water.
- Wear gloves while touching laundry if someone in your home has stomach flu.
- If your child attends a care center, make sure the center has separate and sanitary rooms for changing diapers and preparing or serving food.
- When you're traveling, reduce your risk from contaminated food or water. Use bottled water and avoid undercooked meat and raw food that others have handled.

Strep throat

WHAT IS IT? Strep throat is a bacterial infection of the throat that can make it feel sore and scratchy. It's most common in kids between ages 5 and 15, but it affects people of all ages.

The cause of strep throat is bacteria known as *Streptococcus pyogenes*. This is also known as group A streptococcus. Some people are carriers of strep, which means they can pass the bacteria on to others. But the bacteria aren't making them sick.

SYMPTOM CHECKER Signs and symptoms include:

- Throat pain and difficulty swallowing
- Red and swollen tonsils, sometimes with white patches or streaks of pus
- Tiny red spots at the back of the roof of the mouth
- Swollen, tender lymph glands in the neck
- Fever
- Headache
- Rash
- Stomachache and sometimes vomiting
- Fatigue

A cough and hoarse voice generally aren't associated with strep throat.

WHAT TESTS TO EXPECT A health care provider will usually check your throat for redness, swelling, and white streaks or pus on the tonsils. Laboratory tests to identify strep often include:

- **Throat culture.** A sterile swab is rubbed over the back of the throat and tonsils to get a sample of the secretions. The sample is cultured in a laboratory for the presence of bacteria. Results can take as long as two days.
- **Rapid antigen test.** While waiting for a throat culture, your health care provider may order a rapid antigen test on the swab sample. This test can detect strep bacteria in minutes. But rapid strep tests may miss some strep throat infections. For this reason, many providers use both tests — a rapid antigen test for quick results and a throat culture to confirm the results.

S

TREATMENT The main treatment for strep throat is an antibiotic medication. Drugs commonly prescribed include:

- **Amoxicillin.** It's often a preferred option for children because it tastes better than penicillin and is available as a chewable tablet.
- **Penicillin.** In a young child who is having a hard time swallowing or is vomiting, penicillin can be given by injection.

If you or your child is allergic to penicillin, other options include a cephalosporin such as cephalexin, clarithromycin (Biaxin XL), azithromycin (Zithromax) or clindamycin.

Once treatment begins, you or your child should start feeling better in a day or two, but it's crucial to finish the prescription. Children taking an antibiotic who feel well and don't have a fever can often return to school or child care 24 hours after beginning treatment.

In addition to antibiotics, your provider may suggest a nonprescription pain reliever such as ibuprofen (Advil, Motrin, others) or acetaminophen (Tylenol, others) to relieve throat pain and fever. Because of the risk of Reye's syndrome, aspirin shouldn't be given to young children and teenagers unless your provider specifically prescribes it.

Self-care

In addition to an antibiotic, these tips may help relieve symptoms:

- **Get plenty of rest.** Sleep helps your body fight infection.
- **Drink plenty of water.** Keeping a sore throat moist eases swallowing. Water also helps prevent dehydration.
- **Eat soothing foods.** Foods that are easy on a sore throat include broths, soups, applesauce, cooked cereal, mashed potatoes, soft fruits and yogurt. Very cold foods such as sherbet, frozen yogurt or frozen fruit pops also may be soothing on a sore throat.
- **Gargle with warm salt water.** For older children and adults, gargling several times a day can help relieve throat pain. Mix 1 teaspoon table salt in 8 ounces of warm water. Make sure to tell your child to spit out the liquid after gargling.
- **Use a humidifier.** Moisture keeps mucous membranes in your throat from becoming dry and even more irritated. Choose a cool-mist humidifier and clean it daily, because bacteria and molds can flourish in some humidifiers. Saline nasal sprays also help keep mucous membranes moist.

Stroke

WHAT IS IT? A stroke occurs when the blood supply to part of the brain is interrupted or severely reduced, depriving brain tissue of oxygen and nutrients. Within minutes, brain cells begin to die.

Types

A stroke may result from a blocked artery (ischemic stroke) or the leaking or bursting of a blood vessel (hemorrhagic stroke). Some people experience a temporary disruption of blood flow to the brain without brain cell death. This is called transient ischemic attack (TIA).

Ischemic stroke. About 85% of strokes are ischemic strokes. These occur when the arteries to the brain become narrowed or blocked, causing severely reduced blood flow (ischemia). The most common ischemic strokes include:

- **Thrombotic stroke.** It occurs when a blood clot forms in one of the arteries that supply blood to your brain.
- **Embolic stroke.** It occurs when a blood clot or other debris forms away from your brain — commonly in your heart — and travels through your bloodstream and lodges in a brain artery.

Hemorrhagic stroke. Hemorrhagic stroke occurs when a blood vessel in the brain leaks or ruptures. Brain hemorrhages can result from many conditions, including uncontrolled high blood pressure and weak spots in the blood vessel walls (aneurysms). Types of hemorrhagic stroke include:

- **Intracerebral hemorrhage.** A blood vessel bursts and spills into the surrounding brain tissue, damaging brain cells. Brain cells beyond the leak are deprived of blood and also damaged.
- **Subarachnoid hemorrhage.** An artery on or near the surface of the brain bursts and spills into the space between the surface of the brain and the skull. This type of stroke commonly results from the bursting of an aneurysm.

Transient ischemic attack (TIA). A TIA, also known as a ministroke, is a brief period of symptoms similar to those of a stroke. TIAs often last less than five minutes. Like an ischemic stroke, a TIA occurs when a clot or debris blocks blood flow to part of the brain. But a TIA doesn't leave lasting symptoms because the blockage is temporary. Having a

TIA puts you at greater risk of having a full-blown stroke in the future. And it often indicates an underlying medical condition, so it's important to see your health care provider.

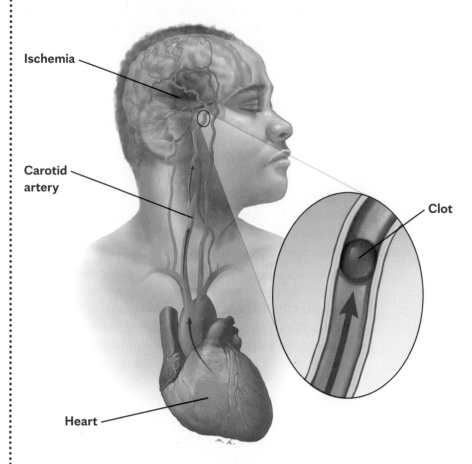

Ischemia

Carotid artery

Clot

Heart

m. k.

Risk factors

Many factors can increase your risk of a stroke. They include being overweight, not getting enough exercise, smoking, excessive alcohol use and use of illicit drugs. Medical conditions such as high blood pressure, high cholesterol, diabetes, cardiovascular disease, obstructive sleep apnea and a previous COVID-19 infection also can increase your stroke risk. A family history of stroke, TIAs or heart attack increase the risk too.

SYMPTOM CHECKER Signs and symptoms may include:

- **Trouble speaking and understanding.** You may experience confusion. You may slur your words or have difficulty understanding speech.

- **Paralysis or numbness of the face, arm or leg.** You may develop sudden numbness, weakness or paralysis in your face, an arm or a leg, especially on one side of your body. Try to raise both your arms over your head at the same time. If one arm begins to fall, you may be having a stroke. Similarly, one side of your mouth may droop when you try to smile.
- **Trouble seeing in one or both eyes.** You may have blurred or blackened vision in one or both eyes, or you may see double.
- **Headache.** A sudden, severe headache, which may be accompanied by vomiting, dizziness or altered consciousness, may indicate you're having a stroke.
- **Trouble with walking.** You may stumble or experience sudden dizziness, loss of balance or loss of coordination.

TREATMENT The treatment you receive will depend on whether you're having an ischemic or hemorrhagic stroke.

Ischemic stroke

To treat an ischemic stroke, health care providers must quickly try to restore blood flow to the brain.

Medication. Treatment is centered around the use of clot-busting medications, which must be administered within about 3 to 4 hours of the start of symptoms — the sooner, the better. Quick treatment not only improves your chances of survival but also may reduce complications. Options include:

- **IV tissue plasminogen activator (TPA).** An injection of TPA is usually given through a vein in the arm. TPA restores blood flow by dissolving the blood clot causing the stroke. Your provider will consider certain risks, such as potential bleeding in the brain, to determine if TPA is appropriate for you.
- **Endovascular therapy.** In some cases, TPA is administered via a slender tube (catheter) inserted into an artery in your groin and threaded to the location in your brain where the stroke is occurring.

Other procedures. Depending on the circumstances, certain procedures may be performed to treat a stroke. They include the following:

- **Mechanical clot removal.** In limited circumstances a catheter is inserted into an artery and threaded to your brain where the device is used to physically break up or grab and remove the clot.

- **Carotid endarterectomy.** To decrease your risk of another stroke or TIA, your doctor may open up an artery in your neck that's become narrowed by fatty deposits (plaques) and remove the deposits.
- **Angioplasty and stents.** A balloon is used to expand a narrowed artery, and a tiny meshlike device (stent) is inserted for support.

Hemorrhagic stroke

Emergency treatment of hemorrhagic stroke focuses on controlling your bleeding and reducing pressure in your brain.

Medication. If you take warfarin (Jantoven) or anti-platelet drugs such as clopidogrel (Plavix) to prevent blood clots, you may be given drugs or transfusions of blood products to counteract the blood thinners' effects. You may also be given drugs to lower pressure in your brain, lower your blood pressure, prevent blood vessel spasms or prevent seizures. Once the bleeding stops, healing is similar to what happens while a bad bruise goes away. If the area of bleeding is large, you may have surgery to remove the blood and relieve pressure on your brain.

Surgery. Surgery may be used to repair damaged blood vessels or blood vessel irregularities and decrease the risk of future strokes.

- **Surgical clipping.** A tiny clamp is placed at the base of an aneurysm to stop blood flow to it. The clamp keeps the aneurysm from bursting, or it can prevent re-bleeding of the aneurysm.
- **Coiling (endovascular embolization).** A surgeon inserts a catheter into an artery in your groin and guides it to your brain. Tiny detachable coils are placed into the aneurysm. The coils block blood flow into the aneurysm and cause blood to clot.
- **AVM removal.** A surgeon may remove a tangle of blood vessels called an arteriovenous malformation (AVM) if it's located in an accessible area of your brain.
- **Stereotactic radiosurgery.** Using multiple beams of highly focused radiation, this procedure may be used to repair some vascular malformations.

Recovery

After emergency treatment, you'll be closely monitored for at least a day. After that, stroke care focuses on helping you recover as much function as possible and return to independent living.

Sty

WHAT IS IT? A sty (also spelled stye) is a red, painful lump near the edge of your eyelid that may look like a boil or a pimple. Sties are often filled with pus, and they usually form on the outside of the eyelid. Sometimes a sty can form on the inner part of the eyelid.

A sty is usually caused by bacteria, especially the bacterium staphylococcus. Touching your eyes with unwashed hands can transfer bacteria to your eyelids. Chronic inflammation of the eyelid caused by a condition called blepharitis also can cause a sty to form.

SYMPTOM CHECKER Signs and symptoms include:

- A red lump on the eyelid that is similar to a boil or a pimple
- Eyelid pain
- Eyelid swelling
- Tearing
- Crusting around the eyelids

Another condition that causes inflammation of the eyelid is a chalazion. A chalazion occurs when there's a blockage in one of the small oil glands at the margin of the eyelid, just behind the eyelashes. Unlike a sty, a chalazion tends to be most prominent on the inner side of the eyelid. It's a chronic problem that's usually painless. Unless a secondary infection is involved, antibiotics usually aren't prescribed.

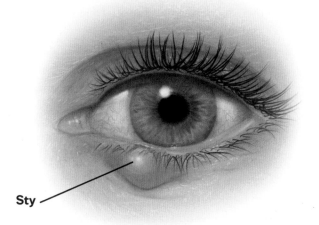

Sty

TREATMENT A health care provider usually can diagnose a sty just by looking at your eyelid. In most cases, a sty doesn't require specific treatment and it often goes away with some basic self-care.

Self-care

Until your sty goes away:

- **Leave it alone.** Don't try to pop the sty or squeeze the pus from a sty. Doing so can cause the infection to spread.
- **Use a warm compress.** To relieve pain, wet a clean washcloth with warm water. Wring out the washcloth and place it over your closed eye. Re-wet the washcloth with fresh warm water when it loses heat. Continue doing this for 10 or 15 minutes, and repeat this process several times each day to encourage the sty to drain on its own.
- **Keep your eye clean.** Don't wear eye makeup, such as mascara and eye liner, until the sty has healed.
- **Go without contact lenses.** It's possible for your contact lenses to become contaminated with bacteria associated with your sty, so go without contacts until your sty disappears.

Treatment

For a sty that persists, your provider may recommend:

- **Antibiotics.** Your provider may prescribe antibiotic eye drops or a topical antibiotic cream to apply to your eyelid. If the infection persists or spreads beyond your eyelid, oral antibiotics may be prescribed.
- **Surgery.** To treat a pus-filled sty that won't rupture or burst on its own, a doctor may choose to lance and drain the sty to relieve pain and pressure.

LIFESTYLE To prevent eye infections or reinfection:

- **Wash your hands.** Wash your hands regularly and keep them away from your eyes.
- **Take care with cosmetics.** Be sure to throw away any eye cosmetics you used when you had a sty or other eye infection and don't share cosmetics with others.
- **Clean your contact lenses.** Always wash your hands thoroughly before inserting your contacts and disinfect them regularly.

Substance use disorder

WHAT IS IT? Substance use disorder, also called drug addiction, affects a person's brain and behavior. People with this disease are unable to control how they use a legal or illicit drug or medication.

Alcohol, nicotine and marijuana use can lead to addiction. If you're addicted to a substance, you may continue using it despite the harm it causes.

WHAT'S THE CAUSE? A person's environment and the traits the person inherits (genetics) both seem to play a role in drug addiction. For example, peer pressure can lead to starting to use or misuse drugs, while genetics may predispose someone to developing an addiction.

Physical addiction seems to occur when repeated use of a drug changes the way the brain feels pleasure. The drug causes physical changes to nerve cells (neurons) in the brain that can remain long after you stop using the drug. Some drugs, such as opioid painkillers, cause addiction faster than others.

As time passes, a person may need more and more of the drug to get high or to feel good. After stopping the drug, the person may have intense cravings and get physically ill.

Anyone can become addicted to a drug. It can start by experimenting with a recreational drug with friends or by taking a medication prescribed by a health care provider.

Certain factors can make addiction more likely to develop or to develop more quickly. Having a difficult family situation, a mental health disorder, or a family member who is addicted to alcohol or drugs increases a person's risk of addiction. People who used drugs at an early age or who take a highly addictive drug are also at greater risk.

SYMPTOM CHECKER Behaviors or symptoms that are "red flags" that you may have a drug addiction include:

- Feeling that you have to use the drug regularly — daily or even several times a day

S

- Having intense urges for the drug that block out other thoughts
- Needing more and more of the drug to get the same effect
- Taking more of the drug and for a longer time than you intended
- Making certain that you have a supply of the drug
- Spending money on the drug even if you can't afford it
- Not meeting obligations or work responsibilities, or cutting back on outside activities because of drug use
- Continuing to use the drug, even though it's causing problems in your life
- Doing things to get the drug that you typically wouldn't do, such as stealing
- Driving or doing other risky activities when you're under the influence of the drug
- Spending a lot of time getting or using the drug, or recovering from its effects
- Being unable to stop using the drug
- Having withdrawal symptoms when you try to stop using the drug

The following may be signs that someone in your family is using drugs:

- Frequently missing school or work, or a drop in grades or work performance
- Lack of energy and motivation, weight change or red eyes
- Lack of interest in clothing, grooming or looks
- Changes in behavior, such as exaggerated efforts by a teenager to keep family members out of the teen's room
- Sudden requests for money that are unreasonable or money or items missing from your home

The signs and symptoms of drug use can vary, depending on what type of drug someone uses.

Marijuana. People use marijuana (cannabis) by smoking, eating or inhaling it. They may be euphoric or paranoid and have red eyes and cravings for foods at unusual times.

Synthetic drugs. Synthetic cannabinoids, also called K2 or Spice, can cause dangerous and unpredictable effects, such as extreme anxiety, agitation or paranoia. These drugs are sprayed on dried herbs and smoked or prepared as an herbal tea. "Bath salts" are mind-altering substances often labeled as other products to avoid detection. A person taking them may have psychotic and violent behavior.

Central nervous system stimulants. Prescription central nervous system depressants such as barbiturates are taken in pills. They can cause drowsiness and slurred speech.

Meth, cocaine and other stimulants. Someone who takes a stimulant such as cocaine may have increased energy, rapid or rambling speech, and dilated pupils. Stimulants can be taken in pills, snorted or smoked

Opioid painkillers. Opioids are pills prescribed to dull a person's sense of pain. They can make you slur your speech and make you confused.

Hallucinogens. Drugs such as LSD and PCP cause hallucinations. Someone taking them may have a rapid heart rate and high blood pressure.

Inhalants. Inhaling substances such as glue, paint thinner or aerosol products can give a person an irregular heartbeat. The person may have a rash around their nose or mouth.

Club drugs. Drugs such as ecstasy that are used at clubs, concerts and parties cause sedation, muscle relaxation, confusion and memory loss. They can make a person hallucinate and lose consciousness.

TREATMENT If your drug use is out of control or causing problems, get help. The sooner you do, the better your chances for a long-term recovery. If you're not ready to approach a health care provider, help lines or hotlines may be a good place to learn about treatment. The U.S. Substance Abuse and Mental Health Services Administration (SAMHSA) operates a national help line at 1-800-662-HELP (4357). You can also go online to find out where to get treatment at *https://findtreatment.gov.*

Seek emergency help if you or someone you know has taken a drug and:

- May have overdosed
- Shows changes in consciousness
- Has trouble breathing
- Has seizures or convulsions
- Has signs of a possible heart attack, such as chest pain or pressure
- Has any other troublesome or psychological reaction

People struggling with addiction usually deny that their drug use is a problem and are reluctant to seek treatment. An intervention by family and friends can give a loved one a structured opportunity to make

S

changes and accept help. The intervention needs to be planned carefully with the help of a doctor or licensed alcohol and drug counselor.

There's no cure for drug addiction. With treatment, a person can overcome addiction and stay drug-free. The treatment depends on the drug involved and whether there's a related medical or health disorder.

Chemical dependence treatment programs

These programs usually offer individual, group or family therapy. They focus on helping people understand the nature of addiction, become drug-free and prevent relapse. Chemical dependence treatment programs can be outpatient, residential or inpatient.

Detoxification

For some people, it's safe to undergo withdrawal (detox) on an outpatient basis. Others may need to be admitted to a hospital or treatment center. Detox may involve gradually reducing the dose of the drug used, temporarily substituting other substances, such as methadone.

Medication for opioid overdose

Someone who overdoses on opioids can be given naloxone by emergency responders, or in some states, by anyone who witnesses the overdose. Naloxone is a drug that temporarily reverses the effects of opioids. It can be given in a nasal spray or injected. Whatever the method of delivery, seek immediate medical care after you receive naloxone.

Self-help groups

Joining a support group can help you cope if you or someone you love has an addiction. Many, though not all, self-help support groups use the 12-step model first developed by Alcoholics Anonymous. A therapist or licensed counselor can help you locate a self-help support group, or you may find one in your community or on the internet.

It takes persistent effort to overcome a drug addiction and stay drug-free. Learning new coping skills and knowing where to find help are essential. Seeing a psychiatrist, psychologist or licensed counselor may give you peace of mind and help you mend your relationships. If you have signs or symptoms of a mental health problem, seek treatment from a qualified mental health provider.

S

Sunburn

WHAT'S THE CAUSE? Sunburn results from too much exposure to ultraviolet (UV) light from the sun's rays or from artificial sources, such as sunlamps.

Signs and symptoms include:

- Skin pinkness or redness
- Skin that feels warm or hot to the touch
- Pain, tenderness or itching
- Swelling
- Small fluid-filled blisters, which may break

See your health care provider if the sunburn is blistering and covers a large portion of your body or is accompanied by a high fever, extreme pain, headache, confusion, nausea or chills.

TREATMENT Treatment won't prevent skin damage, but it can reduce pain, swelling and discomfort. To treat a sunburn:

- **Take a pain reliever.** Ibuprofen (Advil, Motrin IB, others) and naproxen sodium (Aleve) may reduce swelling and pain, especially if you take them soon after sun exposure.
- **Cool the skin.** Apply a compress, such as a towel dampened with cool water, to the affected skin. Or take a cool bath or shower.
- **Soothe the skin.** Apply moisturizer, aloe vera lotion or gel, or hydrocortisone cream to the affected skin. Low-dose (0.5% to 1%) hydrocortisone cream may decrease pain and swelling and speed healing.
- **Drink plenty of fluids.** Sun and heat can cause fluid loss. Adequate fluids, especially water, help your body recover.
- **Don't break blisters.** They serve as a protective layer. Breaking blisters also slows the healing process and increases the risk of infection. If blisters break, gently clean the area with mild soap and water and apply an antibacterial cream.
- **Treat peeling skin gently.** Continue to use moisturizing cream.
- **Control itching.** Corticosteroid creams you apply to your skin can help control itching while your skin is healing.
- **Avoid the sun.** If you have to be in the sun, cover your skin and use sunscreen with an SPF of 30 or greater on exposed skin.

S

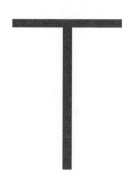

Tendinitis

 WHAT IS IT? Tendinitis is inflammation or irritation of a tendon — one of the thick fibrous cords that attaches muscle to bone. Tendinitis causes pain and tenderness just outside a joint.

The condition is most common around your shoulders, elbows, wrists, knees and heels. Other names for various tendinitis problems include tennis elbow, golfer's elbow, pitcher's shoulder, swimmer's shoulder and jumper's knee.

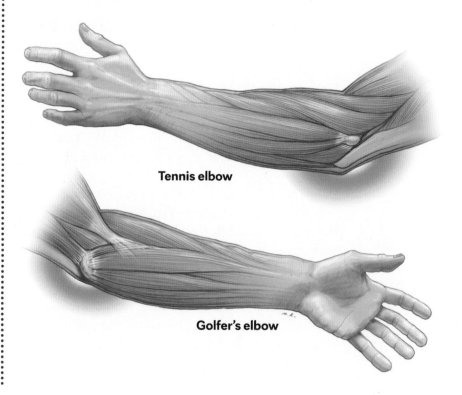

Tennis elbow

Golfer's elbow

The condition is most likely to stem from the repetition of a particular movement over time, which stresses the tendons needed to perform the tasks. Signs and symptoms of tendinitis typically include:

- Pain when moving the affected limb or joint
- Tenderness over the affected tendon
- Mild swelling

TREATMENT Simple self-care may be all that you need. To treat tendinitis at home, remember R.I.C.E. (see page 335).

Medications
Your health care provider may recommend these medications:

Pain relievers. Taking aspirin, naproxen sodium (Aleve) or ibuprofen (Advil, Motrin IB, others) may relieve pain and discomfort. Topical anti-inflammatory creams — popular in Europe and becoming increasingly available in the United States — also may be effective.

Corticosteroids. Sometimes a provider may inject a corticosteroid medication around a tendon to reduce inflammation and ease pain. Repeated injections aren't recommended because they may weaken the tendon and increase the risk of tendon rupture.

Platelet-rich plasma (PRP). This treatment involves taking a sample of your own blood and separating out the platelets and healing factors. The solution is then re-injected into the area of chronic tendon irritation. Though still under investigation, PRP has been shown to be beneficial for many chronic tendon conditions.

Physical therapy
Physical therapy to stretch and strengthen the affected muscle-tendon unit may be helpful in some circumstances.

Surgery and other procedures
Depending on the severity of your tendon injury, surgical repair may be needed, especially if the tendon has torn from the bone. For chronic inflammation, a procedure called focused aspiration of scar tissue (FAST) may be used to remove scar tissue in a tendon. Dry needling, which uses a fine needle to stimulate tendon healing, may be another option.

T

Testicular pain

WHAT'S THE CAUSE? Testicular pain can occur for several different reasons. Causes of testicular pain include:

Testicular torsion

It occurs when a testicle rotates, twisting the spermatic cord that brings blood to the testicle and cutting off blood flow. The condition may result from injury to the scrotum, physical activity or rapid growth of the testes during puberty. Often, the cause isn't known. If blood flow is reduced for too long, the testicle may become badly damaged and need to be removed.

Signs and symptoms of testicular torsion include:

- Sudden or severe pain in the scrotum
- Swelling of the scrotum
- Abdominal pain
- Nausea and vomiting
- A testicle positioned higher than typical or at an unusual angle

Treatment. Surgery is required to correct testicular torsion. In some cases, a medical provider may be able to untwist the testicle by pushing on the scrotum, but you may still need surgery. The surgeon may stitch one or both testicles to the inside of the scrotum to prevent the problem from occurring again. The sooner the testicle is untwisted, the greater the chance it can be saved. The success rate is about 95% when treatment occurs within six hours, but declines steadily to about 20% after 24 hours.

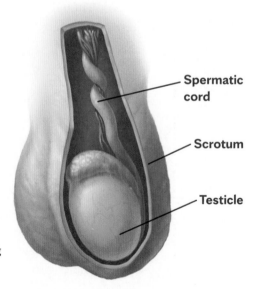

Spermatic cord

Scrotum

Testicle

With testicular torsion, the testicle twists on the spermatic cord, cutting off blood supply to the testicle.

T

Epididymitis

Epididymitis is an inflammation of the coiled tube (epididymis) at the back of the testicle that stores and carries sperm. It's most often caused by a bacterial infection, including sexually transmitted infections such as gonorrhea or chlamydia. Signs and symptoms may include:

- A swollen, red or warm scrotum
- Testicular pain and tenderness, usually on one side
- Painful urination or an urgent need to urinate
- Discharge from the penis
- Painful intercourse or ejaculation
- Enlarged lymph nodes in the groin
- Blood in the semen

Treatment. Antibiotics are used to treat bacterial epididymitis. If the cause is a sexually transmitted infection, your sexual partner also needs treatment. It may take several weeks for the tenderness to disappear. Rest, supporting the scrotum with an athletic strap, applying ice and taking pain medication can help relieve the discomfort. Avoid sexual intercourse until the infection has cleared.

Orchitis

Orchitis is an inflammation of one or both testicles. The condition is usually caused by a bacterial infection or by the mumps virus. Bacterial orchitis that results from epididymitis is called epididymo-orchitis. Orchitis may also occur from bacterial or viral sexually transmitted infections, particularly gonorrhea or chlamydia. Orchitis can affect fertility. Signs and symptoms, which usually develop suddenly, include:

- Swelling in one or both testicles
- Pain ranging from mild to severe
- Tenderness in one or both testicles, which may last for weeks
- Fever
- Nausea and vomiting

Treatment. Antibiotics are needed to treat bacterial orchitis and epididymo-orchitis. If the cause is a sexually transmitted infection, your sexual partner also needs treatment. Self-care measures such as rest, scrotal support, ice packs and pain medication can help relieve discomfort. With viral orchitis, treatment is aimed at relieving symptoms. Most people start to feel better in 3 to 10 days, but it may take longer for the scrotal tenderness to disappear.

T

Tonsillitis

WHAT IS IT? Tonsillitis is inflammation of the tonsils at the back of the throat.

Most cases of tonsillitis are caused by a viral infection. Less often, a bacterial infection is the culprit. Signs and symptoms may include:

- Red, swollen tonsils
- White or yellow coating or patches on the tonsils
- Sore throat and painful swallowing
- Fever
- Enlarged, tender glands (lymph nodes) in the neck
- Bad breath
- Stomachache, particularly in younger children
- Headache

In very young children, signs of tonsillitis may include drooling due to difficult or painful swallowing, refusal to eat or unusual fussiness.

TREATMENT Self-care is generally the first line of treatment and often all that's needed. To reduce symptoms, include:

- **Rest.** Encourage your child to sleep and avoid talking.
- **Adequate fluids.** Give your child plenty of water to keep the throat moist and prevent dehydration.
- **Comforting foods and beverages.** Warm liquids, including broth, and cold treats such as ice pops can soothe a sore throat.
- **Saltwater gargle.** If your child can gargle, mix 1 teaspoon of table salt in 8 ounces warm water. Gargle the solution.
- **Pain relievers.** Ibuprofen (Advil, Motrin, others) or acetaminophen (Tylenol, others) may reduce throat pain and fever.

Antibiotics. For tonsillitis caused by a bacterial infection, antibiotics are generally prescribed.

Surgery. In case of frequently recurring tonsillitis, surgery may be performed to remove the tonsils. Frequent tonsillitis is generally defined as seven or more episodes in one year, five or more episodes a year in each of the preceding two years, or three or more episodes a year in each of the preceding three years.

T

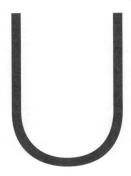

U

Ulcer

WHAT IS IT? Ulcers are open sores that develop on skin or mucous membranes, such as the inner lining of an organ. The term often refers more specifically to peptic ulcers, which include:

- **Gastric ulcers.** These ulcers occur on the inside of the stomach.
- **Esophageal ulcers.** These occur inside the esophagus.
- **Duodenal ulcers.** These occur on the inside of the upper portion of the small intestine (duodenum).

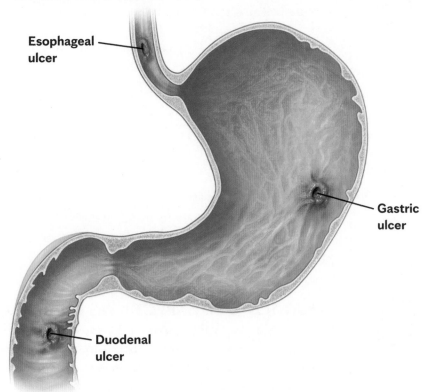

Esophageal ulcer

Gastric ulcer

Duodenal ulcer

WHAT'S THE CAUSE? It's a myth that spicy foods or a stressful job can cause an ulcer. A bacterial infection or sometimes medications are responsible for most peptic ulcers.

H. pylori **bacteria.** *Helicobacter pylori* (*H. pylori*) bacteria can cause inflammation of the stomach's inner layer, producing an ulcer. It's not clear how the bacteria spread. They may be transmitted from close contact, such as kissing. People may also contract *H. pylori* through food and water.

Regular use of pain relievers. Certain nonprescription and prescription pain medications can irritate or inflame the lining of the stomach and small intestine, causing an ulcer. These medications include aspirin, ibuprofen (Advil, Motrin IB, others), naproxen sodium (Aleve) and ketoprofen.

Other medications. Other drugs that can lead to ulcers include those used to treat osteoporosis called bisphosphonates (Actonel, Fosamax, others) and corticosteroids.

SYMPTOM CHECKER Burning stomach pain is the most common symptom of an ulcer. The pain may:

- Be felt anywhere from your bellybutton up to your breastbone
- Be worse when your stomach is empty
- Flare at night
- Be temporarily relieved by eating certain foods that buffer stomach acid or by taking an acid-reducing medication

Some people have no symptoms. Others have severe symptoms, including:

- Vomiting blood, which may appear red or black
- Dark blood in stools or stools that are black or tarry
- Weight loss and appetite changes

 U-V

WHAT TESTS TO EXPECT To find out if you have an ulcer, you may undergo a test called upper endoscopy. It involves passing a slender tube equipped with a lens (endoscope) down your throat and into your esophagus, stomach and small intestine to look for an ulcer. If an ulcer is found, tissue may be removed (biopsied) to determine the cause.

Another diagnostic test involves a series of X-rays of your esophagus, stomach and small intestine. Just before the X-ray, you swallow a white liquid that contains barium. The liquid coats your digestive tract and makes an ulcer more visible.

If *H. pylori* infection is suspected, it can be diagnosed by noninvasive means, including a blood test or breath test.

TREATMENT Treatment for peptic ulcers often includes a combination of medications:

Antibiotics. If *H. pylori* is found in your digestive tract, your health care provider may recommend a combination of antibiotics to kill the bacterium. You also may be prescribed medications to reduce stomach acid.

Proton pump inhibitors. These medications reduce stomach acid by blocking the action of those parts of cells that produce stomach acid. Available by prescription and sold over-the-counter, they include the drugs omeprazole (Prilosec), lansoprazole (Prevacid), rabeprazole (Aciphex), esomeprazole (Nexium) and pantoprazole (Protonix).

Acid blockers. Acid blockers — also called histamine (H-2) blockers — reduce the amount of stomach acid released into your digestive tract, which relieves ulcer pain and encourages healing. Available by prescription or over-the-counter, acid blockers include the medications famotidine (Pepcid AC), cimetidine (Tagamet HB) and nizatidine (Axid AR).

Antacids. Antacids neutralize existing stomach acid and can provide rapid pain relief. Antacids can provide symptom relief, but generally aren't used to heal an ulcer.

Cytoprotective agents. They help protect the tissues that line your stomach and small intestine. Options include the prescription medications sucralfate (Carafate) and misoprostol (Cytotec). A nonprescription cytoprotective agent is bismuth subsalicylate (Pepto-Bismol).

Peptic ulcers that don't heal with treatment are called refractory ulcers. There are many reasons why an ulcer may fail to heal, including the fact that some types of *H. pylori* are resistant to antibiotics. Treatment for refractory ulcers generally involves eliminating factors that may interfere with healing, along with using different antibiotics.

Urinary incontinence

WHAT IS IT? The loss of bladder control (urinary incontinence) is a common problem. Its symptoms range from mild to severe.

Urinary incontinence may result from everyday habits, underlying medical conditions or physical problems. The most common types of urinary incontinence include:

- **Stress incontinence.** Urine leaks when you exert pressure on your bladder by coughing, sneezing, laughing, exercising or lifting something heavy.
- **Urge incontinence.** You have a sudden, intense urge to urinate followed by an involuntary loss of urine. You may also need to urinate often. Urge incontinence may be caused by an infection, but frequently it's associated with overactive bladder contractions related to aging, menopause, or prostate problems.
- **Overflow incontinence.** In this condition, you experience frequent dribbling of urine due to a bladder that doesn't empty completely.

TREATMENT Treatment for urinary incontinence depends on the type of incontinence you have and its severity. A combination of treatments may be necessary. They may include:

Behavioral techniques. Your health care provider may recommend one of the following therapies:

- **Bladder training.** You delay urination after you get the urge to go. Start by trying to hold off for 10 minutes every time you feel an urge to urinate. The goal is to increase the time between trips to the toilet until you're urinating every 2 to 4 hours.
- **Double voiding.** This means urinating, then waiting a few minutes and trying again to empty your bladder more completely.
- **Scheduled toilet trips.** Rather than waiting for the urge to go, you urinate every 2 to 4 hours.
- **Fluid and diet management.** You may need to cut back on or avoid alcohol, caffeine or acidic foods. Reducing how much liquid you consume also may ease symptoms.

Pelvic floor muscle exercises. These exercises are used to strengthen the muscles that help control urination. Also known as Kegel exercises, pelvic floor muscle exercises are especially effective for stress incontinence, but they may help with urge incontinence. To do them, imagine that you're trying to stop your urine flow. Tighten (contract) the muscles you would use to stop urinating and hold the contraction for five seconds, and then relax for five seconds. (If this is too difficult, start by holding for two seconds and relaxing for three seconds.) Work up to holding the contractions for 10 seconds at a time and aim for at least three sets of 10 repetitions daily.

Electrical stimulation. Electrodes are temporarily inserted into your rectum or vagina to stimulate and strengthen pelvic floor muscles. Gentle electrical stimulation can be effective for stress incontinence and urge incontinence. You may need multiple treatments over several months.

Medications. Medications used to treat incontinence include:

- **Anticholinergics.** These drugs can help calm an overactive bladder and may be helpful for urge incontinence. Examples include oxybutynin (Ditropan XL, Oxytrol, others), tolterodine (Detrol), darifenacin, fesoterodine (Toviaz), solifenacin (Vesicare) and trospium chloride.
- **Mirabegron (Myrbetriq).** Used to treat urge incontinence, this medication relaxes the bladder muscle and can increase the amount of urine your bladder can hold. It may also increase the amount you are able to urinate at one time, helping to empty your bladder more completely.
- **Alpha blockers.** These medications are helpful for treating urge and overflow incontinence. They relax bladder neck muscles and muscle fibers in the prostate and make it easier to empty the bladder. Examples include tamsulosin (Flomax), alfuzosin (Uroxatral), silodosin (Rapaflo) and doxazosin (Cardura).
- **Topical estrogen.** Low-dose topical estrogen in the form of a vaginal cream, ring or patch may help tone and rejuvenate tissues in the urethra and vaginal areas, reducing some of the symptoms of incontinence.

Medical devices. Devices to treat incontinence in women include:

- **Urethral insert.** This small, tampon-like disposable device is inserted into the urethra before an activity that can trigger incontinence, such as a game of tennis. The insert acts as a plug to prevent leakage. Then you remove the insert before urination.

U-V

- **Pessary.** This is a flexible silicone ring that you insert into your vagina and wear all day. You don't need to remove it before using the toilet. The device helps hold up your bladder to prevent urine leakage. A pessary may help with incontinence due to a prolapsed bladder or uterus.

Interventional therapies. These treatments include:

- **Bulking material injections.** To treat stress incontinence, a synthetic material may be injected into tissue surrounding the urethra. The bulking material helps keep the urethra closed and reduces urine leakage.
- **OnabotulinumtoxinA (Botox).** Injections of Botox into the bladder muscle may benefit some people with an overactive bladder. Botox helps prevent muscle spasms and it causes the bladder to relax.
- **Nerve stimulators.** Painless electrical pulses are delivered to the nerves involved in bladder control (sacral nerves) by a device resembling a pacemaker that is implanted under your skin or by a removable vaginal device.

Surgery. If other treatments aren't helpful, surgery may help treat the problems causing the incontinence:

- **Sling procedures.** A surgeon creates a pelvic sling around your urethra and the area of thickened muscle where the bladder connects to the urethra (bladder neck). The sling helps keep the urethra closed, especially when you cough or sneeze. This procedure is used to treat stress incontinence.
- **Bladder neck suspension.** This procedure is used to help support the urethra and bladder neck — an area of thickened muscle where the bladder connects to the urethra.
- **Prolapse surgery.** To treat mixed incontinence and pelvic organ prolapse, surgery may include a combination of a sling procedure and surgery to fix the prolapse.
- **Artificial urinary sphincter.** In men, a fluid-filled ring may be implanted around the bladder neck to keep the urinary sphincter tightly shut. When you're ready to urinate, you press a valve implanted under your skin that causes the ring to deflate and allows urine to flow from your bladder. Artificial urinary sphincters are particularly helpful for people whose incontinence is associated with prostate cancer treatment or an enlarged prostate gland.

U-V

Uterine fibroids

WHAT IS IT? Uterine fibroids are noncancerous growths of the uterus that often appear during childbearing years. They aren't associated with an increased risk of uterine cancer and almost never develop into cancer.

Fibroids range in size from seedlings, undetectable by the human eye, to bulky masses that can distort and enlarge the uterus. They may grow slowly or rapidly or remain the same size. Some fibroids shrink on their own.

SYMPTOM CHECKER As many as 3 out of 4 people with a uterus have uterine fibroids at some point. Most are unaware of them because they don't cause symptoms. When signs and symptoms occur, the most common are:

- Heavy menstrual bleeding
- Prolonged menstrual periods
- Pelvic pressure or pain
- Frequent urination
- Difficulty emptying your bladder
- Constipation
- Backache or leg pains

Rarely, a fibroid can cause acute pain. This happens when it outgrows its blood supply.

TREATMENT There's no single best approach to treat uterine fibroids — many treatment options exist. They include:

Watchful waiting. If you aren't experiencing signs or symptoms, watchful waiting could be the best option. Fibroids aren't cancerous and they usually grow slowly, or not at all, and they tend to shrink after menopause.

Medications. Medications target hormones that regulate your menstrual cycle, treating symptoms such as heavy menstrual bleeding and pelvic pressure. They don't eliminate fibroids, but may shrink them. Medications prescribed to treat uterine fibroids include:

U-V

- **Gonadotropin-releasing hormone (Gn-RH) agonists.** Medications called Gn-RH agonists (Lupron Depot, Zoladex, others) treat fibroids by blocking the production of estrogen and progesterone, putting you into a temporary postmenopausal state. Menstruation stops and the fibroids shrink.
- **Progestin-releasing intrauterine device (IUD).** An IUD that releases progestin-can relieve heavy bleeding caused by fibroids. It doesn't shrink fibroids or make them disappear, however.
- **Other medications.** Oral contraceptives can help control menstrual bleeding. Nonsteroidal anti-inflammatory drugs (NSAIDs) may relieve pain. Vitamins and iron may be recommended if you have heavy menstrual bleeding and anemia.

Minimally invasive procedures. These procedures may be used to destroy uterine fibroids:

- **Focused ultrasound surgery (FUS).** This is a newer, noninvasive treatment that preserves your uterus and requires no incision. Once the precise location of the fibroids is determined, an ultrasound transducer is used to focus sound waves into the fibroids to heat and destroy small areas of fibroid tissue.
- **Uterine artery embolization.** Small particles are injected into the arteries that serve the fibroids, cutting off blood flow and causing the fibroids to shrink and die. Complications can occur if the blood supply to your ovaries or other organs is compromised.
- **Radiofrequency ablation.** Radiofrequency energy destroys uterine fibroids and shrinks the blood vessels that feed them. This can be done during a laparoscopic or transcervical procedure. A similar procedure called cryomyolysis freezes the fibroids.
- **Endometrial ablation and resection.** Specialized instruments inserted into your uterus, use heat, microwave energy, hot water or electric current to destroy the lining of your uterus, ending menstruation or reducing your menstrual flow. It doesn't affect fibroids outside the interior lining of the uterus.

Surgery. A surgeon removes the fibroids, either with traditional open surgery or laparoscopic surgery. If the fibroids are small and few in number, laparoscopic surgery may be performed. If you have multiple fibroids, very large fibroids or very deep fibroids, your health care provider may recommend traditional open surgery. The only permanent solution for treating uterine fibroids is surgical removal of the uterus (hysterectomy). Hysterectomy is major surgery, and it ends your ability to bear children.

U-V

UTI (urinary tract infection)

WHAT IS IT? A UTI is an infection in any part of the urinary system — the kidneys, ureters, bladder and urethra. Most infections involve the lower urinary tract, the bladder and the urethra.

UTIs typically occur when bacteria enter the urinary tract through the urethra and multiply in the bladder. Although the urinary system is designed to keep out microscopic invaders, these defenses sometimes fail.

UTIs mainly affect the bladder and urethra in people with female anatomy.

- **Bladder infection (cystitis).** It's usually caused by *Escherichia coli* (*E. coli*), a bacteria commonly found in the gastrointestinal tract. Sexual intercourse may lead to cystitis, but you don't have to be sexually active to develop it. Women are at particular risk of a bladder infection because of the short distance from the urethra to the anus and the urethral opening to the bladder.
- **Urethral infection (urethritis).** A urethral infection may occur when gastrointestinal bacteria spread from the anus to the urethra. Because the urethra is close to the vagina, sexually transmitted infections, such as herpes, gonorrhea and chlamydia, also can cause urethritis.

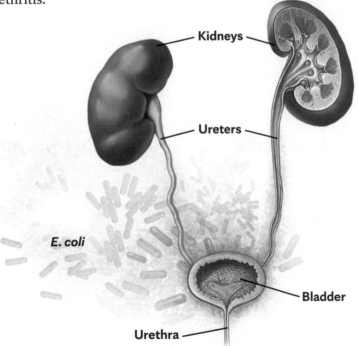

Kidneys

Ureters

E. coli

Bladder

Urethra

U-V

SYMPTOM CHECKER UTIs don't always cause signs and symptoms. When they do, signs and symptoms may include:

- A strong, persistent urge to urinate
- A burning sensation when urinating
- Passing frequent, small amounts of urine
- Urine that appears cloudy
- Urine that appears red, bright pink or cola colored — a sign of blood in the urine
- Strong-smelling urine
- Pelvic pain
- Rectal pain

Being female and being sexually active increase the risk of a urinary tract infection. Using diaphragms for birth control, as well as spermicides, may increase the risk of UTIs. After menopause, UTIs can become more common because reduced estrogen causes changes in the urinary tract, making it more vulnerable to infection. People who need to use a catheter to urinate also are at increased risk of UTIs.

TREATMENT Antibiotics are generally used to treat urinary tract infections. Which drugs are prescribed, and for how long, will depend on your health and the type of bacterium involved.

Drugs commonly recommended for simple UTIs include sulfamethoxazole-trimethoprim (Bactrim, Septra, others), cephalexin, nitrofurantoin (Macrodantin, Macrobid) or ampicillin. For a complicated UTI or kidney infection, your health care provider might prescribe ciprofloxacin (Cipro) or levofloxacin.

Usually, symptoms clear up within a few days of treatment. For an uncomplicated UTI, your health care provider may recommend a shorter course of treatment, such as taking an antibiotic for 1 to 3 days. In other cases, you may need to take antibiotics for a week or more.

If you experience frequent urinary tract infections, your health care provider may recommend a longer course of antibiotics. If your infections are related to sexual activity, another option may be to take a single dose of an antibiotic after sexual intercourse. If you're postmenopausal, your provider may prescribe vaginal estrogen therapy to help reduce the chance of recurrent UTIs.

U-V

LIFESTYLE There's some indication, though unproven, that cranberry juice may have infection-fighting properties and drinking it daily may help prevent UTIs.

It's not clear how much cranberry juice you need to drink or how often you need to drink it to have an effect. If you like cranberry juice and you feel it helps prevent UTIs, there's little harm in drinking it. But don't drink cranberry juice if you're taking the blood-thinning medication warfarin (Jantoven) because it may increase the risk of bleeding.

Other tips to reduce UTIs include:

- **Drink plenty of water.** It dilutes your urine and helps flush out bacteria before infection can begin.
- **Wipe from front to back.** Doing so after urinating or a bowel movement helps prevent bacteria in the anal region from spreading to the vagina and urethra.
- **Empty your bladder soon after intercourse.** This helps to flush out bacteria.
- **Avoid irritating vaginal products.** Use of deodorant sprays, douches and powders in the genital area can irritate the urethra.

KIDNEY INFECTION

Left untreated, a urinary tract infection can lead to a kidney infection. Acute or chronic kidney infections can result in permanent kidney damage, especially in young children, or the bacteria can spread to the bloodstream. Signs and symptoms of a kidney infection include:

- Upper back and side (flank) pain
- High fever
- Shaking and chills
- Nausea
- Vomiting

Treatment usually includes antibiotics. You may need to be hospitalized.

U-V

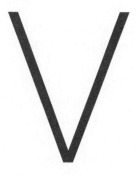

Varicose veins

WHAT IS IT? Varicose veins are enlarged, gnarled veins. Any vein may become varicose, but those most commonly affected are the veins in the legs and feet.

Causes of varicose veins include:

- **Age.** With age, your veins lose elasticity, causing them to stretch, and the valves in your veins weaken. Blood that should be moving toward your heart flows backward and pools in your legs and feet.
- **Pregnancy.** Pregnancy increases the volume of blood in your body, but decreases the flow of blood from your legs to your pelvis. This circulatory change is designed to support the growing fetus, but it can also enlarge the veins in your legs. Hormone changes during pregnancy also may play a role.

Women are more likely than men to develop varicose veins. If any of your family members had varicose veins, there's a greater chance you will, too. Being overweight also increases the risk of varicose veins. Sitting or standing for long periods makes varicose veins more likely to develop as well. Blood doesn't flow as well if you're in the same position for long periods.

SYMPTOM CHECKER Varicose veins usually don't cause any pain. Signs may include:

- Veins that are dark purple or blue in color
- Veins that appear twisted and bulging — like twisted cords underneath your skin

When painful signs and symptoms occur, they may include:

- An achy or heavy feeling in your legs
- Burning, throbbing, muscle cramping and swelling in your lower legs
- Worsened pain after sitting or standing for a long time
- Itching around one or more of your veins
- Skin ulcers near your ankle that can signal a serious form of vascular disease (venous insufficiency) requiring medical attention

TREATMENT For mild to moderate varicose veins, self-care may ease the pain and prevent the problem from getting worse.

Self-care includes getting regular exercise to promote circulation, losing weight, not wearing tight clothes, elevating your legs, and avoiding long periods of standing or sitting.

For more-severe varicose veins, there are several treatment options:

Healthy veins

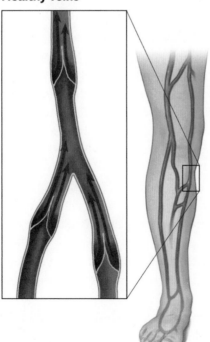

Varicose veins

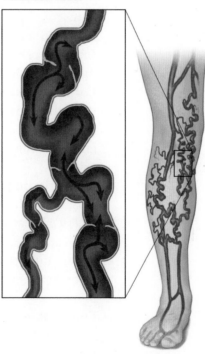

Varicose veins are twisted, enlarged veins under the surface of the skin that are most common in the legs and ankles. They result from stretched veins and weakened valves within the veins.

Compression stockings

Wearing compression stockings is often the first approach to treatment. They steadily squeeze your legs, helping veins and leg muscles move blood more efficiently. The amount of compression varies by type and brand. You can buy compression stockings at most pharmacies and medical supply stores. Prescription-strength stockings also are available.

When purchasing compression stockings, make sure that they fit properly. Use the size chart on the package. Knee-high stockings are generally sufficient. If you have arthritis, getting the stockings on can be difficult. There are devices to make putting them on easier.

Other treatments

If self-care or compression stockings don't improve your condition, or if the problem is more severe, your health care provider may suggest:

- **Sclerotherapy.** Small- and medium-sized varicose veins are injected with a solution that scars and closes the veins. In a few weeks, varicose veins should fade. Sclerotherapy is effective if done correctly.
- **Laser surgery.** It's most effective for smaller varicose veins. Laser surgery works by sending strong bursts of light onto the vein, which makes the vein slowly fade and disappear.
- **Catheter-assisted procedures.** A thin tube (catheter) that heats up at the tip is inserted into an enlarged vein. As the catheter is pulled out, the heat destroys the vein and causes it to collapse and seal shut. This procedure is usually used on larger varicose veins.
- **Vein stripping.** It involves removing a long varicosed vein. Surgically removing the vein won't adversely affect circulation in your leg because veins deeper in the leg take care of larger volumes of blood.
- **Ambulatory phlebectomy.** Smaller varicose veins are removed through a series of tiny skin punctures. Scarring is generally minimal.
- **Endoscopic vein surgery.** It's generally reserved for advanced cases involving leg ulcers. Small incisions are made in the leg and damaged veins are closed and removed.

Varicose veins that develop during pregnancy generally improve without medical treatment within a year after delivery.

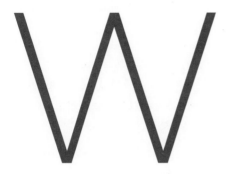

Warts

WHAT IS IT? A wart is a small, rough growth resembling a tiny cauliflower or a solid blister. Warts are caused by the human papillomavirus (HPV). There are more than 100 types of HPV. Different types of the virus cause different types of warts, including:

Common warts. Common warts occur most often on your fingers or hands. They may feature a pattern of tiny black dots, which are small, clotted blood vessels. Common warts are transmitted by touch and are most common in children and young adults.

Common warts are small grainy bumps that are rough to the touch. On white skin, they may be flesh-colored, white, pink or tan. On brown and Black skin, warts may be lighter than the skin color.

Plantar warts. Plantar warts usually appear on the heels or balls of your feet, areas that feel the most pressure. This pressure may cause plantar warts to grow inward beneath a hard, thick layer of skin (callus). The virus enters your body through tiny cuts, breaks or other weak spots on the bottom of your feet.

A plantar wart appears as a small, fleshy, rough, grainy growth on the bottom of the foot. There may be hard, thickened skin (callus) over a "spot" on the skin, where a wart has grown inward. You may experience pain or tenderness when walking or standing.

TREATMENT Common warts and plantar warts often disappear on their own within a year or two. But you may want to treat them for cosmetic purposes, to relieve pain or to prevent their spread.

Self-care

To treat warts at home try these approaches.

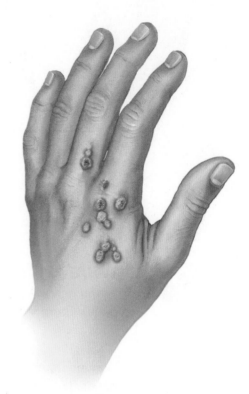

- **Medications.** Look for an over-the-counter solution or patch containing 17% salicylic acid. These products require daily use, often for a few weeks. Soak your wart in warm water for 10 to 20 minutes before applying a solution or patch. File away dead skin between treatments. Stronger solutions also may be prescribed.
- **Duct tape.** Some studies suggest duct tape may help in treating warts. Cover the warts with duct tape for six days, then remove. Soak the warts in warm water and rub them with an emery board or pumice stone. You may need to repeat the process for a couple of months.

Medical care

If self-care isn't effective, see your health care provider. Your provider may recommend one of these options:

- **Freezing (cryotherapy).** Liquid nitrogen is applied to the wart to freeze and destroy it. You may need repeat treatments.
- **Acid treatments.** Bichloracetic or trichloroacetic acid is applied to the wart. Repeat treatments are usually necessary.
- **Minor surgery.** The wart may be cut away or burned with electricity. This is usually reserved for warts that don't respond to other therapies.
- **Immune therapy.** Medications or solutions are used to stimulate your immune system to fight the warts. The substance may be injected into your warts or applied topically.
- **Laser treatment.** Laser treatment burns (cauterizes) tiny blood vessels in the wart. The wart eventually falls off. Evidence on the effectiveness of this method is limited, and it can cause pain and scarring.
- **Vaccine.** The HPV vaccine may be used to treat plantar warts.

Whooping cough

WHAT IS IT? Whooping cough (pertussis) is a highly contagious respiratory tract infection, marked by a severe hacking cough followed by a high-pitched intake of breath that sounds like "whoop."

The condition primarily affects children too young to have completed the full course of vaccinations and teenagers and adults whose immunity has faded.

Whooping cough is caused by a bacterium. Signs and symptoms are usually mild at first and resemble those of a common cold. After a week or two, thick mucus accumulates inside the airways, causing uncontrollable coughing. Some people don't develop the characteristic whoop sound, but have a persistent hacking cough.

TREATMENT Antibiotics can kill the bacteria causing whooping cough and help speed recovery.

Unfortunately, not much is available to relieve the cough. Nonprescription cough medicines have little effect and are discouraged. These tips may help reduce symptoms while you're recovering:

- **Get plenty of rest.** Rest helps your body fight the infection.
- **Drink plenty of fluids.** Water, juice and soups are good choices. In children, especially, watch for signs of dehydration, such as dry lips, crying without tears and infrequent urination.
- **Eat smaller meals.** To avoid vomiting after coughing, smaller, more-frequent meals are better than large ones.
- **Clean the air.** Keep your home free of irritants that can trigger coughing spells, such as tobacco smoke.

Vaccination

The best way to prevent whooping cough is with the pertussis vaccine, which is often combined with vaccines against diphtheria and tetanus. The pertussis vaccine is administered during infancy and early childhood. Because immunity tends to wane by age 11, booster shots are recommended at that age and again later in adulthood. A booster shot is also recommended in pregnancy, between weeks 27 and 36, to provide the baby with protection in early life.

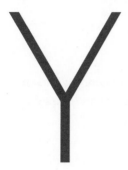

Yeast infection (vaginal)

WHAT IS IT? A vaginal yeast infection is an inflammation or irritation of the vagina and the tissues at the opening of the vagina (vulva) that causes itchiness and vaginal discharge.

Also called vaginal candidiasis, vaginal yeast infection is very common. As many as 3 out of 4 women experience the condition at some point in their lifetimes.

A vaginal yeast infection is caused by the fungus candida that interferes with the natural balance of yeast and bacteria in the vagina. Disruption of this healthy balance results in an overgrowth of yeast, leading to a yeast infection. Overgrowth may result from:

- Antibiotic use, which can change your natural pH balance, allowing yeast to overgrow
- Pregnancy
- Uncontrolled diabetes
- An impaired immune system
- Douching or irritation from inadequate vaginal lubrication

SYMPTOM CHECKER Yeast infection signs and symptoms can range from mild to moderate and include:

- Itching and irritation in the vagina and vulva
- A burning sensation, especially during intercourse or urination
- Redness and swelling of the vulva
- Vaginal pain and soreness
- Thick, white vaginal discharge with a cottage cheese appearance

W-Z

You might have a more complicated yeast infection if you experience extensive redness or itching that causes tears, cracks or sores, or if you've had four or more yeast infections in a single year.

TREATMENT For mild to moderate symptoms and infrequent episodes of yeast infection, a vaginal or oral medication is the most common treatment.

Short-course vaginal therapy. A one-time application or a 1- to 3-day regimen of an antifungal cream, ointment, tablet or suppository effectively clears a yeast infection in most cases. This includes the azole medications butoconazole, clotrimazole, miconazole (Monistat 3) and terconazole, which are available by prescription or over the counter.

Single-dose oral medication. Your health care provider might prescribe a one-time single dose of the antifungal medication fluconazole (Diflucan).

Treatment for a complicated yeast infection might include:

Long-course vaginal therapy. An azole medication is prescribed for a longer period — 1 to 2 weeks.

Multidose oral medication. Two or three doses of fluconazole are taken by mouth. This isn't recommended during pregnancy.

Maintenance therapy. For recurrent yeast infections, your provider may recommend a plan to keep yeast overgrowth in check and prevent future infections. Maintenance therapy starts after the initial treatment clears the yeast infection, and it may include fluconazole tablets taken once a week for six months. Some health care providers prescribe the suppository clotrimazole used weekly instead of an oral medication.

LIFESTYLE To reduce your risk of vaginal yeast infection:

- Don't douche.
- Wear cotton underwear.
- Avoid tight-fitting underwear, pantyhose, pants or shorts.
- Change out of wet clothes, such as swimsuits or workout attire, as soon as possible.
- Avoid hot tubs or very hot baths.

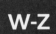

Additional resources

Looking for more information beyond these pages? MayoClinic.org is a good place to start. Try the resources listed here for other reliable health information. If you have specific questions, talk with your health care provider.

988 Suicide and Crisis Lifeline
988 or 800-273-8255 • https://988lifeline.org

American Cancer Society
800-227-2345 • www.cancer.org

American Heart Association
800-242-8721 • www.heart.org

Centers for Disease Control and Prevention
800-232-4636 • www.cdc.gov

HealthyChildren.org – From the American Academy of Pediatrics
https://healthychildren.org

International Diabetes Federation
www.idf.org

National Alliance on Mental Illness
800-950-6264 • www.nami.org

National Institute of Diabetes and Digestive and Kidney Diseases
800-860-8747 • https://niddk.nih.gov

National Institute on Aging
800-222-2225 • www.nia.nih.gov

National Tobacco Quitline
800-784-8669 • www.cdc.gov/tips

Office on Women's Health
800-994-9662 • https://womenshealth.gov

Substance Abuse and Mental Health Services Administration
800-662-4357 • www.samhsa.gov

Index

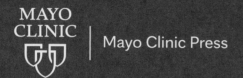
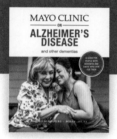
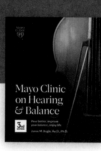
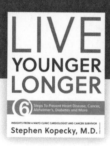
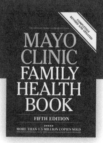
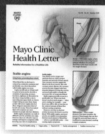